FUNDAMENTALS OF CARDIAC PACING

THE INTERNATIONAL CARDIAC PACING SOCIETY

DEVELOPMENTS IN CARDIOVASCULAR MEDICINE

VOLUME 3

1. C.T. Lancée. *Echocardiology*. 1979. ISBN 90-247-2209-8.
2. J. Baan, A.C. Arntzenius, E.L. Yellin. *Cardiac Dynamics*. 1979. ISBN 90-247-2212-8.
3. H.J.Th. Thalen, C.C. Meere. *Fundamentals of Cardiac Pacing*. 1979. ISBN 90-247-2245-4.

FUNDAMENTALS OF CARDIAC PACING

edited by

HILBERT J.TH. THALEN
Groningen

and

CLAUDE C. MEERE
Montreal

1979

MARTINUS NIJHOFF PUBLISHERS

THE HAGUE / BOSTON / LONDON

The distribution of this book is handled by the following team of publishers:

for the United States and Canada

Kluwer Boston, Inc.
160 Old Derby Street
Hingham, MA 02043
USA

for all other countries

Kluwer Academic Publishers Group
Distribution Center
P.O. Box 322
3300 AH Dordrecht
The Netherlands

Library of Congress Cataloging in Publication Data

Main entry under title:

Fundamentals of cardiac pacing.

(Developments in cardiovascular medicine: v. 3)
Bibliography: p.
Includes index.
1. Pacemaker, Artificial (Heart) I. Thalen, H.J.Th. II. Meere, Claude C. III. Series.
RC 684.P3F86 617'.412 79-9449

ISBN-13: 978-94-009-9336-5 e-ISBN-13: 978-94-009-9334-1
DOI: 10.1007/978-94-009-9334-1

CONTENTS

Foreword VII

Acknowledgement VIII

Contributors IX

1. History of cardiac pacing 1
HILBERT J.TH. THALEN

2. Anatomy and pathology of the conduction system of the human heart 23
THOMAS N. JAMES

3. Current indications of pacemaker therapy 57
GUY FONTAINE

4. Electrophysiology related to cardiac pacing techniques. 79
BERNDT LÜDERITZ

5. Pacing modes and related haemodynamics. 109
ANTHONY F. RICKARDS

6. Surgical techniques in cardiac pacing 127
CLAUDE MEERE and JACQUES LESPÉRANCE

7. Electrodes, leads and interface problems 171
MARIUSZ J. STOPCZYK

8. Pacemaker technology 181
DAVID L. BOWERS

9. Energy sources 189
WILSON GREATBATCH

10. Detection of pacemaker malfunction. 211
HARRY G. MOND, LYNDEL SUTTON, and J. GREAME SLOMAN

11. A review of pacemaker surveillance, 1978 237
VICTOR PARSONNET, GEORGE H. MYERS, and MARJORIE MANHARDT

Index of subjects 257

FOREWORD

The VIth World Symposium on Cardiac Pacing in Montreal 1979 opened with a course, meant to be an introduction for newcomers and an updating refresher and link between the various fields of knowledge needed by experienced persons for cardiac pacing. Invited guest lecturers were selected for their world recognized expertise in the individual subjects.

This book is a collection of the various presentations on historical, clinical, electrophysiological and technical aspects of cardiac pacing. Together they cover the fundamentals of cardiac stimulation.

We hope that this book may become an introductory guide to the field of cardiac pacing and that it may contribute to a better understanding of the pacemaker system and a better treatment of the pacemaker patient.

Claude C. Meere
Hilbert J.Th. Thalen

ACKNOWLEDGEMENT

The editors of 'Fundamentals on Cardiac Pacing' acknowledge the understanding and support of their families, during the long nocturnal hours and weekends during which this book was prepared.

A special note of appreciation is extended to our secretaries, especially Mrs. Carolyn Gaarenstroom-Arriëns and Miss Katrien Schuurman for their 'emergency typing' and Miss Lynn Bacon and Mr. Boudewijn Commandeur from Martinus Nijhoff Publishers, who succeeded in completing the book in time for the Montreal meeting. Only those involved are able to realize the importance of their contribution.

CONTRIBUTORS

David L. Bowers, B.S.E.E., Vitarel Inc. San Diego, California, U.S.A.
Guy Fontaine, M.D., Groupe Hospitalier, Pitié-Salpétrière, Paris, France.
Wilson Greatbatch, F.I.E.E.C., Wilson Greatbatch Inc., Clarence, New York, U.S.A.
Thomas N. James, M.D., Dept. of Medicine, University of Alabama in Birmingham, Birmingham, Alabama, U.S.A.
Jacques Lespérance, M.D., Dept. of Radiology, University of Montreal, Medical School, Montreal, Canada.
Berndt Lüderitz, M.D., Ludwig Maximilians Universität, Klinikum Grosshadern, München, F.R. Germany.
Marjorie Manhardt, Pacemaker Center, Newark, Beth Israel Hospital, Newark, New Jersey, U.S.A.
Claude Meere, M.D., Dept. of Surgery, Montreal Heart Institute, Montreal, Canada.
Harry G. Mond, M.D., Dept. of Cardiology, The Royal Melbourne Hospital, Melbourne, Australia.
George H. Myers, Ph.D., Pacemaker Center, Newark Beth Israel Hospital, Newark, New Jersey, U.S.A.
Victor Parsonnet, M.D., Dept. of Surgery, Newark Beth Israel Hospital, Newark, New Jersey, U.S.A.
Anthony F. Rickards, M.D., National Heart Hospital, London, England.
J. Greame Sloman, E.D., Dept. of Cardiology, The Royal Melbourne Hospital, Melbourne, Australia.
Mariusz J. Stopczyk, M.D., Polish Academy of Sciences, Institute of Biomedical Engineering, Warsaw, Poland.
Lyndell Sutton, Dept. of Cardiology, The Royal Melbourne Hospital, Melbourne, Australia.
Hilbert J.Th. Thalen, M.D., Dept of Cardiology, University Hospital, Groningen, the Netherlands.

1. HISTORY OF CARDIAC PACING

HILBERT J.TH. THALEN

The first drawing of the heart known to mankind was made 50,000 years before Christ in a grotto in Altamira in Spain. The drawing not only pictures the heart roughly as we know it today, but it also was positioned well in the body of the animal. This was no coincidence. The people who made the drawing were hunters, and they had to know where to hit the animal most effectively. The heart was known to be important. The Greeks called it the 'Acropolis of the body'. Galen, a famous medical researcher and practitioner in Roman times, analysed the function of the heart and the correlation between the various heart compartments. His – partly incorrect – concept of the function of the heart and the peripheral pulse dominated the medical scene for over fifteen centuries. This persisted until 1628 when William Harvey in England wrote his famous *De motu cordis* that brought us the modern concepts of circulation and the heart.

ANCIENT HISTORY

It is not only the anatomy and physiology of the heart, but also the analysis of the peripheral pulse that plays an important role in the history of cardiac pacing. The Greeks, and even before them, the Chinese often attempted to explain the origin and variations of the pulse. As early as 280 B.C. Wang Chu Ho in China wrote ten books on the pulse. The pulse in Greek is *sphygmos* and sphygmology is the knowledge of the peripheral pulse. It was again Galen, who in Roman times, in his *Opera omnia*, interpreted the various pulses. He thought, as did a lot of the people during that time, that every organ had its own pulse and pulse frequency, and every disease had its own pulse pattern. It was again the important work of Harvey in 1628 that outlined our concepts of circulation and peripheral pulse. In the analysis of the pulse at that time there was one problem. It was very difficult to count the pulse: pulse counting was done in relation to the respiration of the patient or of the doctor himself. The Greeks and Romans worked with a water clock, and it was Galileo who saw a candelabrum swinging in the dome of Pisa and found that the frequency of this candelabrum was exactly the frequency of this own pulse. He constructed a device called the *pulsilogon*, with a heavy ball on a cord. By arranging the ball such that the swing correlated with the patient's

FIGURES 1A-E. THE RECORDINGS.

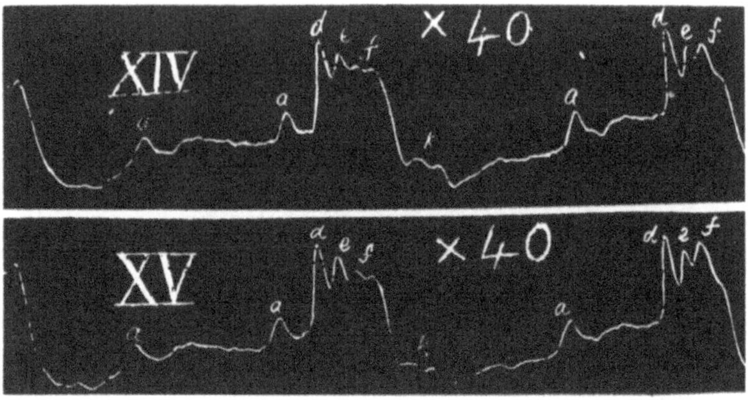

Figure 1A. Sphygmographic recording of heart block in 1875 by Galaban, who did not recognize the significance.

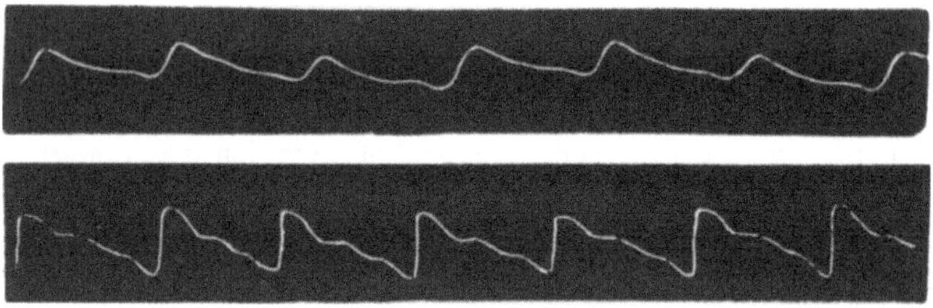

Figure 1B. Sphygmographic records by Beard in 1891, showing a normal pulse (upper) and alterations provoked by galvanization of faradization of cervical sympathetic nerves in normal subjects (lower).

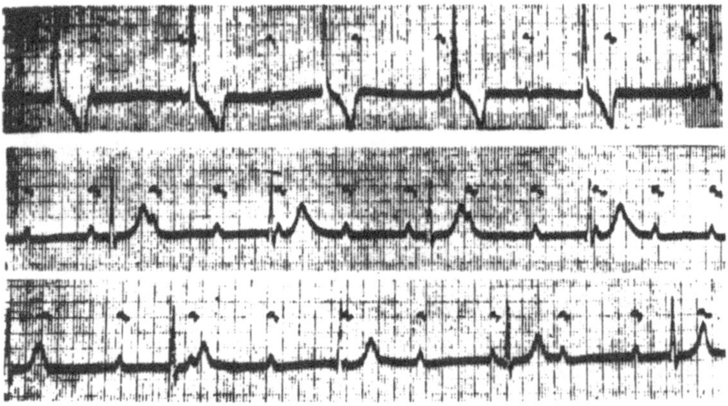

Figure 1C. The first electrocardiogram of experimental and clinical heart block from Einthoven's classic 1906 paper.

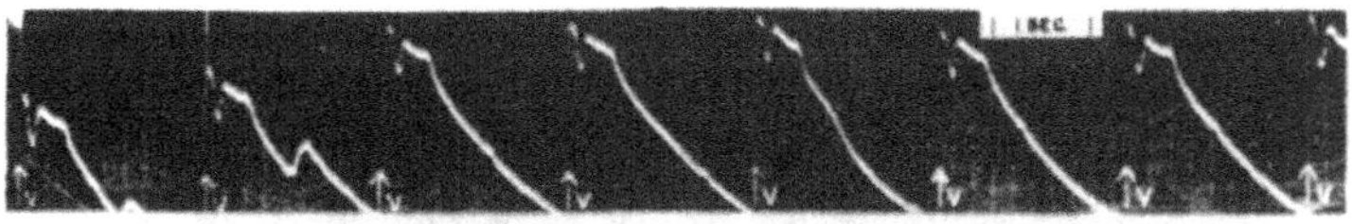

FIGURE 1. *Electrocardiogram (Lead I) Taken during External Electric Stimulation at a Rate of 32 per Minute in Case 1. The moment of electric stimulation is marked by a large, rapid, upward deflection and a wide displacement of the baseline. On all the electrocardiograms the time of electric stimulation is indicated by an arrow, and the ventricular response to it by a "V". A ventricular deflection (broad inverted QRS complex and upright T wave) follows each stimulus regularly, demonstrating the dependence of the ventricular beats on the external electric pulses. P waves of dissociated auricular rhythm are also present.*

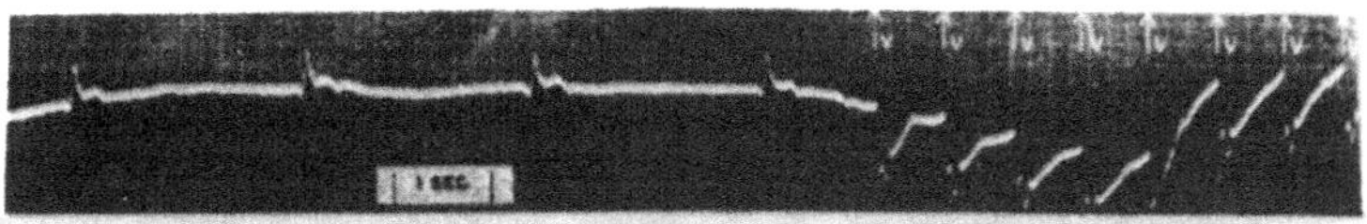

FIGURE 6. *Electrocardiogram (Lead 3) in Case 2, Showing Interruption of Inadequate Idioventricular Rate of 38 per Minute by Ventricular Responses (V) to Artificial Pacemaker (Arrow) at a Rate of 85 per Minute.*

Figure 1D. Electrocardiogram showing interruption of inadequate idioventricular rate of 38 per minute by ventricular responses to artificial pacemaker at a rate of 85 per minute (lower) from Zoll's 1952 paper in the New England Journal of Medicine.

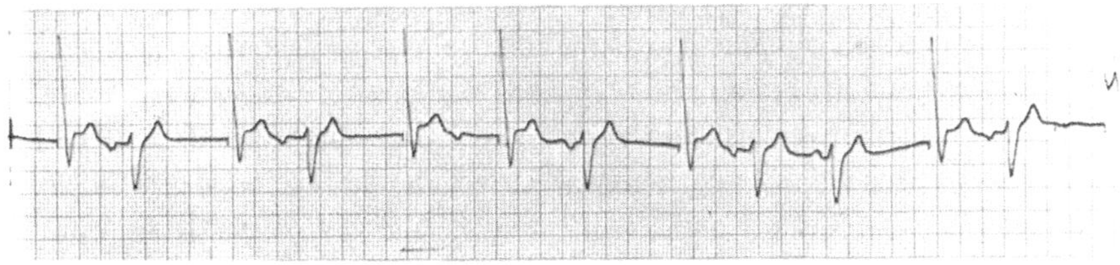

Figure 1E. Electrocardiogram of the now generally used R-wave inhibited pacemaker.

heartbeat, one could read of the frequency of the heart from the altitude of the ball. It was this that initiated the use of the pendulum and ended up in 1657 with Christian Huygens making his first pendulum clock, but his pendulum was not accurate enough form pulse counting. It was not until 1707, when Floyer in England introduced what he called the 'physician's pulse watch', that accurate counting of the pulse became possible. By the end of the eighteenth century, people were able to count the pulse, and they knew especially because of Harvey's contributions how the circulation functioned.

At this same time people also started to record the pulse with special devices. These systems, called sphygmographs, produced the first recordings of heart block in 1875 bij Galaban, who did not recognize the phenomenon at that time however.

When one starts counting the pulse, one soon finds out that some heart rates go fast and some go slow. These changes in pulse frequency were mostly thought to be caused bij emotions. Bradycardia was thought to be due especially to mental depression and also melancholia. In 1719 Gerbezius in Italy published a very accurate clinical survey of the pulse. In some of his patients he thought the pulse abnormalities were due to hypochondria. John Cheyne in England, known from the Cheyne-Stokes attacks, also had the same theory. The concept of hypochondria and melancholia as the cause of bradycardia lasted until 1761 when Giovanni Morgagni in Italy published a careful and thorough research in a case of bradycardia with a priest from Padua. He described the combination of bradycardia and epileptiform attacs and stated that changes in the brain caused the pulse arrhythmias.

EARLY HISTORY

By the nineteenth century, interest in the study of heart disease in relation to diet and body habitus arose. In 1827 Robert Adams did a postmortem on a 60-year-old army officer, and he changed Morgagni's thesis and for the first time mentioned that perhaps the brain was not the cause of bradycardia, but suggested that the fatty degenerated heart which he found in this general was the cause of the bradycardia and also of the cerebral disease. He was attacked by a lot of people: Mayo from England, Addison, etc. These criticisms were reviewed in 1846 by William Stokes. He had his own experiences and went to the literature and concluded that Adams's concept was correct and that the heart was the cause of the bradycardia. Some years later in a publication in 1890 and in his famous textbook on cardiology from 1899 Huchard in France described the syndrome of bradycardia and syncopal attacks caused by the diseased heart and proposed to name this disease *la maladie de Adams-Stokes*, or Stokes-Adams disease.

Thus, the relation between circulation, pulse abnormalities, and disease had been found. However, the real anatomical substrate was not yet discovered. In Greek times, Aristotle had watched the heart of chicken embryos. He registered various heart movements and already was able to make a distinction between the atrial and the ventricular contractions. Galen, the Roman, evaluated these findings further and found that the right atrium was the first part of the heart where the contractions started, *primum oriens*, and also the last part which stopped beating, *ultimum moriens*. Harvey in 1628 described in his studies the complete sequence of the now generally accepted cardiac cycle. In the nineteenth century Stannius and Gaskel showed that it was possible to make an interruption between the atria and the ventricles. Physiologists continued this research and John McWilliams in England wrote in 1807, 'The contraction arises from the heart, the first contraction most probably at the terminal portions of the great veins or close to it'.

The physiologists had made their recordings but still there was no anatomic substrate. Of course in 1839, Purkinje in Brno had found his Purkinje fibres, but further discoveries of the conduction system of the heart had to wait until 1893 when His in Germany published his anatomical studies on a rabbit heart where he had found a tissue connection between the atria and the ventricles, the bundle of His. The picture of the anatomy cleared further in 1896 when Aschoff and Tawara described the AV node and Tawara traced that the AV node was connected with the Purkinje system via the various bundle branches. In 1907, Keith and Flack in England found what they called the *primum mobile*, where everything starts, exactly where the physiologist McWilliams had thought it to be, the sinus node. The atrial pathways were discussed and described during the first half of our century.

The disease we speak about, atrioventricular block, was already mentioned by His in 1894. He postulated that since the AV bundle connects the atria and ventricles, it could be the cause of the Adams-Stokes attacks when interrupted. He dit not publish it at that time but only in 1933 and by that time the electrocardiograph had been developed. The first electrocardiographic tracing of total AV block was made in 1906 bij Einthoven in Leiden. From these tracings, Lewis and other people in England became aware that the AV conduction system was the origin of AV block and Stokes-Adams disease.

How did people treat this disease? It was known since the eighteenth century that you could stimulate the heart. In 1804 Aldini described studies in Turin in which the hearts of decapitated criminals were stimulated with the column of Galvani and Volta. Electricity was used in the eighteenth century and was applied especially for indirect stimulation of various organs, for instance to speed up the heart frequency. Galvanization became popular, and various devices were developed in the eighteenth and nineteenth centuries. It was known that through stimulation of the sympathetic nerves the heart rhythm could be influenced, as a sphygomograph recording of that time by Beard demonstrated. There were even special clinics in the eighteenth and nineteenth century for electrical treatment and cardiac stimulation, like that of Charcot in Paris. These clinics were rather popular and originated the development of various devices like sophisticated units for a doctor's office and also special patient devices to use in their own homes.

RECENT HISTORY

The techniques of direct stimulation of the heart and also of stimulation of the arrested heart as in the investigations of Aldini were difficult however. Perhaps acupuncture, already made popular in the nineteenth century, by, among others, the father of the famous French composer Berlioz, started an-

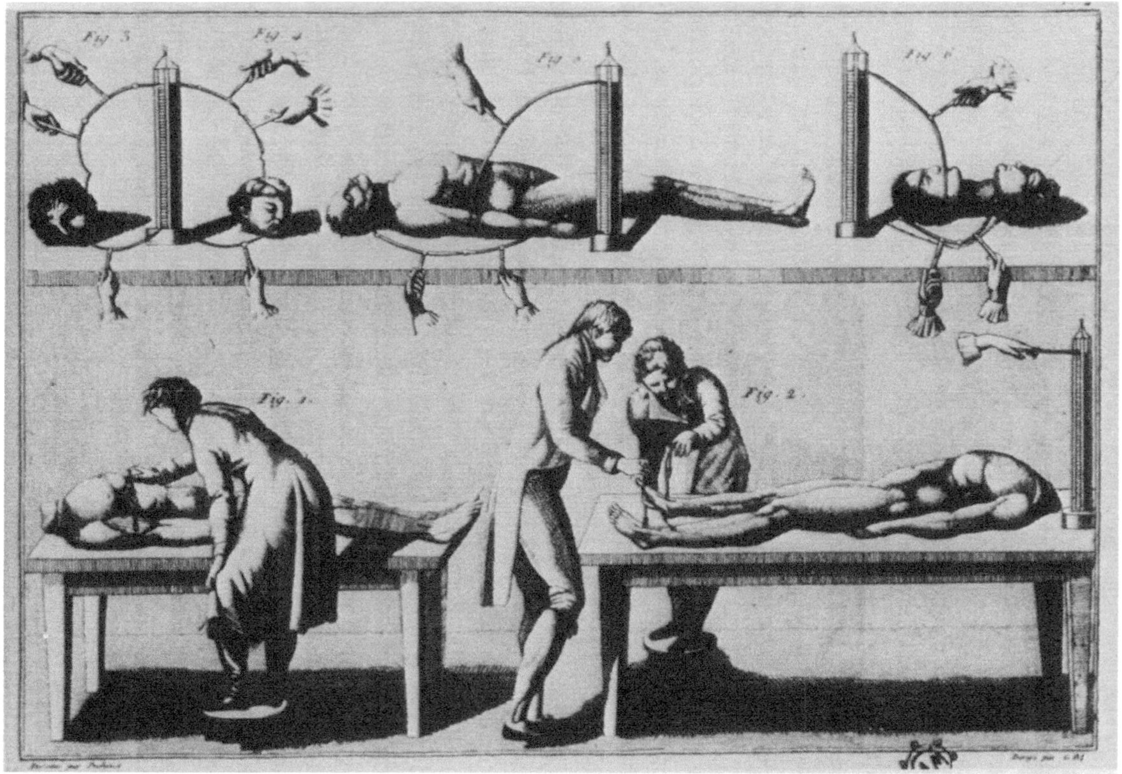

Figure 2A. Studies with electrical stimulation with Galvani's collum on decollated criminals by Vassali et al. in Turin and reported by Aldini in 1804.

FIGURES 2A-D. THE PATIENTS.

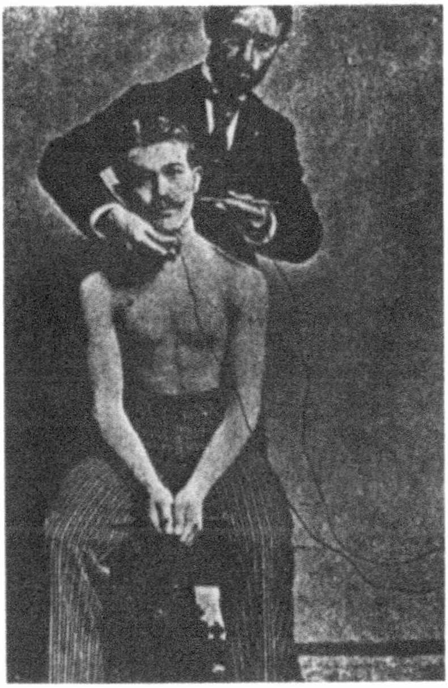

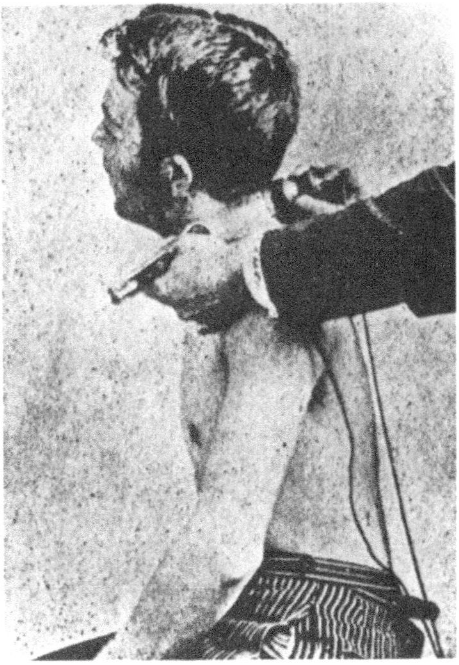

Figure 2B. Stimulation of vagal and cervical sympathetic nerves as practiced at the end of the 19th century.

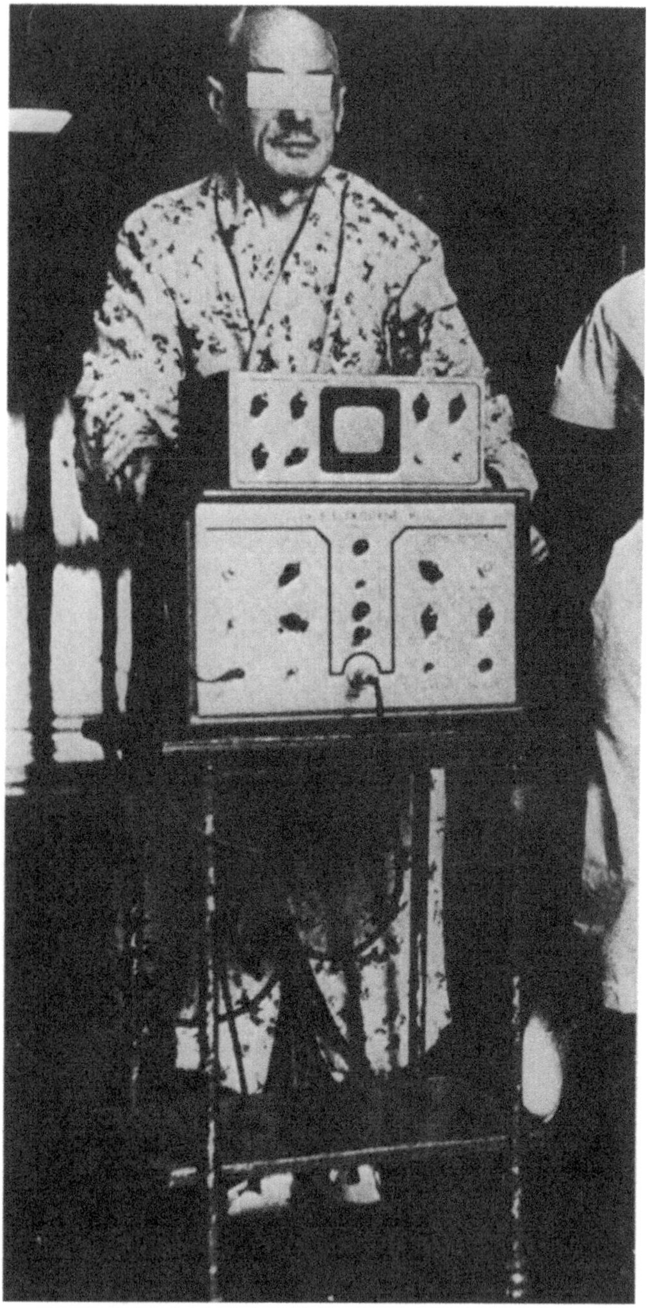

Figure 2C. The first patient who underwent transvenous pacing in 1958 in New York from Furman's publication. The electrode carried current from the 'internal' output of the pacemaker monitor. A 15 m. extension cord allowed ambulation with the patient supported by and pushing the pacemaker on a mobile cart.

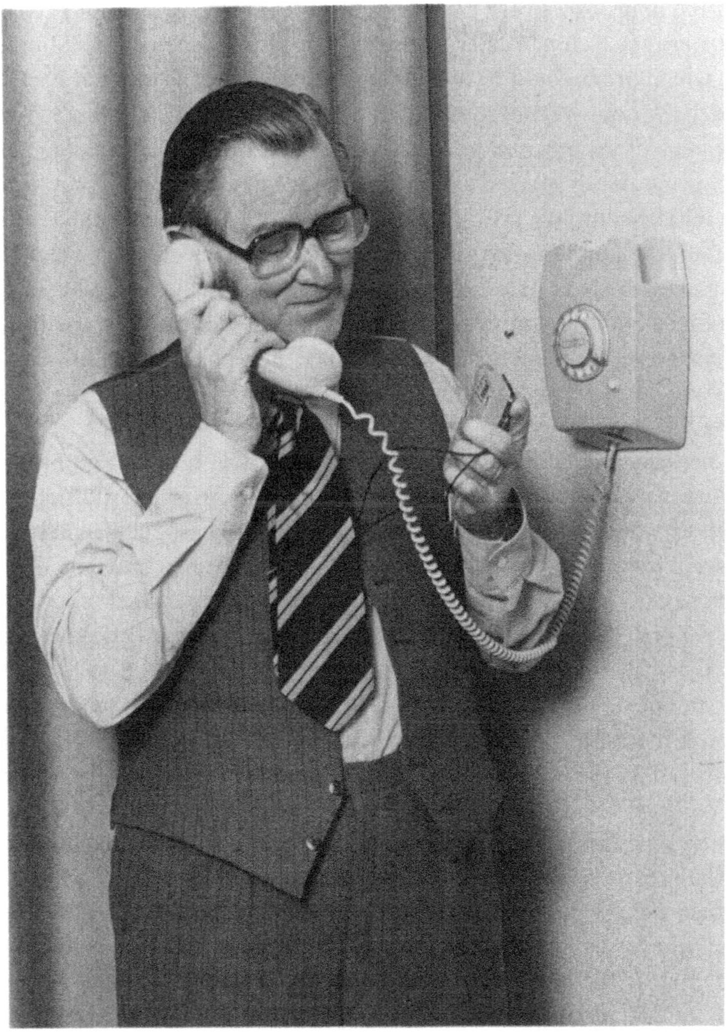

Figure 2D. Ir. Arne Larsen, the first patient to receive an implantable pacemaker in october 8th, 1958, by Ir. Elmqvist and Dr. Senning in Stockholm, checking his 23rd pacemaker during a visit at the Pacemaker Clinic of the University Hospital of Groningen.

other direct approach to the heart: a needle electrode driven into the heart through the intact chest. Later the needle was replaced by a hollow needle through which drugs could be introduced into the heart. Hyman in New York analysed the various ways of stimulation of the heart in 1932 and concluded that most probably it was not the drug that stimulatd a stopped heart but the needle puncture per se. He developed a device with a needle electrode that could be put through the chest into the heart and which produced interrupted pulses and not galvanic current as used earlier. The device had a spring mechanism which had to be rewound every six minutes. This enabled him to save the lives of at least two patients for 24-48 hours in 1932. Hyman, the man who really started cardiac pacing, also gave it its name, as he wrote: 'Since this apparatus is a substitute for the non-functioning normal sinus nodal pacemaker, it is called the artificial pacemaker'.

Zoll knew Hyman, who died in 1972, and described him during the Boston colloquium in 1976: 'He used to sit in the front row at the heart meetings. With his impressive manner, grey moustache and Vandyke beard, he would stand up and object to many of the so-called new advances that were presented'. Hyman's approach to cardiac stimulation had resulted in five units, called 'hearttticklers' in a New York Times article, and in the search for a more effecient way to energize the unit. He tried to replace the spring motor that had to be rewound every six minutes by a battery-powered unit and was negotiating for a special battery with the German Siemens company. Unfortunately the last Hyman unit was destroyed in the Siemens factory during the bombing of Dresden in the Second World War.

After the war, Zoll in Boston coordinated the ideas of Hyman and the work of two Canadians, Bigelow and Callaghan from Toronto. They presented in 1950 at the meeting of the American College of Surgeons in Boston their results of stimulation of canine hearts with one electrode in the oesophagus and a second one over the precordium. Two years later Zoll published in the New England Journal of Medicine an article on 'Resuscitation of the heart in ventricular standstill by external electric stimulation' his first results with an external stimulator connected to two skin-electrodes. The work of Hyman and Zoll did not receive great acclaim from colleagues and medical institutions. Hyman was in one comment on his work accused of 'fooling around with dead patients' and Zoll's application for a US $ 5000 grant from the United States Public Health Service was turned down.

Zoll and many others were not discouraged however and went on with their research and twenty years later, in 1973, Zoll was honoured for his contribution to the field of cardiac arrhythmias with the Wenckebach Memorial Lecture at the Fourth World Meeting on Cardiac Pacing in Groningen, in front of an audience with representatives from 48 countries.

Initially in the early fifties, research was focused on the development of internal long-term electric pacemakers, but it failed, among other reasons because of stimulation threshold in the days after implantation of the electrodes. This problem was also met by Lillehei's group in Minneapolis with their newly-developed intramural suture electrodes, placed in the myocardium.

In a meeting in 1959 at the Rockefeller Institute in New York the discussion on long-term pacing also encountered the electrode problem. As with many other problems, it is attacked by various groups and sooner or later a solution comes around the corner. In this case Zoll met it in the corridors after the meeting. He writes almost twenty years later: 'After the meeting Dr. John Schwedel told me that a young surgical house officer working in the catheterization laboratory at the Montefiore Hospital, a fellow named Seymour Furman, had developed a technique for long-term stimulation of the heart by passing an endocardial catheter electrode into the right ventricle. I went with him to the hospital late that afternoon and observed the patient, who was indeed being stimulated repeatedly for days in this way.' And although Zoll reports: 'I recognized this experience as the beginning of long-term electric stimulation of the heart', Furman too met great criticism when he wanted to publish his early results.

Not only in the United States but also in Europe, research on cardiac pacing had produced positive results. In Stockholm Elmqvist and Senning had not only worked on the electrode problem and found a solution in an epicardial disc electrode but they had also constructed a small implantable pacemaker by using the newly-developed trasistors. Transistors are small and efficient but most of all function at a low voltage and can be combined with small batteries. On 8 october 1958, they implanted their first unit in a patient. This man, an engineer, Arne H.W. Larsson, is still alive and presented in early May 1978 the opening address at the first European Symposium on Cardiac Pacing in London, almost 20 years after he received the first of 23 pacemakers that enabled him to lead his active life as chairman of the Swedish Society of Heart Patients.

MODERN HISTORY

In the last two decades cardiac pacing has become a widely accepted electrotherapy in cardiology. About 2000 participants are expected at the Sixth World Meeting on Cardiac Pacing in Montreal. This does not only illustrate that more persons are getting involved in the care of pacemaker patients but also that cardiac pacing is still changing and improving during the recent years.

To discuss the recent progress of cardiac pacing it is reasonable to divide the pacemaker unit into three parts: electrode, electrode lead, and generator with circuit and batteries.

Electrode

The skin-electrode of Zoll was replaced by the epicardial or intramural electrode that had to be implanted on the heart by thoracotomy. This electrode, although initially used in many patients, has been replaced by the transvenous electrode, initiated by Furman and Schwedel in the United States and Lagergren in Sweden. In 1976 at the Tokyo Pacemaker World Meeting 93.4% of the reported 15,000 electrodes implanted in 1975 were transvenous endocardial electrodes. This great acceptance of the endocardial electrode is due to the less complicated way of implantation for patient and doctor and due to improvements made especially in this type of electrode.

Although the intramural corkscrew electrode, which can be implanted through the Sauerbruch approach – *pericardiotomia inferior longitudinalis* – has recovered some of the intramural electrode applications, the disadvantages of the endocardial electrodes, such as dislocations and high energy consumption, have decreased. The dislocation ratio has improved by better medical training and by improvements in electrode design such as electrode barbs and tines. Also special fixation mechanisms like hooks and coils have decreased the 4-9 percent dislocation ratio met with standard electrodes and procedures. The efficiency has also improved by decrease of the electrode surface area. Originally electrodes with surface areas of 50mm^2 have been used. About ten years ago the surface area decreased to 20-28mm^2, the last five years to 10-12mm^2, and recently electrodes with special tip design like the ring-shape electrode with a surface area of 5-8mm^2 have been applied. This has resulted in a decrease of energy consumption from the batteries from 25-30 μA. to 2-4 μA.

Electrode lead

The electrode lead still poses a great problem. Of the pacemaker emergencies 15-18 percent are due to lead problems such as insulation defects or wire fractures. The failure mode – mostly 'sudden failure' with complete interruption of stimulation – has great consequences for the patient. Research is now focusing on this problem and on solutions such as redundancy systems and, especially, improved wires (wire diameter, coil diameter, and coil speed are very important parameters) are now in clinical evaluation.

Generator

Great improvements have been made in the technical field which have resulted in improved generators both for circuit design and for batteries. Because of the cumulated knowhow on components and construction highly reliable pacemakers have been produced with standard components. The application of integrated circuits is the most recent improvement, and this has enabled the construction of smaller, more complicated, but still efficient, pacemakers. In some cases the circuit consumes only ten percent of the energy that was necessary in the early designs.

The lifetime of the pacemakers is not only determined by the decreased current consumption of the electrode and electronic circuit but also by the available energy in the pacemakers. The first implantable Swedish pacemaker used nickel-cadmium batteries with an energy of 60 mAh that could be recharged inductively. The first American implantable pacemaker, developed by Chardack and Greatbatch in 1960 in Minneapolis, used mercury oxide-zinc batteries with 1200 mAh. These 12-gram, 3-cm^2 batteries produce about 1.3 volts. Depending on the pacemaker type, 3-5 batteries are used to create pacemaker lifetimes of initially 2-3 years, but now 3-4 years. Recently great improvements have been made by the use of lithium batteries, which do not contain an electrolyte but are solid-state batteries. Contrarily to the mercury-zinc batteries there is no gas development during the chemical process and this enables the construction of completely hermetically-sealed pacemakers so that no body fluid can enter the battery and circuit. With this type of battery and circuit, and also by the replacement of the epoxy insulation by the metal can, life expectancies of 4-6 years and even over ten years seem possible. The lithium battery that in 1970 was brought into the field of pacing by its developer Mr. Schneider in Baltimore and by Greatbatch and in France by Lehman's group in Poitiers was applied clinically in a pacemaker for the first time in November 1972 and is now the most commonly used battery type. Nowadays six types of lithium batteries are in use or in research projects. The lithium-lithium iodine and the lithium-silver chromate are the most used types, but also the lithium-lead iodine, the lithium-thirylchloride, lithium-copper sulphide and the lithium-bromide are applied in the modern pacemakers. All of these units have their own end-of-life characteristics that are used with the various circuits and that should be known by the responsible doctor and engineer. These improvements in generator design have resulted in a decrease of the pacemaker volume from about 60-70 cm^3 to 30-35 cm^3 and of the pacemaker weight from about 130-140 to 40-45 grams.

The types of generators have kept up with the technical improvements, Besides the fixed rate units; the by far most used R-wave-controlled units (about 97 percent of all implanted pacemakers), with the R-wave-inhibited and in some cases R-wave-triggered types; and the hemodynamically optimal design; the atrial-triggered unit, there has been an extensive development in units such as atrial-on-demand, bifocal-demand, and so on, and the programmable pacemaker that enables external programming of parameters like impulse frequency, impulse duration, output current/voltage, refractory period, etc. Further developments try to work out parameters that will program the pacemaker automatically, whereas another line of new development focuses on pacemakers that

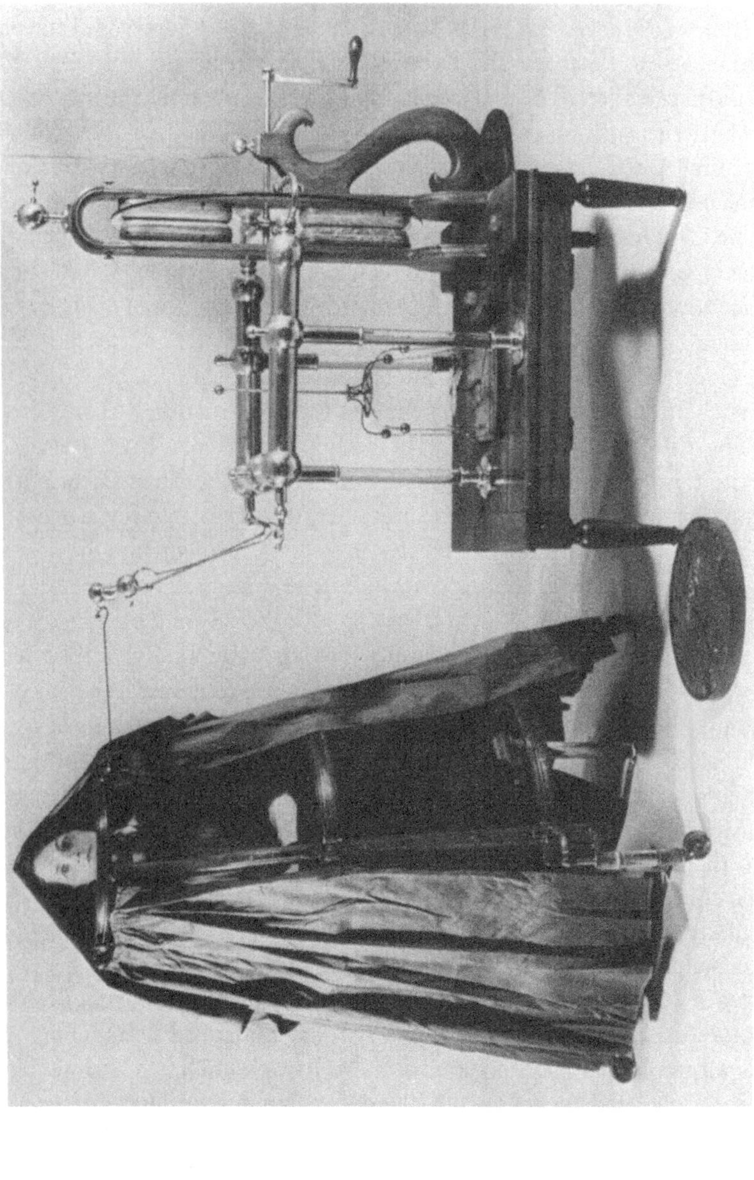

Figure 3A. Faradic stimulator used at the end of the 19th century. There was in these times an extensive discussion that the heartrate of the patient did not increase because of the faradic influence but because of the patients' agony.

FIGURES 3A-E. THE STIMULATORS.

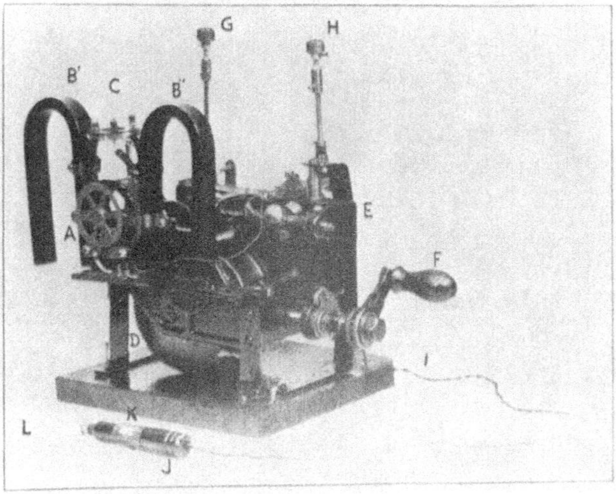

Figure 3B. The 7.2 kg artificial pacemaker by Hyman used in 1932 in New York.

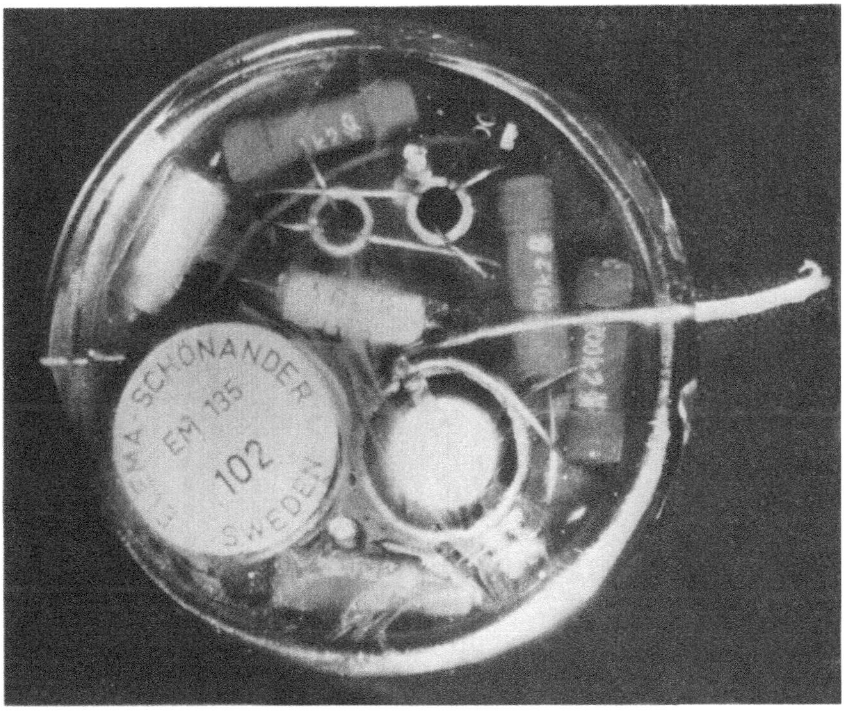

Figure 3C. The first implantable pacemaker developed in 1958 by Elmqvist and Senning in Stockholm, that had to be recharged inductively.

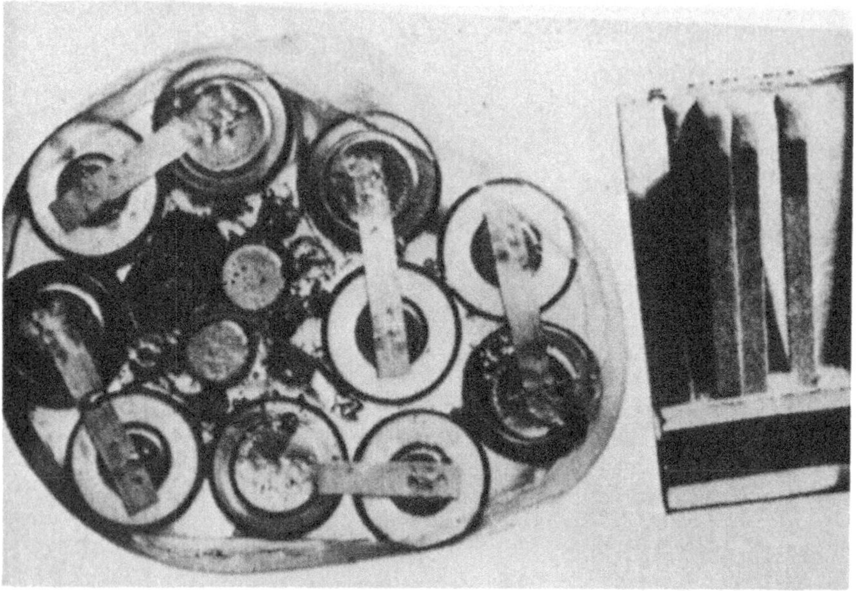

Figure 3D. The first implantable pacemaker developed in the USA by Chardack, Gage and Greatbatch in 1960.

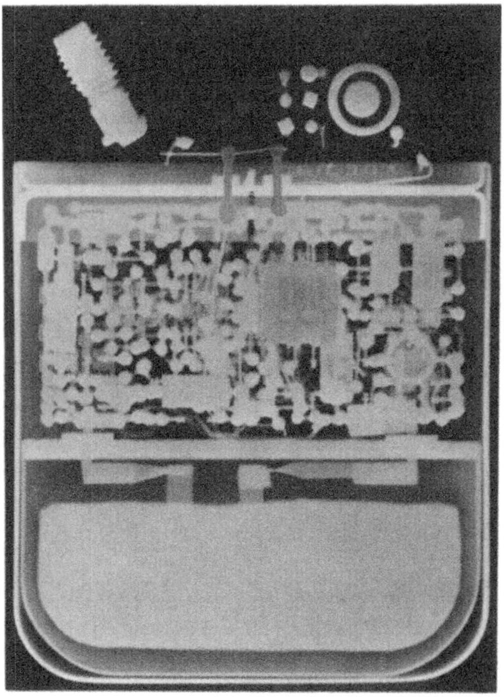

Figure 3E. Röntgenpicture of the now generally applied lithium powered pacemaker with hybrid circuit, in an hermetically sealed can.

will record and store data and will pı ovide the data to print-out systems at the pacemaker clinic.

Pacemaker clinic

The abovementioned improvements have resulted in longer-lasting, more reliable pacing systems that have been implanted in an increasing number of patients. It is now estimated that every year, worldwide, about 200,000 patients are treated with an implantable pacemaker. Due to the technical improvements pacemaker replacements are far less frequent and include now about 20 percent of the overall pacemaker procedures in our clinic, whereas only four years ago they comprised 50 percent of our interventions. This enables medical assistence for more patients with the same effort and about the same costs. These new patients are especially patients with the so-calles sick sinus syndrome, who form an increasing percentage of the pacemaker patients. From only a few percent some years ago they now account for 30-40 percent of the new pacemaker implants. This group of patients can be traced especially by dynamic electrocardiography, a technique also developed during the last decade. The increasing numbers of patients, with different etiology and various types of pacemakers, need constant medical support. This has resulted in pacemaker follow-up clinics, where pacemaker performance is analysed. This special follow-up was initiated, particularly in Europe, in 1967, with ECG, vector analysis, and photoanalysis as the techniques used. With these systems pacemaker impulse and pacemaker function could be checked. With the development of more reliable pacemakers this intensive follow-up, necessitating visits by the pacemaker patient to a clinic, became less productive, and some of the clinical visits were replaced by analysis over the telephone, a technique initiated in the United States and now being introduced slowly in Europe.

Pacemaker societies

With the increasing number of pacemaker patients the number of persons involved with the treatment of such patients also increased. At the First World Meeting on Cardiac Pacing in New York (1964) about 100 persons participated, mostly from the United States. The basis for international coordination was established five years later during the second meeting, also in New York. The initiative of Furman and Esscher was followed in Europe by Dodinot and Faivre (Monaco, 1970) and Thalen and Nieveen (Groningen, 1973). At this last meeting 1250 participants from 48 countries discussed the development in the field of cardiac pacing. During the fifth meeting in Tokyo (1976) the 1500 participants decided to organize themselves into the International Pacing Society and started an international journal, Pacing and Cardiac Electrophysiology (PACE), that,

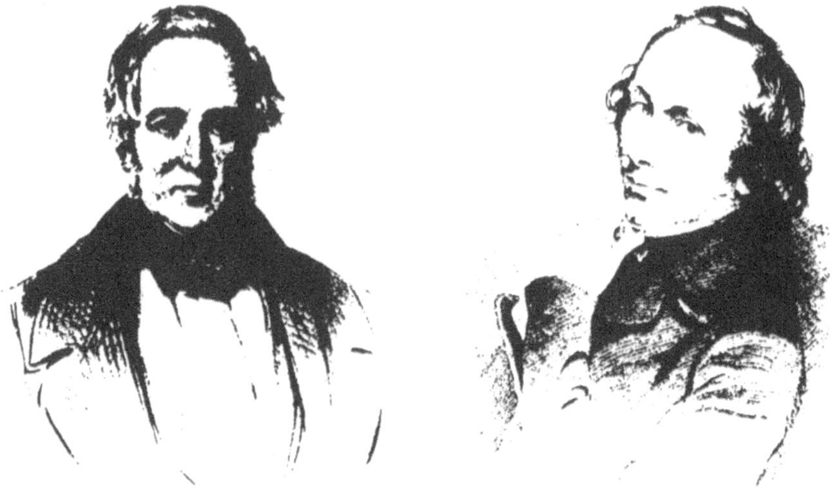

Figures 4A-B. Robert Adams (L) and William Stokes (R), who combined the symptoms and aetiology of heart block at the end of the 19th century.

especially due to the efforts of Seymour Furman, has become a great success in the two years of its existence.

The international activities were reflections of local initiatives. In Europe national pacing societies originated in various countries and were brought together in 1976 in the Working Group on Cardiac Pacing of the European Society of Cardiology. In 1978, 18 countries paricipated in the first European Symposium on Cardiac Pacing in London. In South America also various national societies were initiated whereas last year in the United States the first steps were taken to organize an American Pacing Society.

These groups will all meet at the Sixth Symposium on Cardiac Pacing in Montreal, that has developed into a five-day meeting with about 2000 participants. Besides reports about the recent technical developments the agenda of the meeting now includes the standardization of terminology, pacemaker identification and pacemaker tests; the pacemaker patient identity card; legal aspects of pacing; coordination in failure reporting; and the very crucial subject of pacemaker reconditioning for reimplantation.

This last subject clearly illustrates the tremendous progress of pacemaker technology in the last forty years: from the external pacemaker of Hyman that had to be rewound every six minutes to the small implantable units that outlast most of their patients, a progress made possible by cooperation between engineers, doctors, technicians, and many others – a group that receives new members every year. Especially for these new members we have started this volume *Fundamentals of cardiac pacing* with an historical outline to illustrate that cardiac

FIGURES 4A-F. THE DOCTORS.

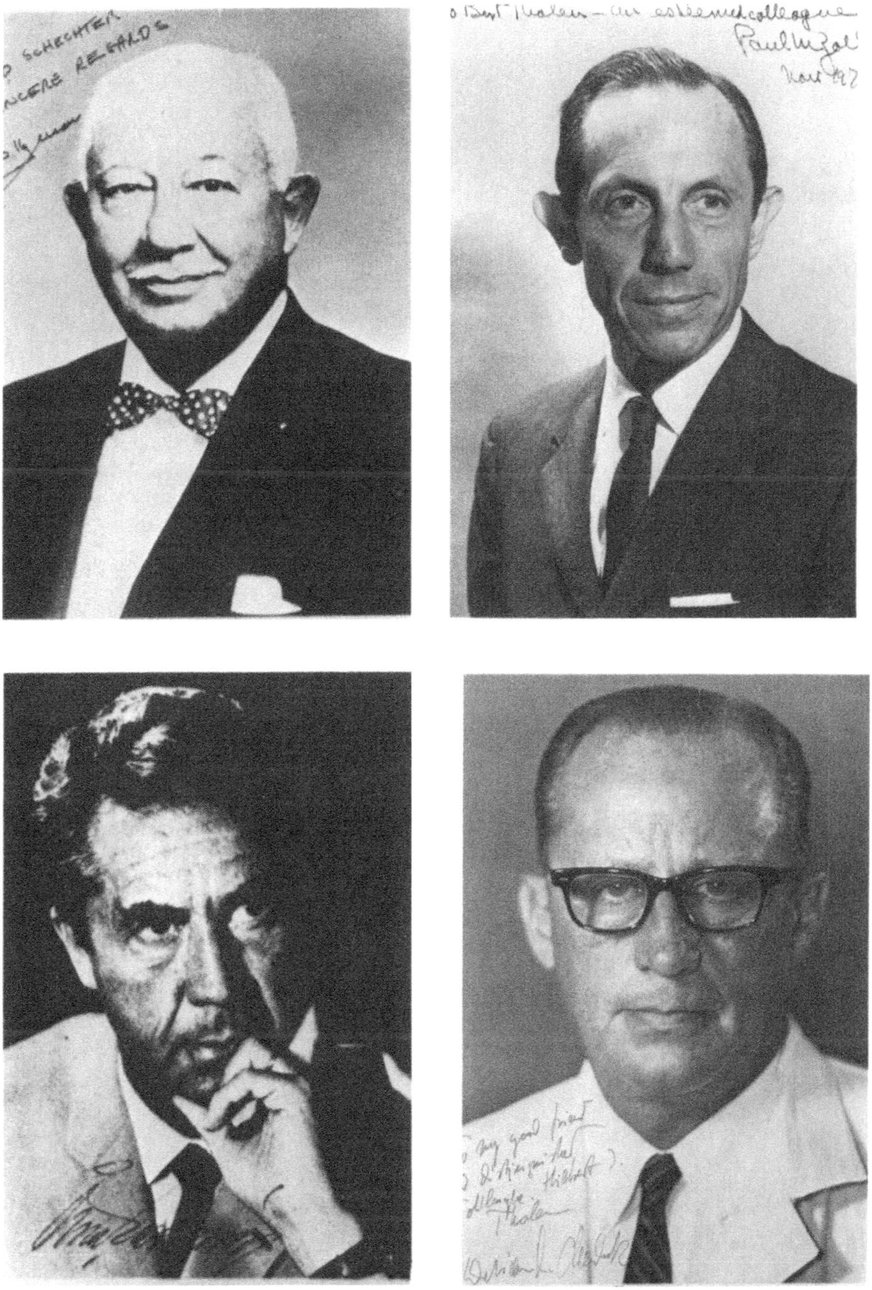

Figures 4C-F. Albert Hyman (top L), who produced the first artificial cardiac pacemaker in 1932 and Paul Zoll (top R), who initiated with his activities in 1952 the modern developments of cardiac pacing. Åke Senning (bottom L) and William Chardack (bottom R) the two cardiac surgeons who implanted the first pacemaker in resp. Europe and the USA (1958-1960).

FIGURES 5A-D. THE ELECTRODES.

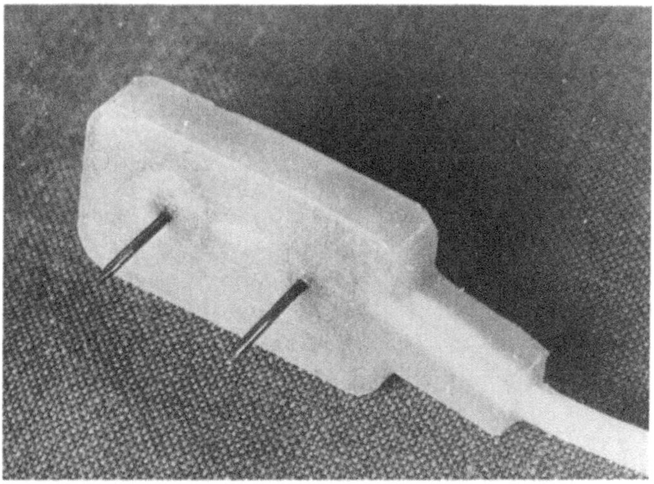

Figure 5A. The first bipolar intramural electrode with two stainless steel pin electrodes with a length of 7.5 mm. as developed by Hunther et al. in 1959.

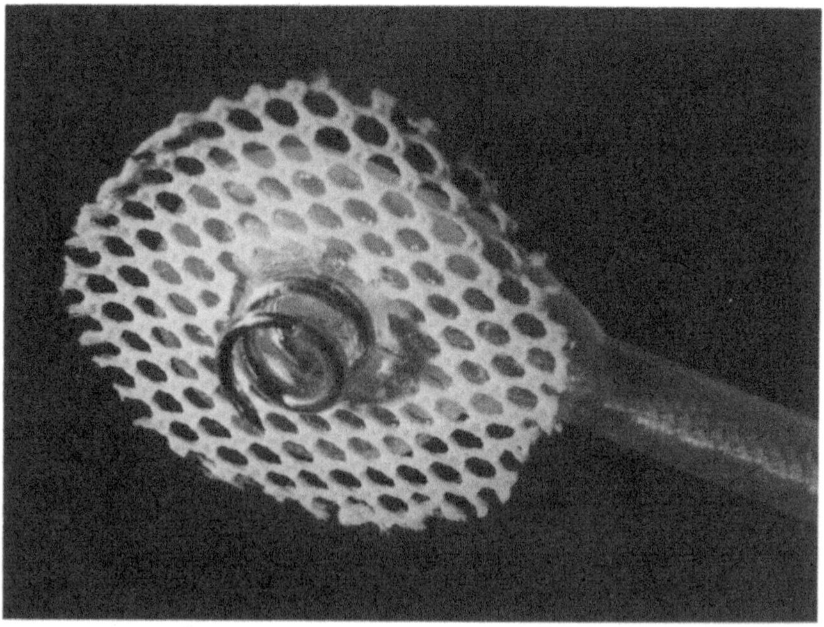

Figure 5B. The most recent variant of the intramural electrodes, the corkscrew electrode developed by Hunther et al. in 1973.

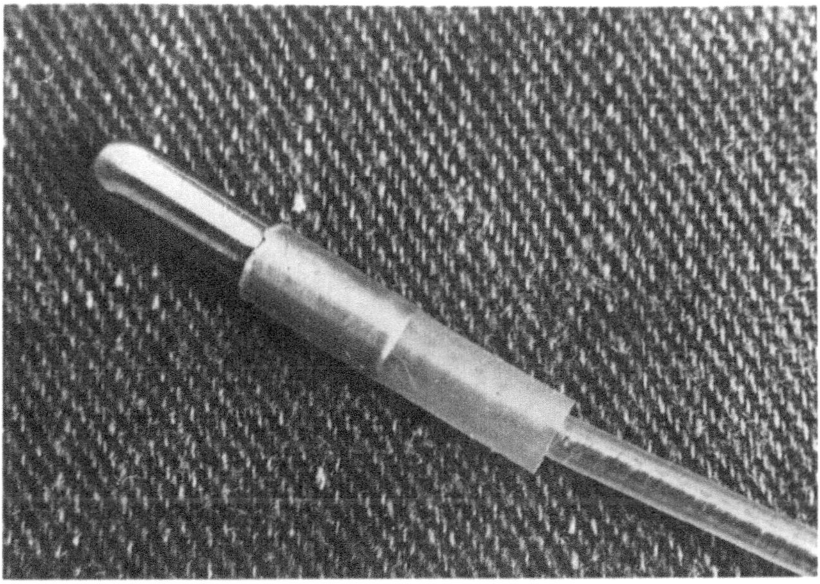

Figure 5C. The first transvenous electrode developed by Lagergren and Johansson in 1963 with a surface area of 48 mm^2.

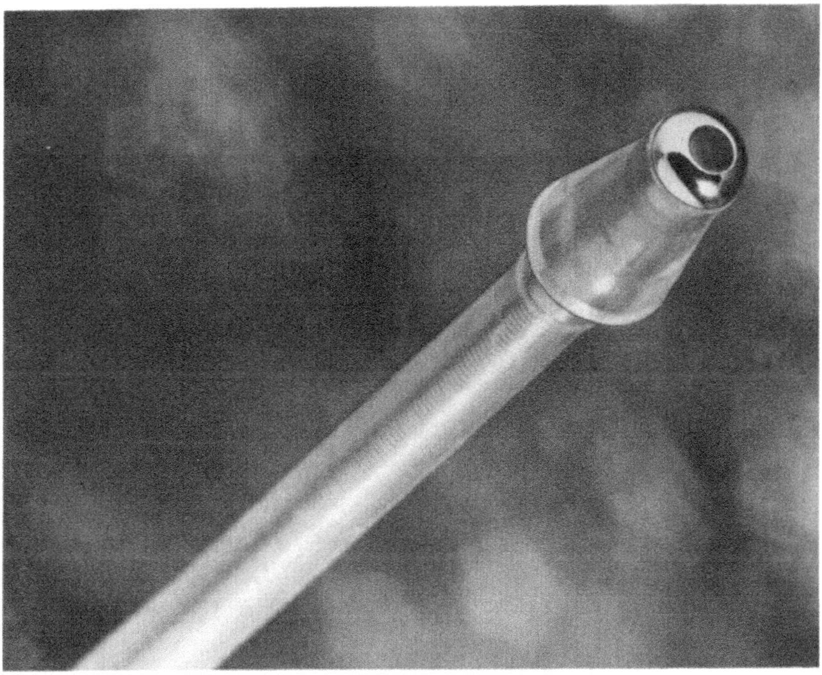

Figure 5D. A recent variant of the transvenous electrode, the ring tip electrode with a surface area of 7.6 mm^2 developed by Thalen in 1973.

pacing has come a long way and that Montreal will be another step on the way to improve the quantity and the quality of life for the increasing number of pacemaker patients.

ACKNOWLEDGEMENTS

This article is condensed from a monograph entitled *The artificial cardiac pacemaker history*, by David Chas. Schechter (New York Medical College) Dennis Stillings (Museum of Electricity in Life, Minneapolis), and Hilbert J.Th. Thalen (University Hospital, Groningen), to be published by Martinus Nijhoff Medical Division, The Hague, The Netherlands as part of a series on various aspects of cardiac pacing. Data for the publication have been collected at the library of the New York Academy of Medicine, the museum of Electricity in Life (Minneapolis), the Francis A. Countway Library of Medicine (Boston), the Teyler Museum (Haarlem), and the Museum of the University of Groningen. Selected references by the above authors on the history of cardiac pacing are included in the reference list (1, 2, 3, 4). Further information on developments is to be found in the proceedings of the five international symposia (5, 6, 7, 8, 9).

REFERENCES

1. Schechter DC, Lillehei CW, Soffer: History of heart block. *Diseases of the chest* 55 (suppl 1), 1969.
2. Schechter DC: Origins of electrotherapy. *New York State J Med* 71: 11-12, 1971.
3. Schechter DC, Background of clinical cardiac electrostimulation. *New York State J Med* 71-72, 1971-1972.
4. Thalen HJTh, van den Berg JW, Homan van der Heide JN, Nieveen J: *The artificial cardiac pacemaker, its history, development and clinical application*, Assen, Van Gorcum, 1969 (3rd printing 1975).
5. Glenn WWL (ed): Cardiac pacemakers. *Ann New York Ac Sciences* 11 (3): 813-1122, 1964.
6. Furman S (ed): Advances in cardiac pacemakers. *Ann New York Ac Sciences* 167 (2): 515-1075, 1969.
7. Dodinot B (ed): Clinical aspects of long-term cardiac pacing. *Ann de Cardiol et d'Angéiol* 20 (4): 281-557, 1971.
8. Thalen HJTh (ed): *Cardiac pacing: proceedings of the fourth international symposium*, Assen, Van Gorcum, 1973.
9. Watanabe Y (ed): *Cardiac pacing: proceedings of the fifth international symposium*, Amsterdam, Excerpta Medica, 1977.

2. ANATOMY AND PATHOLOGY OF THE CONDUCTION SYSTEM OF THE HUMAN HEART

THOMAS N. JAMES

In the normal rhythm of the human heart an electrical impulse originates within the sinus node and courses by way of internodal pathways to the AV (atrio-ventricular) junction where it enters the AV node and passes to the His bundle for distribution through its right and left bundle branches to the ventricular myocardium. To describe the normal and abnormal anatomy of the responsible structures I will use the same sequence in which electrical activation occurs. When disturbances of either rhythm or conduction occur, the physiological sequence of activation can and often does vary, but the normal arrangement and its understanding is still the fundamental basis for unraveling how these disturbances originate and behave.

THE SINUS NODE

Normal anatomy

Keith and Flack were the first to describe a special structure lying between the superior vena cava and the free wall of the right atrium just beneath the epicardium and to suggest that it was the origin of the heart beat (1). There is little to add to the accuracy and clarity of their original report, as concerns the gross and light microscopic anatomy; however, electron microscopy and new electrophysiologic technics have greatly expanded our knowledge of just how the sinus node is organized and functions. Although Keith and Flack considered the blood supply of the human sinus node as an arterial circle, it is actually provided by a single conspicuous atrial branch (2, 3) of either the right (55%) or left circumflex (45%) coronary artery. There is always anastomosis between the sinus node artery and neighboring atrial coronary arteries, but there is no true circle. It is rare for more than one major atrial artery to serve as the sinus node branch, and the sinus node artery is nearly always the largest and thereby most important of all atrial coronary branches.

Lying as it does just beneath the epicardium, the sinus node (Figure 1) is susceptible to injury or disease by any process affecting the pericardium. Its anterior margin rarely extends beyond the crest formed by the right atrial appendage at its juncture with the superior vena cava, and this crest (4) can be used as an anatomical landmark indicating the anterior edge of the sinus node. From that point the flattened body of the sinus node extends parallel to the sulcus terminalis and lies just over the crista terminalis if viewed from within the right atrium. Histologically, the sinus node is completely organized about a centrally located artery within it and normally contains a distinct collagen framework within which the cells of the sinus node are disposed in an interweaving meshwork. There is no true head or tail for the sinus node, despite the popular use of these terms.

Within the sinus node there are two types of special myocardial cells. There are also numerous nerves, although ganglia are predominantly outside the node near its posterior margin. The two cell types are a slender elongated one and another which is round or ovoid. The slender one is called a *transitional cell* and probably functions as the distributor system from the sinus node. The round or ovoid one is called a *P cell* and is probably the site of impulse formation (2, 5, 6), although it seems likely that multiple such cells are responsible for the origin of a normal sinus impulse. P cells are grouped in grape-like clusters predominantly within the deeper or central portions of the sinus node, where interweaving transitional cells attach to them and then serve as the exclusive bridge for connection to other types of myocardial cells. P cells thus connect only to each other or to transitional cells, while the latter connect to all types of myocytes. There is a regrettable tendency to refer to 'nodal cells' as if they are a single type. Anatomically, there are at least two distinct types of myocardial cells within every human sinus node, and *both* are true nodal cells.

Abnormal anatomy

There are several useful ways to consider the pathological changes which may afflict the sinus node. It is a subepicardial structure full of collagen and is organized about a central artery, so that any disease of the pericardium (7), or of collagen (8, 9) (Figure 1) or of small arteries (8, 10-12) can cause damage to the sinus node. On the other hand, every systemic disease which affects the heart can include the sinus node and examples include amyloidosis (13), lupus erythematosus (8) and Whipple's lipodystrophy (14). Hemachromatosis for some reason seems to spare the sinus node although it does damage other parts of the conduction system (15).

Vascular diseases merit special discussion as they relate to the sinus node. Atherosclerosis is the most frequent cause of vascular injury or ischemic damage. However, this is always the consequence of significant narrowing or occlusion of a main coronary artery proximal to the origin of the sinus node branch, and not due to atherosclerotic narrowing of the latter. During acute myocardial infarction, the new onset of an atrial arrhythmia is a useful clinical clue that the responsible coronary obstruction is proximal to the origin of the sinus node

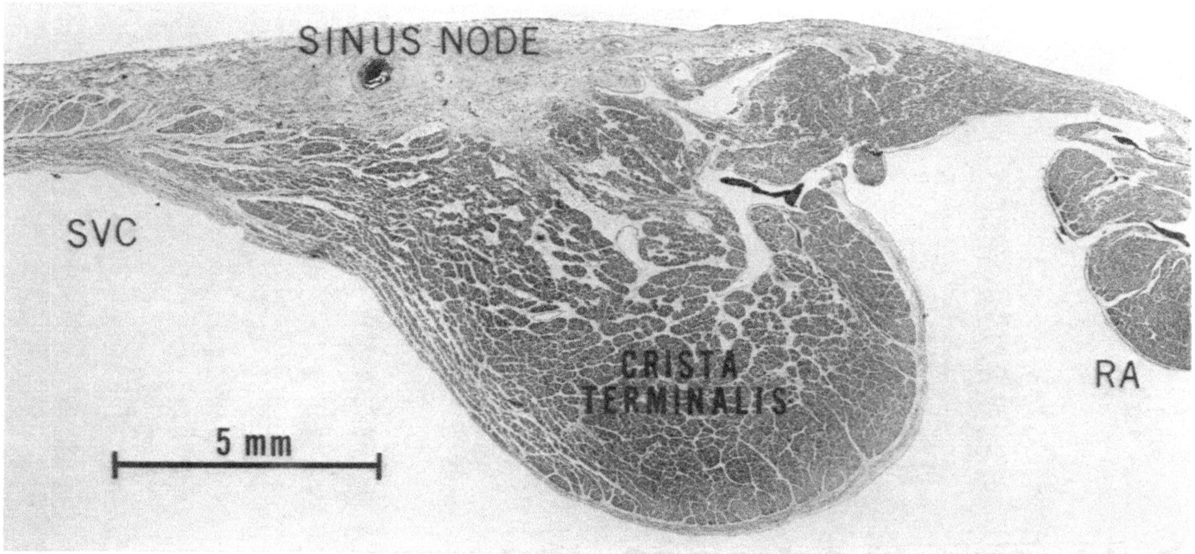

Figure 1A.

Figure 1. These three photomicropraphs illustrate the histological appearance of the human sinus node. The panels A and B are both normal sinus nodes at two different magnifications (indicated by reference bars) from two different hearts. The panel C illustrates scirrhous fibrosis of the sinus node from a patient with scleroderma heart disease; the light colored tissue is collagen, the relative proportion of which is much greater in scleroderma heart disease. For the normal sinus node seen at low magnification note its proximity to the epicardium above, and its location at junction of superior vena cava (SVC) and free wall of right atrium (RA); the crista terminalis here was cut in cross section. Goldner trichrome stain in these and subsequent photomicrographs, except as indicated.

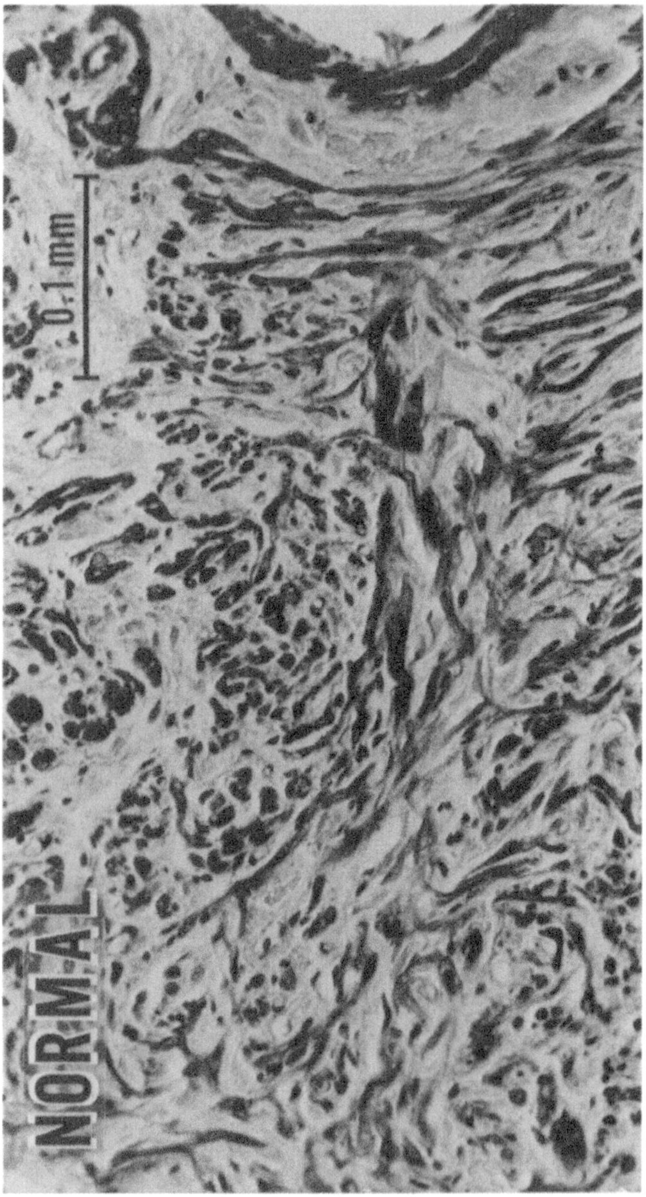

Figure 1B.

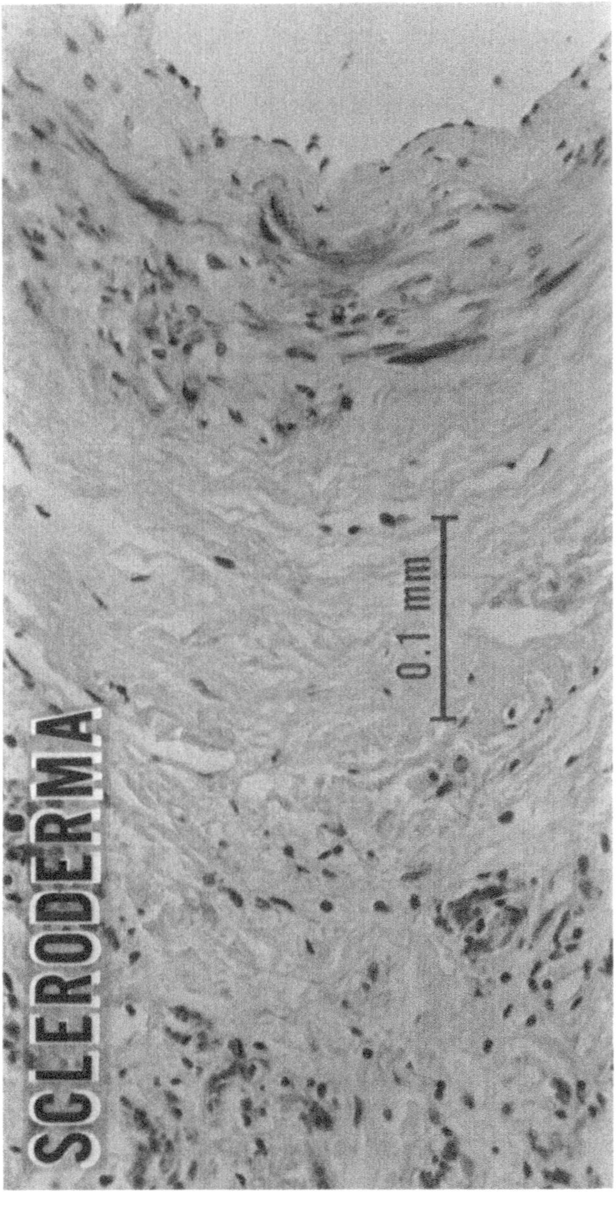

Figure 1C.

artery (16). Those diseases which produce arteritis or obliteration of small arteries elsewhere can and do involve the sinus node artery directly, two examples being polyarteritis nodosa (11) and lupus erythematosus (8). Finally, disorders of coagulation will sometimes produce transient or permanent thrombotic occlusion of the sinus node artery, examples including thrombotic thrombocytopenic purpura (17), disseminated intravascular coagulation (18) and congenital homocystinuria (19).

Rarer abnormalities of the sinus node include its involvement by tumors and the occurrence of congenital malformations. Although a variety of cancers have been shown to metastasize to or directly invade the sinus node, this is nearly always but one component of widespread dissemination, making the clinical significance of atrial arrhythmia or similar complications of less significance than they might be under different circumstances. Little is known of congenital malformations of the sinus node, although it can logically be anticipated that absence of the right superior vena cava or presence of an abnormal left superior vena cava (20) could influence the embryogenesis of the structures, such as the sinus node, to which they are normally so closely related. The rich opportunity to investigate this question among the large spectrum of various congenital cardiovascular malformations could provide us with especially useful information about malposition, malformation or analogous distortions of the developmental anatomy and subsequent malfunction of the sinus node.

THE INTERNODAL PATHWAYS

Normal anatomy

From the sinus node the normal cardiac impulse travels via three pathways (Figure 2) to the AV node (21). None of these is shielded or isolated by collagen sheaths, and none is composed of any single type of myocardial cell. All three pathways mingle with adjacent ordinary atrial myocardium, but they do exist as distinct and easily identified gross anatomical structures in the form of muscle bundles. Within these muscle bundles the cells (22) include ones which resemble Purkinje cells, some resembling ordinary atrial myocardium, some like slender transitional cells (especially in the regions near either the sinus node or AV node), and ones which appear to be the same as the P cells thought to be the site of origin of the sinus impulse within the sinus node. The relative predominance of these four types of cells varies from heart to heart and certainly between species, but the Purkinje-like cells and the ones resembling ordinary working myocytes are the most abundant and intermingle with each other.

Arrangement of the three internodal pathways is in a centrifugal fashion from the sinus node and centripetal to the AV node, at least when considered in relation to the route of spread of the normal sinus impulse. The *anterior inter-*

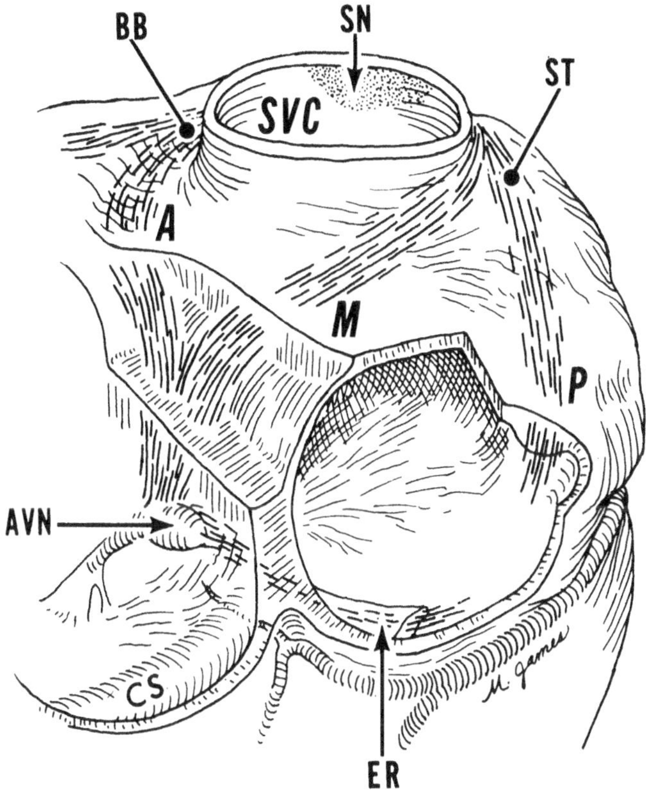

Figure 2. In this drawing the course of the three internodal pathways is shown for the human heart. View of the heart is from above and behind the left atrium, which is cut away along with a slice into the upper portion of the interatrial septum. BB is Bachmann's bundle, from which the anterior internodal pathway (A) descends back into the interatrial septum where it joins with fibers from the middle internodal pathway, marked M. The third internodal pathway from the sinus node (SN) to the AV node (AVN) is the posterior, marked P and coursing initially within the crista terminalis which is seen from the surface as the sulcus terminalis (ST). The terminal portion of the posterior internodal pathway enters the AV node from above the coronary sinus (CS), just after it passes through the eustachian ridge (ER), cut across in this schematic drawing as part of the window opening into the right atrium in the region of the inferior vena cava.

nodal pathway leaves the sinus node to course forward around the superior vena cava and enter the anterior interatrial myocardial band known as Bachmann's bundle. Near its midpoint Bachmann's bundle divides into one portion continuing toward the left atrium and a second major component of fibers which descends posteriorly into the interatrial septum toward the crest of the AV node (Figure 2). The *middle internodal pathway* leaves the posterior margin of the sinus node and immediately sweeps around the superior vena cava to cross toward the upper margin of the interatrial septum. There it soon joins fibers from the anterior internodal pathway as they jointly descend toward the crest of the AV

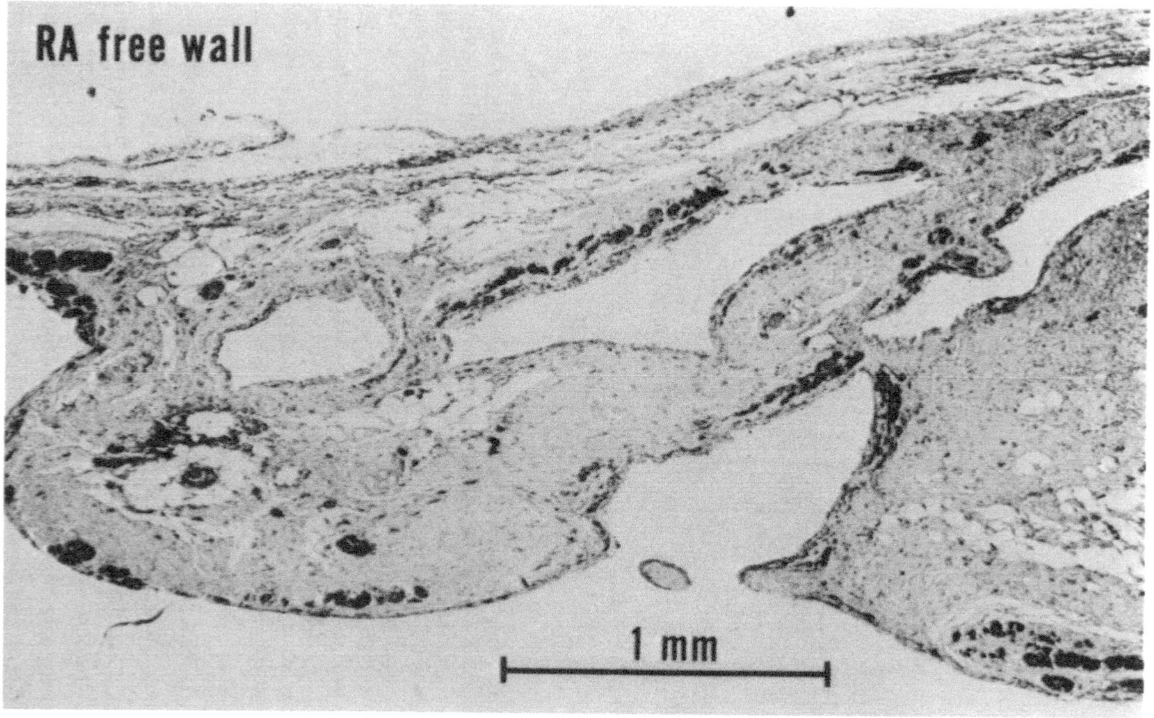

Figure 3A.

Figure 3. These two photomicrographs illustrate extensive fibrotic degeneration of unknown cause involving portions of the right atrium in a patient with a recurring variety of atrial arrhythmias.

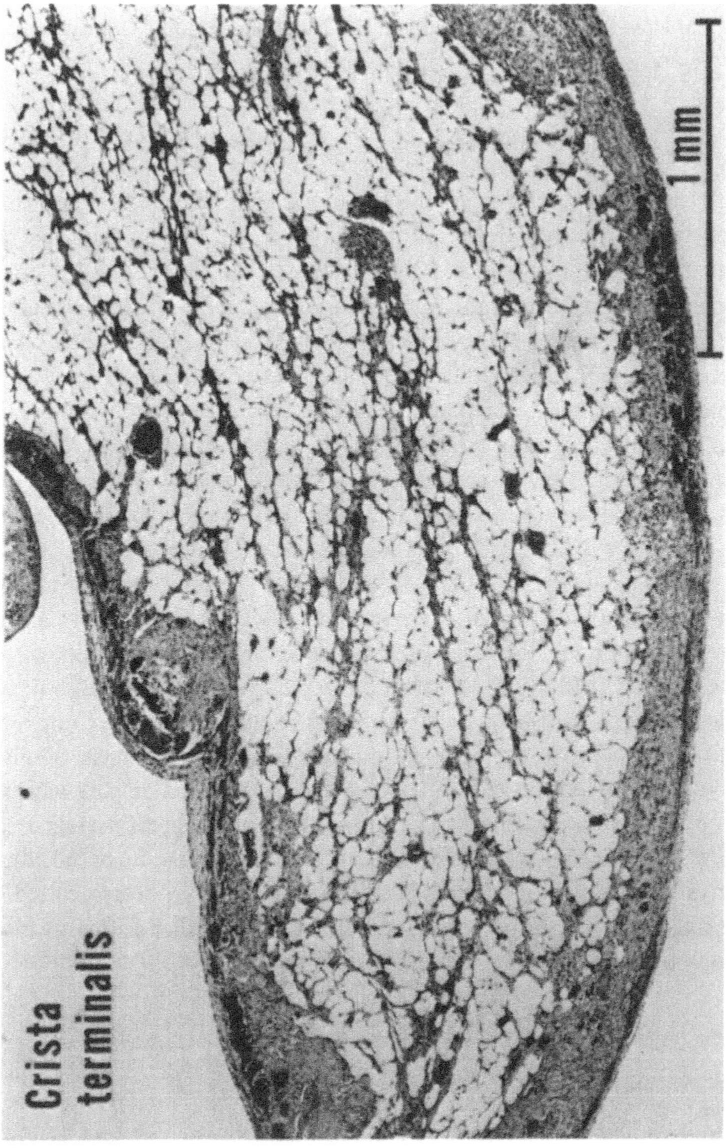

Figure 3B.

node. This juncture of anterior and middle internodal pathway fibers forms the torus Loweri, an easily identified gross anatomic landmark lying anterior to the fossa ovalis. The *posterior internodal pathway* also leaves the posterior margin of the sinus node but does not veer across the sinus intercavarum, continuing instead within the crista terminalis toward the inferior vena cava. There it passes beneath the inferior vena cava and over the ostium of the coronary sinus, being recognizable at this location as within the Eustachian ridge, finally entering the posterior and subendocardial margins of the AV node.

Abnormal anatomy

Because there are three of them and because they are not isolated or discretely shielded structures, the internodal pathways are quite often found to contain focal anatomical abnormalities. However, these need to be especially numerous and widespread to become functionally important, in other words, focal fibrosis or destruction of any type in one internodal pathway would still permit spread of the sinus impulse through either or both of the two other pathways. There are examples of widespread destruction of all the three internodal pathways (Figure 3) both in human (23) and canine (24) hearts, associated with instability of sinus rhythm and intermittent or sustained atrial arrhythmias.

Selective impairment of internodal conduction in only one of the internodal pathways may be of little clinical significance except in the anterior pathway and its interatrial component. There, it is possible for interatrial conduction to become sufficiently distorted to broaden the P wave of the electrocardiogram and perhaps facilitate either the disorganization of atrial excitation or the production of atrial fibrillation. There is now impressive experimental evidence (25) that the internodal pathways form important components of the route by which atrial flutter propagates its circus movement. Surgeons have increasingly come to appreciate the importance of preserving the internodal pathways during certain operations associated with transposition of the great vessels or during cardiac transplantation; conversely, destruction of one or more of the internodal pathways during such operations has been recognized to be associated with a higher incidence of postoperative arrhythmias and other forms of electrical instability of the heart.

THE AV NODE

Normal anatomy

In the human heart the AV node is a small elliptical structure lying just beneath the right atrial endocardium, just anterior to ostium of the coronary sinus, just above the septal attachment of the tricuspid valve, and having a concave surface resting on the central fibrous body or the septal anchor of the mitral annulus

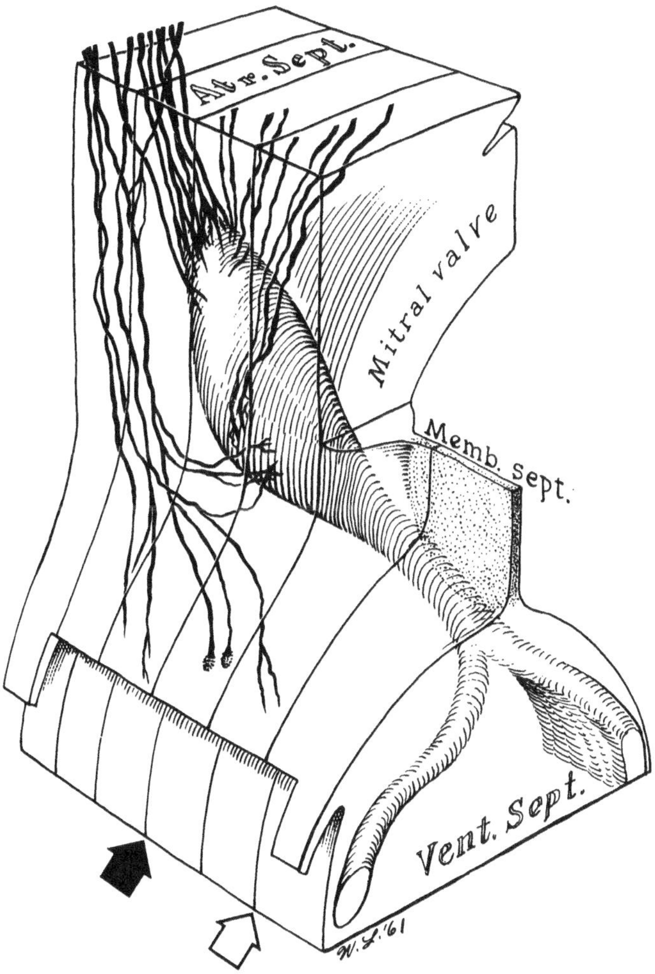

Figure 4. This drawing of a human AV node shows fibers from the three internodal pathways entering the crest and convex surface of the node. From the anterior inferior margin of the AV node the His bundle veers centrally to course just behind and beneath the membranous interventricular septum and then divide into a slender single right bundle branch and a broad sheet of left bundle branch (see Figure 10). The black arrow indicates the plane of sectioning of AV node illustrated in the photomicrograph of Figure 7A, while the open arrow marks the plane of sectioning of His bundle as illustrated in Figures 6B, 8A and 11.

(26). These anatomic features (Figure 4) are slightly different in the dog (27) and very different in the rabbit (28), and it is important for experimental physiologists to understand these differences. Following the route of normal distribution of the sinus impulse, the functional anatomy of the human AV node may be thought of as receiving a span of fibers from the three internodal pathways which enter predominantly into the nodal crest. After passing through the AV node, the

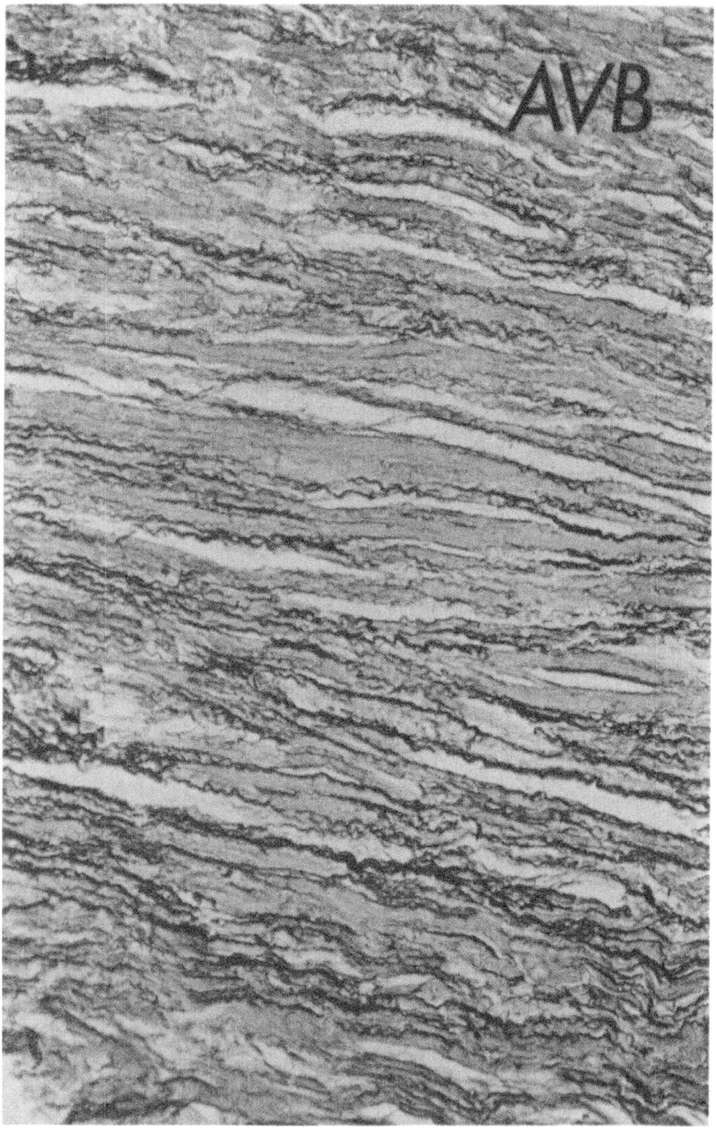

Figure 5A.

Figure 5. The purpose of these two photomicrographs is to contrast the interweaving histological organization of fibers of the human AV node with the longitudinally parallel orientation of fibers in the His bundle (AVB). The van Gieson stain used causes a black appearance of collagen for photography, accentuating accurate depiction of the collagen framework which in turn is an accurate

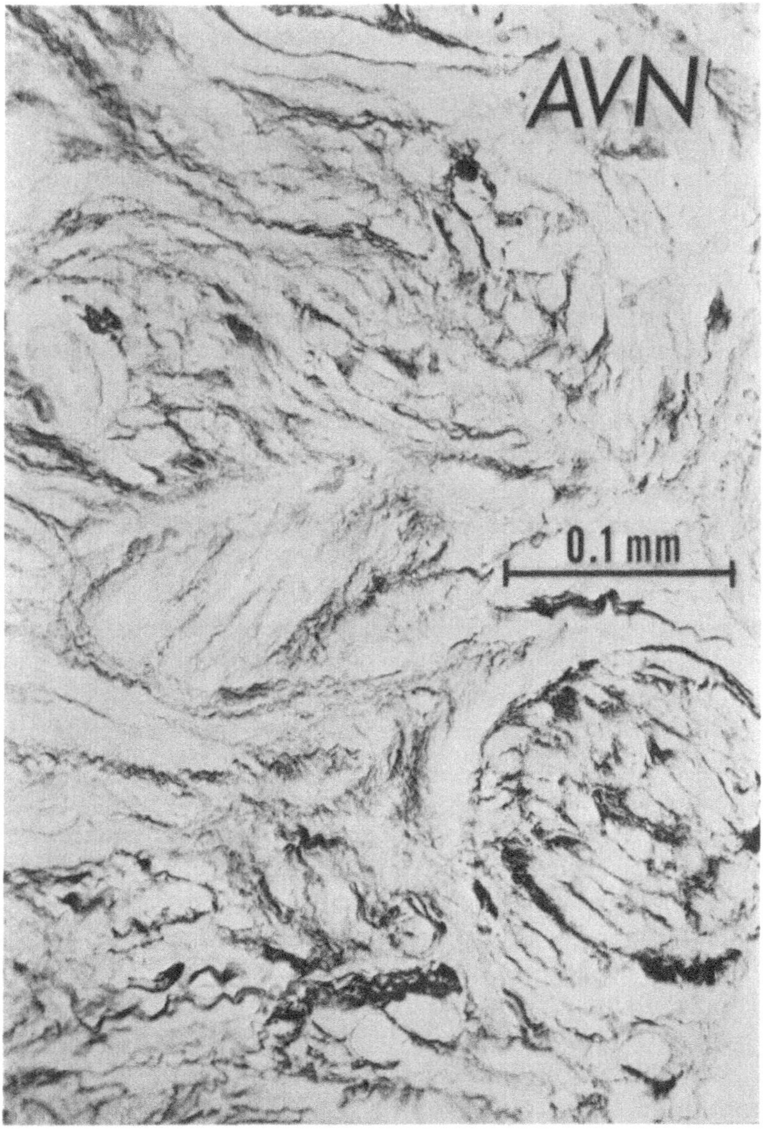

Figure 5B.

indirect indicator of orientation of the myocardial fibers. For both of these pictures the sectioning plane of the AV node and His bundle was sagittal rather than the more usual frontal plane illustrated with diagrammatic slices in Figure 4. Magnification is the same in both these panels.

sinus impulse would then exit into the His bundle which is directly continuous from the anterior inferior margin of the AV node (Figure 4).

Normal input into the AV node is not only at its crest, however, but also occurs all along its convex surface which faces the right atrial endocardium. Some of these latter fibers anatomically bypass (26) the body of the AV node to enter its anterior and inferior margin close to the region where it is beginning to form the His bundle. It has been suggested (29) that this bypass tract could serve as the route of early excitation of the His bundle thought to be responsible for the Lown-Ganong-Levine syndrome. In association with other distortion of conduction within or near the His bundle, the bypass tract could also be responsible for some examples of ventricular pre-excitation and the Wolff-Parkinson-White syndrome (30).

Since the bypass tract just described exists in every normal human heart, one of the puzzles is why ventricular pre-excitation is not seen more frequently. The answer to this question may lie in a fuller understanding of the histologic organization of the AV node and, if more precisely considered in terms of the exact cells responsible, just where it is that the normal delay occurs during conduction through the AV node. Recent experimental studies shed some light on this cellular locus (31, 32), but it is not the place for fuller discussion of that problem here. However, in addition to the normal bypass tracts of the human AV node, there are some rare examples of bypass fibers coursing directly from the atrial septum through the central fibrous body to enter the distal AV node or even proximal His bundle, and these are also potential participants in ventricular pre-excitation (33, 34). Such bypass fibers lie on the opposite side of the AV node from the normal bypass, and it is to be emphasized that they are exceptionally rare and probably represent an important developmental fault (35).

Although Purkinje cells and ordinary working myocytes abound at all margins of the AV node, the former being particularly prominent in the bypass tract (36), the substance of the AV node is composed predominantly of two myocardial cell types. These are the slender transitional cells and P cells. Individual characteristics of these cells bear close resemblance to the same cells found in the sinus node, although the predominance of slender transitional cells is much greater in the AV node. Conversely, P cells appear sparsely distributed in the AV node except at its anterior inferior margin where it begins to form the His bundle; at that site the P cells tend to occur in small clusters. The usual overall appearance of the adult human AV node is rather uniform and is comprised predominantly of slender interweaving fibers (Figure 5) formed by the transitional cells.

Blood supply to the human AV node and His bundle is provided primarily by the AV node artery, which originates from the apex of a turn penetrating from the right coronary artery (90% of human hearts) or the left circumflex (10%) into the junction between interatrial and interventricular septa (3, 26). There is supplemental or collateral supply provided to this region by arterial branches ascending toward the His bundle from the first septal perforating branch of the left anterior descending coronary artery (37), and this source is especially important for the distal His bundle and proximal portions of the two bundle branches. The septal artery is an even more important source of primary blood supply to this region in the heart of the dog (38), but this species difference should not be confused in considering coronary supply to the human AV node and His bundle.

Abnormal anatomy

Every form of vascular, focal inflammatory or infiltrative disease which was discussed for the sinus node is also to be found in the human AV node. Hemachromatosis seems to have a special affinity for the AV node and His bundle within the conduction system (15), whereas it tends to spare the sinus node. Furthermore, the AV node is not so conspicuously a periarterial structure, having its blood supply more diffusely distributed, so that arterial and periarterial diseases may be more destructive in the sinus node than in the AV node. Amyloidosis is a good example of this, often completely destroying the sinus node while affecting the AV node to lesser degree (13). Similarly, the greater predominance of collagen in the sinus node, where it forms a unique framework structure, seems to make the sinus node especially vulnerable to certain collagen diseases such as scleroderma (9) and lupus erythematosus (8), which tend to damage the AV node less. Finally, because the AV node is not normally located near the epicardium, pericarditis does not damage it as it does the sinus node.

There is one type of vascular pathology of the AV node which deserves greater recognition as a possible cause of slowly progressive heart block, and this is focal fibromuscular dysplasia of the AV node artery (39). Although focal fibromuscular dysplasia of the sinus node artery may also be important, particularly since it has been observed in association with sudden unexpected death under a variety of circumstances (10, 40), there may be a more straightforward effect of progressive narrowing of the lumen of the AV node artery. Study of the AV node of a boy who died several years after treatment with a pacemaker for heart block demonstrated that there was not only virtual obliteration of the AV node artery by focal fibromuscular dysplasia (Figure 6), but there was also a dense scirrhous fibrosis which nearly destroyed the His bundle which it supplied. This makes more plausible the functional significance of lesser degress of AV nodal or His bundle fibrosis which are more often seen with such arterial lesions, since the difference in degree of scirrhous destruction may simply be a reflection of how long the arterial perfusion deficit had existed.

Congenital heart block is most often associated with an anatomical discontinuity between the internodal pathways and the AV node (41), although the gap or fault may also occur at the site of junction of AV node and His bundle. In

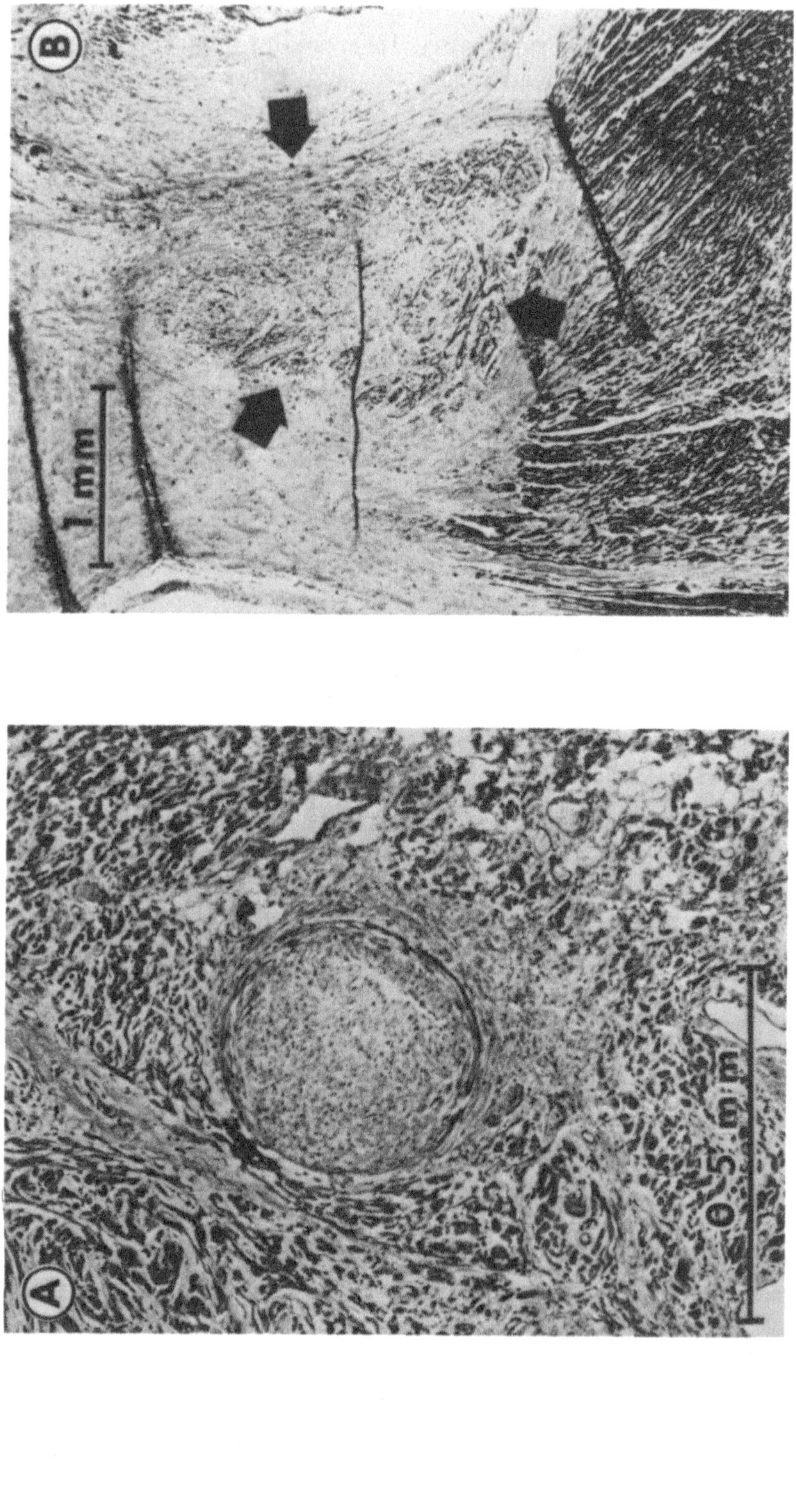

Figure 6. These two photomicrographs illustrate fibromuscular dysplasia causing marked narrowing of the lumen of the AV node artery in *A*, and dense fibrotic destruction of the His bundle (three black arrows in *B*) normally perfused by this vessel. Case discussed in text.

addition to gross anatomical discontinuities of this type, there are more sublte but nevertheless important distortions of the AV node which occur as part of a normal postnatal molding and shaping of this region (42-44). In the human fetus and early in postnatal life, both the AV node and His bundle are relatively large and shaggy structures with indistinct margins, many of which protrude into the contiguous central fibrous body. As part of the normal postnatal morphogenesis of the heart, these protruding fronds of AV nodal or His bundle tissue are slowly destroyed and resorbed, leaving the more distinct demarcation between AV node or His bundle margins and central body which is characteristic of the adult heart. However, in some hearts this form of fetal dispersion of the AV node or His bundle throughout the central fibrous body persists much later into life (43) and forms potential routes for re-entrant AV junctional tachycardias or the site of origin for parasystolic or other ectopic automatic rhythms.

Finally, there are at least two primary tumors which may be found in the region of AV node and His bundle and they deserve special comment. These are a fibroma of the central fibrous body (45), sometimes compressing the His bundle or AV node, and the benign congenital polycystic tumor of the AV node (46) most familarly described as a mesothelioma. There are few clinical clues to the presence of a fibroma, but it has been found in association with otherwise unexplained sudden death (45). The polycystic tumor of the AV node (Figures 7 and 8), on the other hand, is nearly always associated with some degree of heart block which may be slowly progressive over a period of decades. The escape AV junctional rhythm in such cases is impressively stable in most patients and syncope or similar symptoms surprisingly infrequent. Benign congenital polycystic tumors of the AV node are thus a fascinating paradox: they may be associated with long and useful life without significant cardiac symptoms, but eventually they may cause sudden death. One special caution in such cases concerns the possible hazard of electronic pacing, and more will be said of this later.

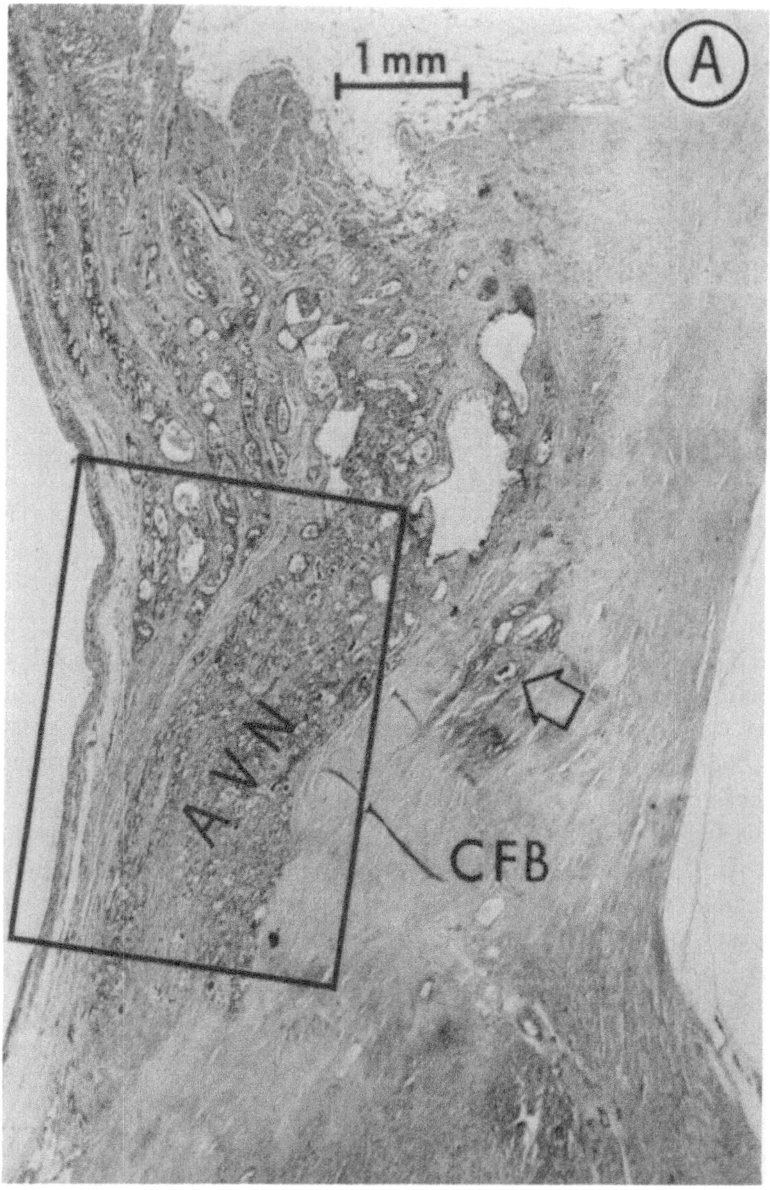

Figure 7A.

Figure 7. These photomicrographs are of the AV node from a patient with longstanding complete heart block. The region boxed in *A* is seen at higher magnification in *B*. Although general *outline* of the node here is entirely normal, virtually all the *Substance* of the AV node has been replaced by a

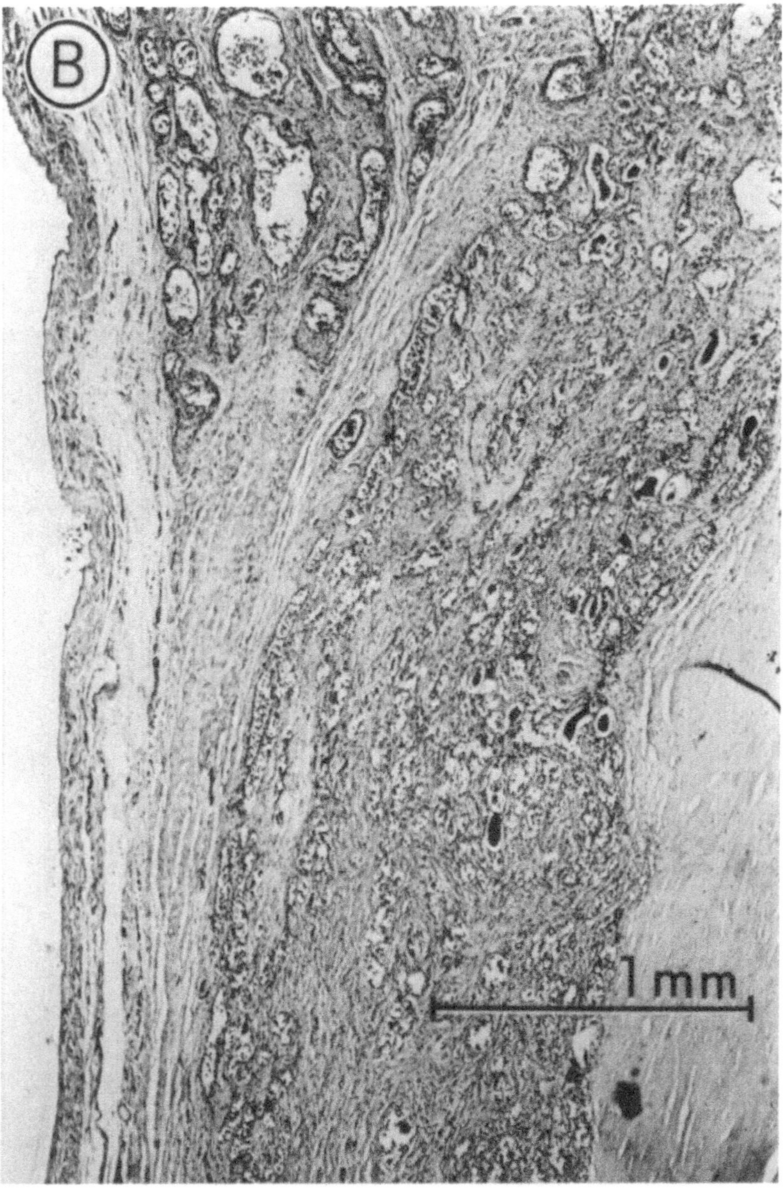

Figure 7B.

congenital polycystic benign tumor of the type usually called a mesothelioma. Open arrow indicates a small fragment of AV node also represented by tumor within the central fibrous body.

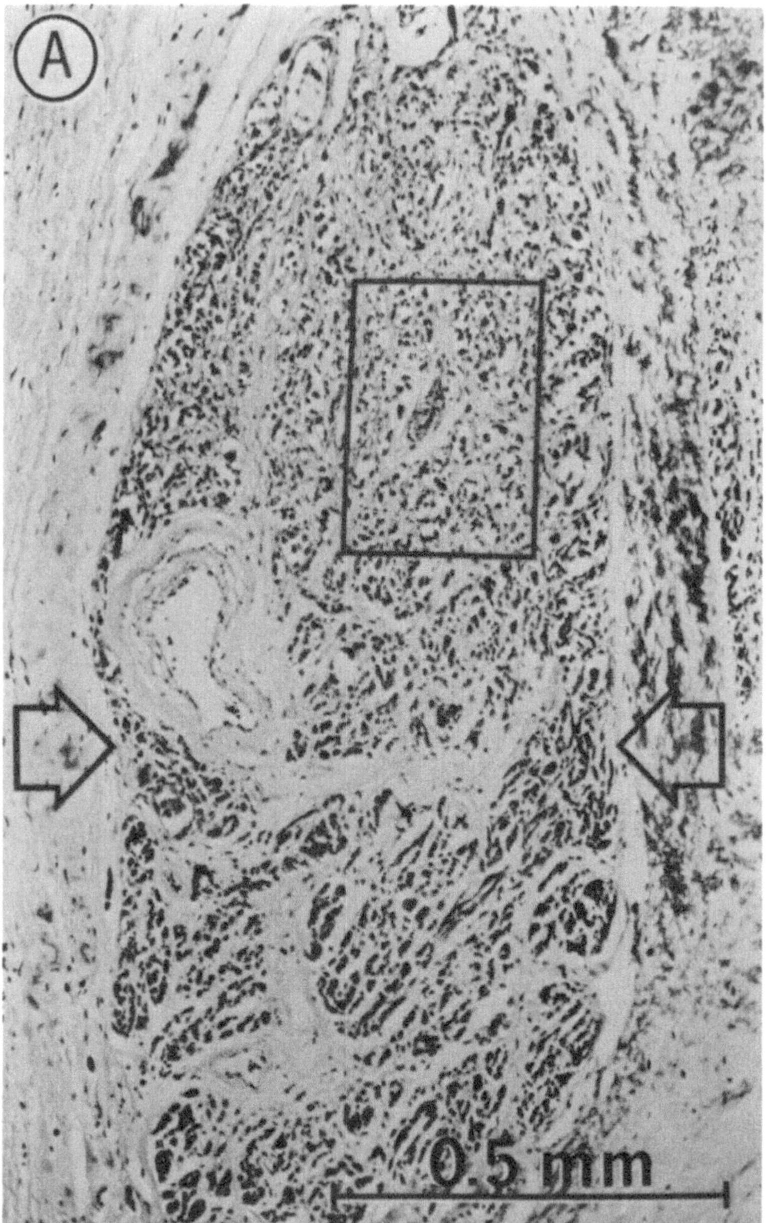

Figure 8A.

Figure 8. His bundle of the same heart seen in Figure 7 has complete replacement by tumor above the

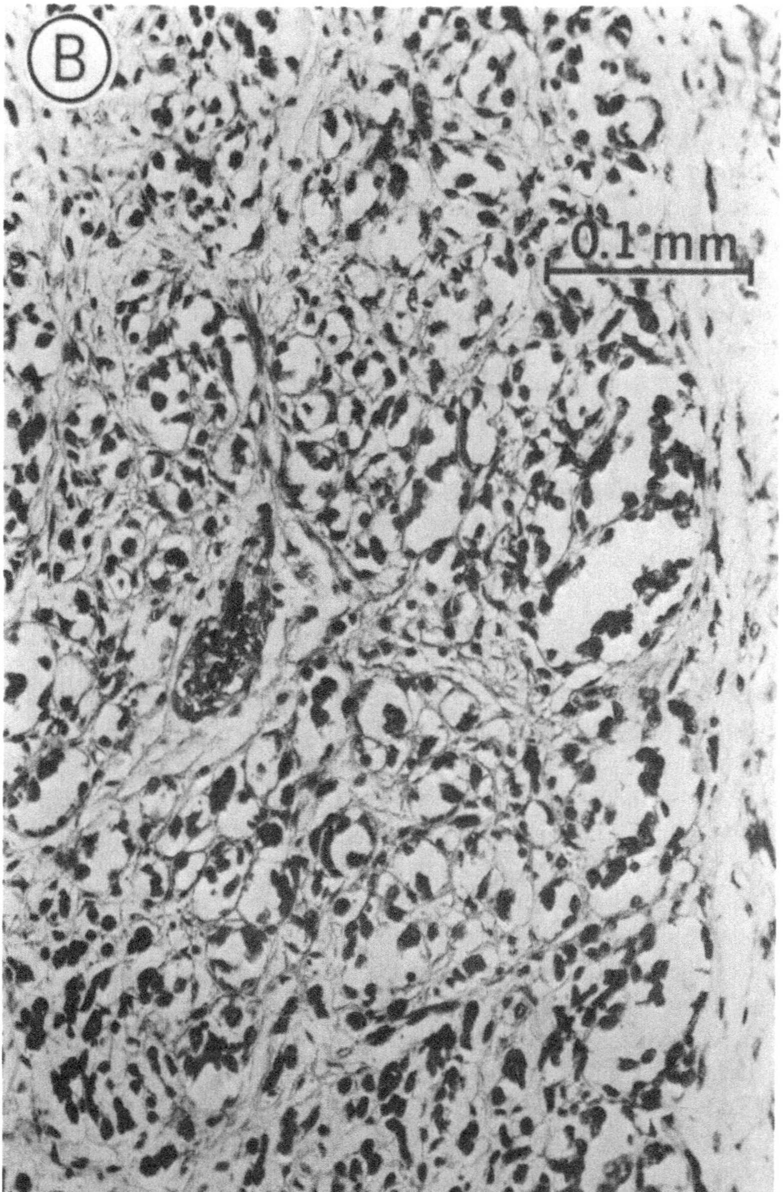

Figure 8B.

line indicated by open arrows in *A*. Area boxed is seen at higher magnification in *B*.

THE HIS BUNDLE AND ITS BRANCHES

Normal anatomy

Arising from the distal portion of the AV node, the human His bundle normally courses along the posterior inferior margin of the membranous interventricular septum to reach the crest of the muscular septum (Figures 4 and 9). In this course it gradually moves from right to left, giving off a slender single right bundle branch and an undivided sheet of left bundle branch. In about 15% of normal human hearts the His bundle courses predominantly along the right side of the septal crest and only gives rise to the left bundle branch at its anteriormost portion (47). In such hearts the origin of the left bundle branch is by a narrow stalk 1 mm or so in maximal dimensions instead of continuous sheet 10 to 22 mm in width. Although the origin of the right bundle branch is normally a narrow stalk, the unusual origin of left bundle branch in this fashion may be less safe in an electrophysiological sense, perhaps making it more vulnerable to focal disease which would, in turn, influence the activation process to the main pumping chamber of the heart. However that may be, focal lesions of a narrow origin left bundle branch have been observed in cases of sudden unexpected death (48). Since this anatomic variation is not rare, occurring in 15% of normal human hearts, its potential functional significance deserves wider appreciation.

From its narrow cylindrical origin the right bundle branch remains an ensheathed slender tube as it courses toward the moderator band on the right side of the interventricular septum, from where it spreads in the endocardium to the remainder of the right ventricle. Much of its septal course is near the endocardium, but the right bundle branch sometimes courses deep within the septal myocardial for a distance of several millimeters or more as it leaves the His bundle. Although popularly fancied as dividing into two distinct fascicles, the human left bundle branch does not do this (47). Instead it originates as a thin sheet of fibers which remains undivided for at least 20 to 30 mm along the left septal endocardium (Figure 10). Thereafter, it splits into a wide variety and totally unpredictable array of configurations, with many interconnections, as it sprads toward the two papillary muscles and remaining endocardium of the left ventricle.

In its course toward the crest of the interventricular septum, the human His bundle is encased in the collagen of the central fibrous body. Although it does rarely give rise to small slips of tissue (so-called Mahaim fibers) connecting it directly to the subjacent septal myocardium, these are rare. It is actually more accurate to think of the His bundle as lying within a sea of collagen, however, rather than as having collagen sheath of its own. When it leaves the AV node, the His bundle still contains an array of slender transitional cells which quickly merge to form typical larger Purkinje cells. Simultaneously, the histologic organization of fibers changes from a thickly interwoven meshwork into discrete,

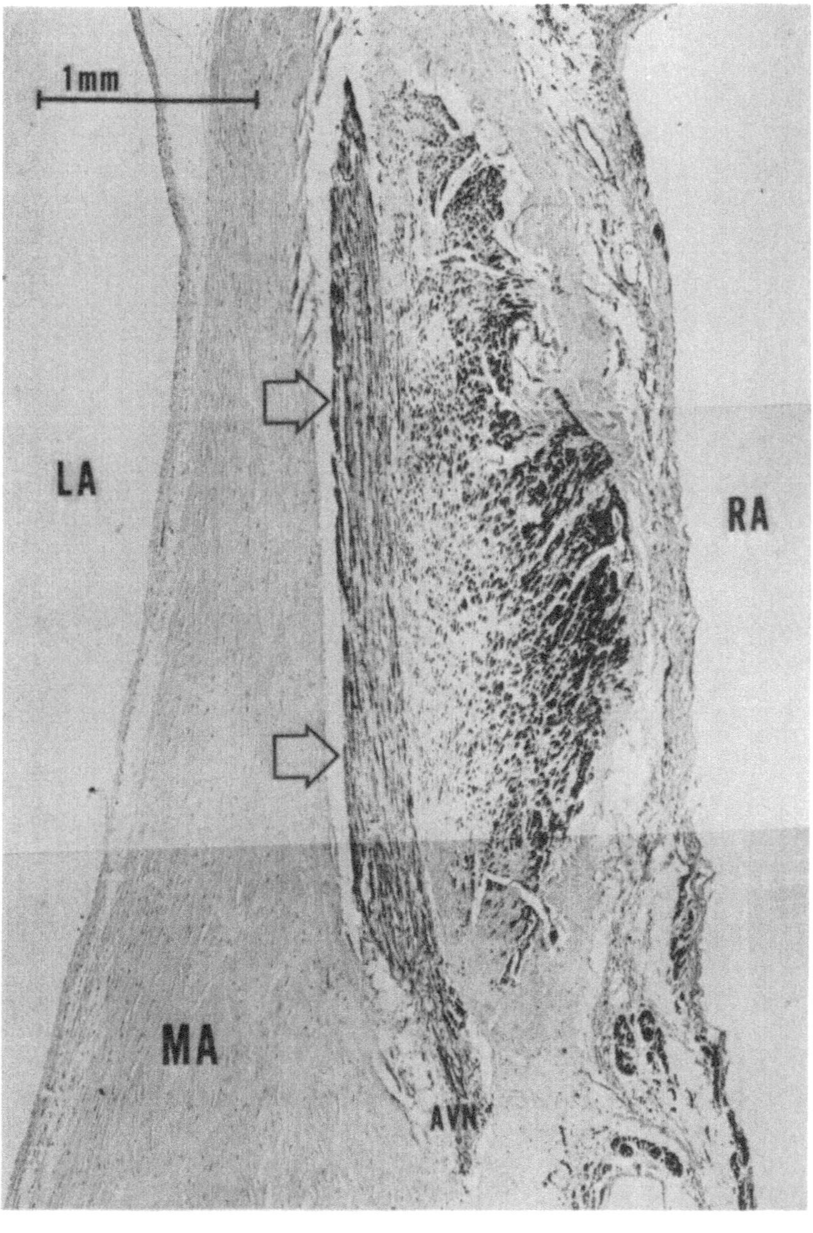

Figure 9. This low power photomicrograph of human His bundle is from a section prepared in an unconventional plane for such studies: the cut is parallel to the two AV valve rings and is thus a horizontal plane section. It illustrates the longitudinal partitioning (see also Figure 5) of the His bundle (two open arrows) by collagen as the bundle passes from right to left through the central fibrous body and to the left of the crest of the muscular interventricular septum. LA and RA are left and right atrium, MA is mitral annulus which is continuous with the collagen of central fibrous body, and AVN marks the anterior tip of the AV node from which the His bundle proceeds forward.

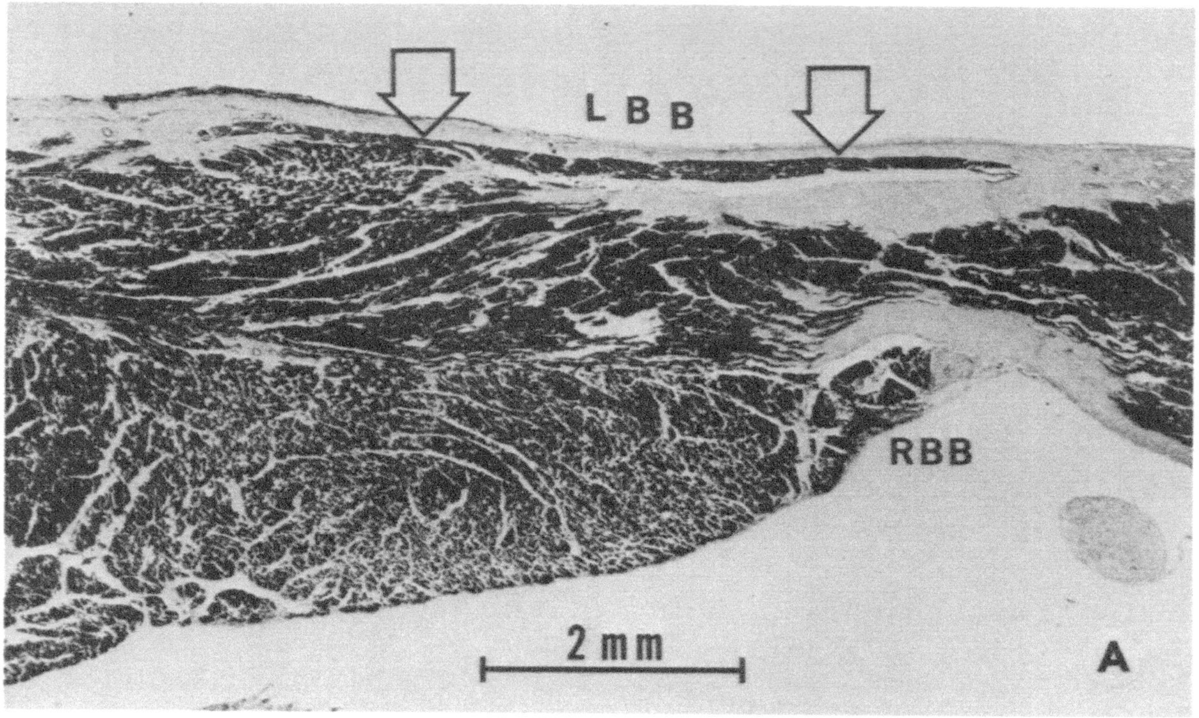

Figure 10A.

Figure 10. These two photomicrographs are from sections prepared in the same plane as that of the His bundle in Figure 9, but they are at two different levels below (i.e. toward the apex of the heart) the His bundle. From the His bundle the normal human left bundle branch (LBB and open arrows) descends as an undivided sheet lying just beneath the left septal endocardium, while the right bundle branch (RBB and black arrow) is a slender cylindrical tube.

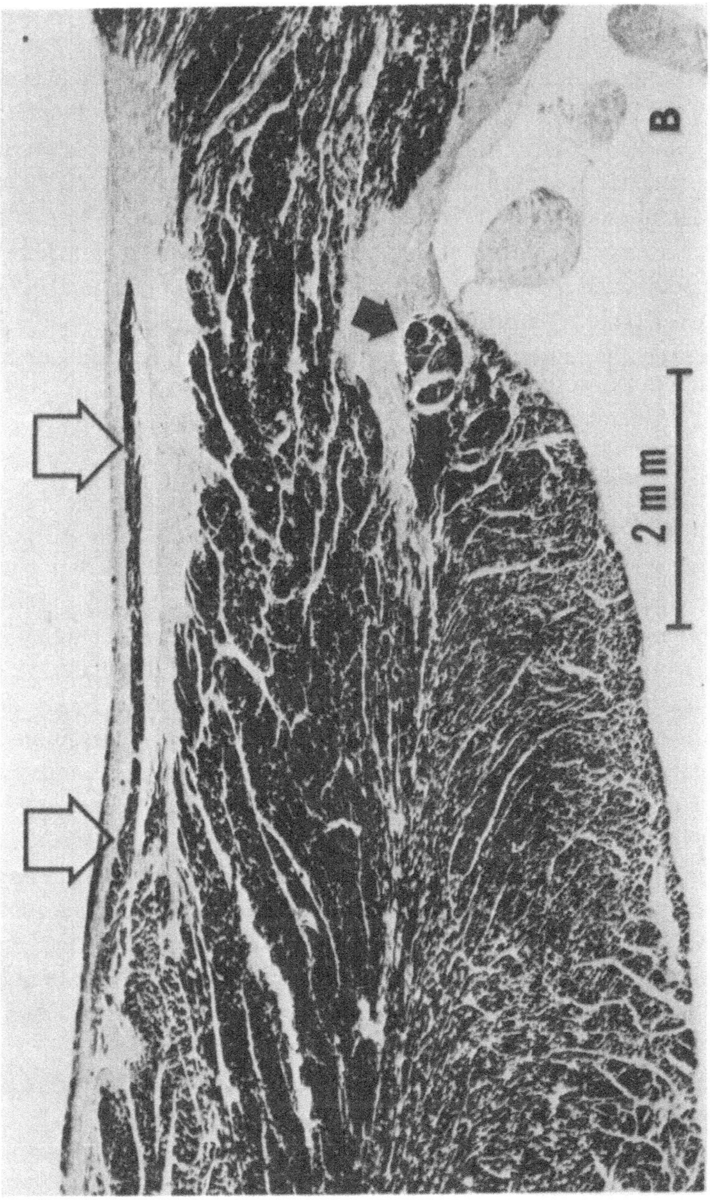

Figure 10B.

longitudinally arrayed fibers coursing parallel to each other. This longitudinal organization (Figures 5 and 9) is further enhanced by fine collagen septa which outline strands containing one or more Purkinje fibers to give the His bundle a histologic appearance resembling multiple shielded parallel cables. The separation is not total, a few small fibers crossing from one longitudinal strand to another, but the prevailing pattern of parallel array is distinctive. Orientation of fibers and composition of cells differs between the left and right bundle branches in the human heart. Just as in the His bundle, the cells in the left bundle branch are predominantly of the Purkinje type but not entirely so. There are occasional working myocytes and even slender transitional cells. Furthermore, the longitudinal orientation into parallel strands separated by collagen as seen in the His bundle also persists in the proximal portion of the left bundle branch, but tends to disappear much more than 10 mm down the septal endocardial course. By contrast, cell types are much more heterogenous within the right bundle branch, and there the fibers interweave without any distinctive longitudinal orientation (49).

Abnormal anatomy

Many of the same diseases and malformations discussed for the AV node also apply for the His bundle, as indicated previously. The normal variation in which a 'right-sided' His bundle gives origin to its left branch by a very thin stalk can hardly be considered an abnormality, but it is a normal variation which must be considered to be associated with greater risk of significant disruptive disease than is true for the usual left bundle origin which is so much larger. Another feature of normal anatomy of the His bundle which introduces an important functional consideration is the parallel orientation of Purkinje strands and their tendency for longitudinally-oriented shielding by collagen septa (Figures 5 and 9). Even though there are some sparse crossovers between these strands, a focal lesion within one or a few longitudinal Purkinje strands may alter the pattern of the electrical wavefront propagated through the His bundle. This would represent a true anatomic counterpart for longitudinal dissociation so long considered physiologically by electrocardiographers. Consequently, a variety of abnormalities of the QRS complex could have their origin in abnormal conduction within the His bundle itself.

There are three concepts worth separate comment and they are Lenegre's disease, Lev's disease and the concept of bilateral bundle branch block. Lenegre first described a type of non-inflammatory and unexplained degeneration of the His bundle or its proximal branches (50). We have recently introduced evidence for a familial basis for Lenegre's disease with the suggestion that it may represent some form of genetically programmed degeneration of special myocytes in this location (51), although why this should happen is unknown. Lev's disease is characterized by destructive fibrosis of the His bundle or its proximal branches (52), without any recognized preceding primary degeneration, thus differentiating it from Lenegre's disease. Lev's disease has been attributed to aging and local trauma from cardiac motion or compression by scar, with or without calcification in the adjacent cardiac valves. On the other hand, it is known that there is true bone in these regions of the hearts of some animals (53), with a conspicuous absence of any associated fibrotic destruction of adjacent His bundle or branches. It seems more plausible to suspect that the dynamic cytological interplay and interface of fibroblasts in the central fibrous body with the cells of the His bundle sometimes leads to a tilt in favor of proliferation by the fibroblasts, which then actively destroy portions of His bundle. It will be recalled that this type of molding and shaping of the His bundle is an ubiquitous normal process in the postnatal period and is responsible for the transformation of the large shaggy His bundle of the fetus into the smooth cylinder which is seen in the human adult heart (Figures 9 and 11). Failure of this normal process to occur and then terminate sometimes ends in persistent fetal dispersion of the adult AV node or His bundle throughout the central fibrous body (Figure 11). An opposite type of failure would be for the resorptive degeneration to become excessive, at any period of adolescence or early adulthood, and thus produce what appears as destructive fibrosis. At older ages, much of the destructive fibrosis by occlusive coronary disease, involving large or small coronary vessels or both.

Bilateral bundle branch block is a vexing anatomical concept, particularly in attempts to relate structural findings to electrocardiographic interpretations. There have been too many careful studies in which the anatomical block was on the 'wrong' side for one to be comfortable with the other anatomical correlative examples in which structural and electrocardiographic findings were concordant. If one accepts the anatomical evidence for longitudinal dissociation being a normal process in the human His bundle, then a necessary corollary would be that any form of distortion of ventricular activation could just as logically be attributed to a lesion in the His bundle as in one of its branches. This would include any degree of either right or left bundle branch block. What is lacking in nearly all studies concerning the anatomical substrate for 'bundle branch block' is an appropriate appreciation of the potential importance of and sufficiently careful search for lesions within the His bundle rather than only within its branches. In some reports which have included photomicrographs of His bundle in such cases there are striking abnormalities which are virtually never discussed as they may relate to bundle branch block. Granted that we do not know that such lesions truly do cause bundle branch block electrocardiographically defined in man, nor do we know in which portion of the His bundle to look as an explanation for left compared to right bundle branch block, still it seems a narrow view of the question not to consider these possibilities.

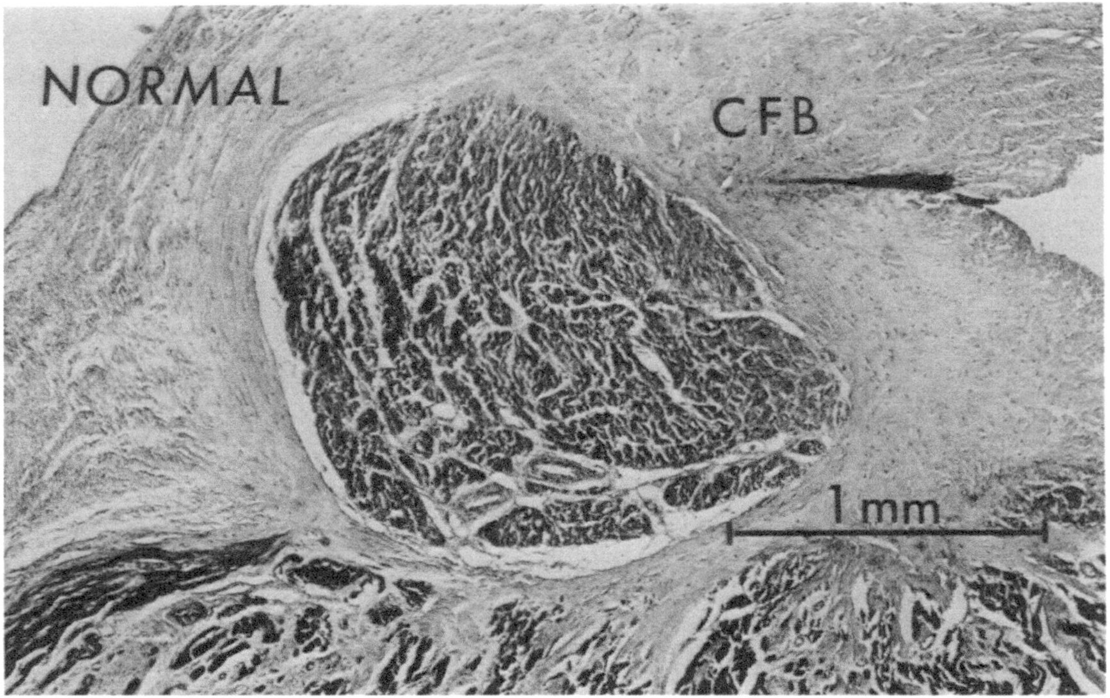

Figure 11A.

Figure 11. In the normal adult human heart the His bundle in cross section appears as a sharply outlined cylinder with smooth margins. However, in some hearts there is delay in the morphogenesis by which this appearance is achieved, so that both the AV node and His bundle persist in having an irregular outline with multiple fronds, loops and protrusions into the central fibrous body (CFB). This latter appearance is normal in the human fetus and during early postnatal life, but such fetal dispersion is abnormal at older ages. Small arrows point to one linear fragment descending from the interatrial septum toward some of the dispersed His bundle tissue.

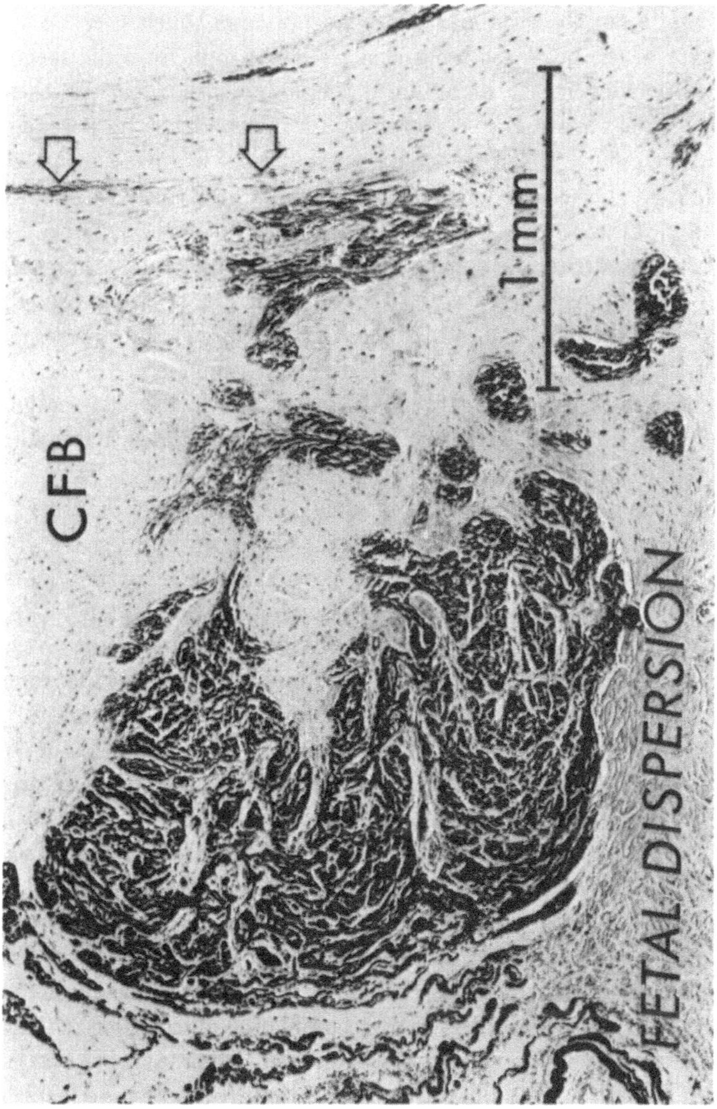

Figure 11B.

DISCUSSION

Much of what is appropriate to discuss in a review such as this has been presented in the sections dealing separately with the sinus node, internodal pathways, AV node, His bundle and its branches. However, there are some aspects of abnormal anatomy which need be discussed in a more general fashion in order to provide an appropriate overview relative to clinical decisions about pacing of the heart. Paramount among these is the fact that most diseases which affect the conduction system of the heart are multifocal, as is apparent from the spectrum of etiologies included in the preceding discussions. Thus, most causes for abnormality of the sinus node may also affect the internodal pathways and the AV node or His bundle. It is this multiplicity of sites of involvement which is responsible for the electrical instability so often associated with sinus node dysfunction. If that were not so, then failure or default of the sinus node should always be succeeded by the emergence of a slower but usually quite effective escape rhythm originating within the AV junction (54, 55). Similarly, if structural disease of the sinus node and of the AV node coexists and is responsible at both places for erratic automaticity, then the structural disease in the AV node may also be responsible for impaired AV conduction which could be significant during sinus rhythm and even more important if one of the escape rhythms is a tachycardia, of whatever origin.

While multiple sites of structural abnormality in the conduction system are the rule, there are single or isolated lesions which can be devastating. This is probably more true of the AV node or His bundle rather than of the sinus node, since interruption of AV conduction has obvious hemodynamic and related consequences. However, we do not yet know what all the functional consequences of local disease in the sinus node may be. For example, it is possible that some form of feedback control essential to the normal stability of cardiac rhythm (56) would be lost.

There is one isolated lesion of the AV node which is especially important to include in any differential diagnosis of newly discovered heart block at any age. This is the benign congenital polycystic tumor of the AV node, or so-called mesothelioma. When during life these tumors will lead to heart block is completely unknown, although available evidence indicates that they are probably present in some form and of some size even at birth. Whether later progression to greater degrees of heart block should be attributed to cellular growth of the tumors, or to expansion of their size by accumulation of secretions in their many tubules, or to some other explanation is unknown. What is known (46) is that a number of patients later found to have such a tumor of the AV node died either during diagnostic pacing studies, or some time shortly after the placement of an electronic pacemaker. This seems a bizarre paradox, since complete heart block due to most other causes is so successfully treated and readily responsive to electronic pacing. Whether the irregular forward extension of the tumor in the region of His bundle (Figure 8) somehow distorts the pattern of response from an electronically paced signal, or whether the tumor in some way causes abnormal competitive automaticity, or failure of any automaticity, are still other speculative possibilities. Whatever the explanation, those who study patients with heart block and who may plan to treat them with an electronic pacemaker should be aware that in some cases with tumor of the AV node, the results have been catastrophic. Since it is not known how many patients with heart block and successful electronic pacing may have an unprovable tumor of the AV node, it is possible that the bad results are not representative of all such patients. Nevertheless, cautious consideration of the possibility is warranted.

ACKNOWLEDGEMENT

The following figures originally appeared in Circulation as indicated, and are reproduced with permission of the American Heart Association: Figure 3 first was published in reference number 23, Figure 5 in reference number 36, Figure 6 in reference number 39, Figures 7 and 8 in reference number 46, and Figures 9 and 10 in reference number 47.

REFERENCES

1. Keith A, Flack M: The form and nature of the muscular connections between the primary divisions of the vertebrate heart. *J Anat Physiol* 41: 172, 1907.
2. James TN: The sinus node. *Am J Cardiol* 40: 965, 1977.
3. James TN: Anatomy of the Coronary Arteries. Hagerstown, Maryland, Harper and Row, Inc, 1961.
4. Hudson REB: The human pacemaker and its pathology. *Brit Heart J* 2: 153, 1960.
5. James TN, Sherf L , Fine G, Morales AR: Comparative ultrastructure of the sinus node in man and dog. *Circulation* 34: 139, 1966.
6. Woods WT, Urthaler F, James TN: Spontaneous action potentials of cells in the canine sinus node. *Circ Res* 39: 76, 1976.
7. James TN: Pericarditis and the sinus node. *Arch Intern Med* 110: 301, 1962.
8. James TN, Rupe CE, Monto RW: Pathology of the cardiac conduction system in systemic lupus erythematosus. *Ann Intern Med* 63: 402, 1965.
9. James TN: De Subitaneis Mortibus. VIII. Coronary arteries and conduction system in the scleroderma heart disease. *Circulation* 50: 844, 1974.
10. James TN, Marshall TK: De Subitaneis Mortibus. XVII. Multifocal stenoses due to fibromuscular dysplasia of the sinus node artery. *Circulation* 53: 736, 1976.
11. James TN, Birk RE: Pathology of the cardiac conduction system in polyarteritis nodosa and its variants. *Arch Intern Med* 177: 561, 1966.
12. James TN: Small arteries of the heart. The 36th George E. Brown MEmorial Lecture. *Circulation* 56: 2, 1977.
13. James TN: Pathology of the cardiac conduction system in amyloidosis. *Ann Intern Med* 65: 28, 1966.

14. James TN, Haubrich WS: De Subitaneis Mortibus. XIV. Bacterial arteritis in Whipple's disease. *Circulation* 52: 722, 1975.
15. James TN: Pathology of the cardiac conduction system in hemachromatosis. *New Eng J Med* 271: 92, 1964.
16. James TN: Myocardial infarction and atrial arrythmias. *Circulation* 24: 761, 1961.
17. James TN, Monto RW: Pathology of the cardiac conduction system in thrombotic thrombocytopenic purpura. *Ann Intern Med* 65: 37, 1966.
18. James TN, Marshall ML, Craig MW: De Subitaneis Mortibus. VII. Disseminated intravascular coagulation and paroxysmal artrial tachycardia. *Circulation* 50: 395, 1974.
19. James TN, Carson NAJ, Froggatt P: De Subitaneis Mortibus. IV. Coronary vessels and conduction system in homocystinuria. *Circulation* 49: 367, 1974.
20. James TN, Marshall TK, and Edwards JE: De Subitaneis Mortibus. XX. Cardiac electrical instability in the presence of a left superior vena cava. *Circulation* 54: 689, 1976.
21. James TN: The connecting pathways between the sinus node and A-V node and between the right and left atrium in the human heart. *Am Heart J* 66: 498, 1963.
22. Sherf L, and James TN: Fine structure of cells and their histological organization within the internodal pathways of the heart. *Am J Cardiol* in press.
23. James TN, Puech P: De Subitaneis Mortibus. IX. Type A. Wolff-Parkinson-White syndrome. *Circulation* 50: 1264, 1974.
24. James TN: Congenital deafness and cardiac arrhythmias. *Am J Cardiol* 19: 627, 1967.
25. Pastelin G, Mendez R, Moe GK: Participation of atrial specialized conduction pathways in atrial flutter. *Circ Res* 42: 386, 1978.
26. James TN: Morphology of the human atrioventricular node with remarks pertinent to its electrophysiology. *Am Heart J* 62: 756, 1961.
27. James TN: Anatomy of the AV node of the dog. *Anat Rec* 148: 15, 1964.
28. James TN: Anatomy of the cardiac conduction system in the rabbit. *Circ Res* 20: 638, 1967.
29. Durrer D: Electrical aspects of human cardiac activity: A clinical-physiological approach to excitation and stimulation. *Cardiovasc Res* 2: 1, 1968.
30. Lev M, Fox SM III, Bharati S, Greenfield JC Jr, Rosen KM, Pick A: Mahaim and James fibers as a basis for a unique variety of ventricular preexcitation. *Am J Cardiol* 36: 880, 1975.
31. James TN: Selective experimental chelation of calcium in the AV node and His bundle. *J Mol Cell Cardiol* 8: 361, 1976.
32. James TN, Isobe JH, Urthaler F: Correlative electrophysiological and anatomical studies concerning the site of origin of escape rhythm during complete atrioventricular block in the dog. *Circ Res* in press.
33. Lev M, Leffler WB, Langendorf R and Pick A: Anatomic findings in a case of ventricular preexcitation (WPW) terminating in complete atrioventricular block. *Circulation* 34: 718, 1966.
34. Brechenmacher C: Atrio-His bundle tracts. *Brit Heart J* 37: 853, 1975.
35. James TN, Spencer MS, and Kloepfer JC: De Subitaneis Mortibus. XXI. Adult onset syncope, with comments on the nature of congenital heart block and the morphogenesis of the human atrioventricular septal junction. *Circulation* 54: 1001, 1976.
36. James TN and Sherf L: Ultrastructure of the human AV node. *Circulation* 37: 1049, 1968.
37. Frink RJ and James TN: The normal blood supply to the human His bundle and proximal bundle branches. *Circulation* 47: 8, 1973.
38. James TN, Bear ES, Frink RJ, Lang KF, Tomlinson JC: Selective stimulation, suppression or blockade of the AV node and His bundle. J Lab Clin Med 76: 240, 1970.
39. James TN, Hackel DB, Marshall TK: De Subitaneis Mortibus. V. Occluded AV node artery. *Circulation* 49: 772, 1974.
40. James TN, Froggatt P, Marshall TK: Sudden death of young athletes. *Ann Intern Med* 67: 1013, 1967.
41. Lev M, Silverman J, Fitzmaurice FM, Paul MH, Cassels DE, Miller RA: Lack of connection between the atria and the more peripheral conduction system in congenital atrioventricular block. *Am J Cardiol* 27: 481, 1971.
42. James TN: Cardiac conduction system: Fetal and postnatal development. *Am J Cardiol* 25: 213, 1970.

43. James TN, Marshall TK: De Subitaneis Mortibus. XVIII. Persistent fetal dispersion of AV node and His bundle within central fibrous body. *Circulation* 53: 1026, 1976.
44. James TN: Sudden death in babies: New observations in the heart. *Am J Cardiol* 22: 479, 1968.
45. James TN, Carson DJL, Marshall TK: De Subitaneis Mortibus. I. Fibroma compressing His bundle. *Circulation* 48: 428, 1973.
46. James TN, Galakhov I: De Subitaneis Mortibus. XXVI. Fatal electrical instability of the heart associated witn benign congenital polycystic tumor of the atrioventricular node. *Circulation* 56: 667, 1977.
47. Massing GK, James TN: Anatomical configuration of the His bundle and bundle branches in the human heart. *Circulation* 53: 609, 1976.
48. James TN, Schlant RC, Marshall TK: De Subitaneis Mortibus. XXIX. Randomly distributed focal myocardial lesions causing destruction in the His bundle or a narrow-origin left bundle branch. *Circulation* 57: 816, 1978.
49. James TN, Sherf L, Urthaler F: Fine structure of the bundle branches. *Brit Heart J* 36: 1, 1974.
50. Lenegre PJ: Les lésions du système de His-Tawara dans les blocs auriculoventriculaires d'un haut degré. *Cardiologia* 46: 261, 1965.
51. James TN, McKone RC, Hudspeth AS: De Subitaneis Mortibus. X. Familial congenital heart block. *Circulation* 51: 379, 1975.
52. Lev M: The Conduction System. In: *Pathology of the Heart*, Gould SE (ed.), Springfleld, CC Thomas, 1960, p. 132.
53. James TN: Anatomy of the sinus node, AV node and os cordis of the beef heart. *Anat Rec* 153: 361, 1965.
54. Urthaler F, Katholi CR, Macy J Jr, James TN: Mathematical relationship between automaticity of the sinus node and the AV junction. *Am Heart J* 86: 189, 1973.
55. Urthaler F, Katholi CR, Macy J JR, James TN: Electrophysiological and mathematical characteristics of the escape rhythm during complete AV block. *Cardiovasc Res* 8: 173, 1974.
56. James TN: The sinus node as a servomechanism. *Circ Res* 32: 307, 1973.

3. CURRENT INDICATIONS OF PACEMAKER THERAPY

GUY FONTAINE

The indications of pacemaker therapy have greatly increased as a result of the findings in longitudial studies of large series of patients (1, 2) showing not only that the Stokes-Adams syncope and the associated risk of sudden death may be prevented on a long-term basis, but also that the quality of life of the patients may be improved by sparing them the unpleasant symptoms caused by bradycardia (3). This has been allied with technical innovations which have increased the reliability of both the power units and their leads. The implantation of permanent pacemakers has become a well-regulated and almost always successful procedure in trained hands. When problems do arise (lead dislodgement, infection) simple remedies applied in time are nearly always effective.

The success of this technique has led to the extension of the indications in atrioventricular block, based on more general concepts such as bundle branch block associated or not with atrioventricular conduction defects or the analysis of the sequence of intracardiac activation (measurement of H-V intervals). These conditions are not necessarily in relation to atrioventricular block but they may herald it. In this new field the indications for permanent pacing are therefore debatable and management may vary from centre to centre.

Pacing has also been used in cases of bradycardia with or without syncope. In some of these patients the arrhythmia is no longer a result of a conduction defect but of an abnormality in sinus node activation. This group has significantly increased the number of pacemaker patients and currently accounts for about 30 percent of the total.

Pacemakers have also been used 'paradoxically' in the treatment of certain tachycardias, either to terminate or prevent them.

In this chapter we propose to review the main indications at the present time for permanent pacing in the most frequently encountered situation of patients in sinus rhythm.

1. INDICATIONS OF PACEMAKER THERAPY IN PAROXYSMAL ATRIOVENTRICULAR BLOCK

As the first syncope of a patient with paroxysmal atrioventricular block may be mortal the tendency is to institute pacemaker therapy at an earlier stage of the disease. The main difficulty arises in deciding when this should be undertaken. Clinical examination and surface electrocardiography (4, 5) have recently been complemented by endocavitary electrocardiology (6), sometimes with pharmacodynamic stress testing to increase its sensitivity and continuous ambulatory electrocardiography: Holter monitoring (7). The information obtained by all these methods is taken into account but the clinical history of the patient is of the utmost importance and may in itself be decisive.

The patient may present a wide range of cardiac arrhythmias as will be seen. However for clarity, they have been classified into two groups, 'symptomatic' patients with syncope, dizziness, fainting, lightheadness, and so on, and 'asymptomatic' patients, who usually display an abnormality of activation or conduction on routine ECG, raising the question in prophylactic permanent pacing.

1.1. Symptomatic patients

Some typical cases may be identified from their clinical histories. In general they are over 50 years old and have symptoms suggestive of permanent or paroxysmal atrioventricular block. The previously mentioned features of Stokes-Adams syncope are always asked after attentively. However, it should be remembered that besides the classical loss of consciousness without warning described by patients after their first attack, patients who have had several syncopes may experience a malaise just before losing consciousness. Although classically these syncopes are short-lived and recovery is rapid and complete with flushing of the face, in other cases syncope is followed by attacks of palpitations, malaises or disturbance of consciousness which may last several minutes with gradual recovery afterwards. Finally, minor forms with symptoms which do not immediately suggest cardiac pathology may be encountered (vertigo, transient malaises, tinnitus, visual disturbances, and so on). The progressive nature of the condition should be recognized, the attacks becoming more severe over a period of months or years, despite their capricious and unpredictable character.

It is often useful to go over the history after allowing the patient time for reflection as more information may be obtained regarding questions which were initially answered negatively. The circumstances in which the syncope occurred are very important and particular attention must be paid to points which may orient one away from an arrhythmogenic cause, such as:

- sudden rotation of the head, suggestive of acute vertebro-basilar insufficiency;
- a severe bout of coughing, suggestive of cough syncope;
- standing still for a long time, suggestive of orthostatic hypotension;
- progressive syncope accompanied by nausea, pallor, and sweating, suggestive of vasovagal syncope;

- after shaving, in patients with hypersensitive carotid sinus syndrome.
- biting of the tongue and postictal state of epilepsy;
- effort syncope of severe aortic stenosis;
- and, of course, symptoms caused by cardiac arrhythmias other than atrioventricular block, such as sinus bradycardia: dizziness when getting up, anorexia, and tiredness (8).

1.1.1. Paroxysmal advanced atrioventricular block. When a patient with typical or atypical syncope has an ECG documenting complete atrioventricular block, cardiac arrest by ventricular standstill or *torsades de pointes* (9) are the most apparent mechnisms and pacemaker therapy is indicated from the outset.

The same reasoning applies in both types of second-degree atrioventricular block, whether 2/1 or greater: type II (frequently referred as Mobitz II), when the conducted impulses show constant conduction times; and type I (Wenckebach), where the blocked impulse is preceded by prolongation of the conduction time relative to the first conducted impulse.

1.1.2. Partial or imcomplete atrioventricular block. In cases of partial or incomplete atrioventricular block the nature of the symptomatology and the precise type of atrioventricular (AV) or intraventricular (IV) block are all-important:

A). Pacemaker therapy may be indicated from the outset:

- when the syncopes are typical Adams-Stokes attacks with documented ECG 2/1 second-degree block (this block cannot be classified as Type I or Type II because there are no consecutive PR intervals to show prolongation of the conduction time);
- when the symptoms are less typical but ECG shows:
  - alternating bundle branch block (right bundle branch block alternating with left bundle branch block, sometimes on the same tracing),
  - permanent right bundle branch block with alternating left anterior and left posterior hemi-block (so-called trifascicular block),
  - right bundle branch block associated with extreme left axis deviation leading to progressive widening of the QRS complex resulting in a pattern of complete left bundle branch block (Figure 1).

B). The decision to implant an pacemaker will depend on the results of complementary investigations providing there is no non-cardiac cause for the symptomatology:

- when the symptoms are typical and ECG shows only complete left bundle branch block, or bifascicular block with or without a long PR interval or an isolated prolongation of the PR interval, or isolated left axis deviation. In this group, the special case of patients with typical Stokes-Adams attack with no atrioventricular or intraventricular block on ECG may be encountered (10).

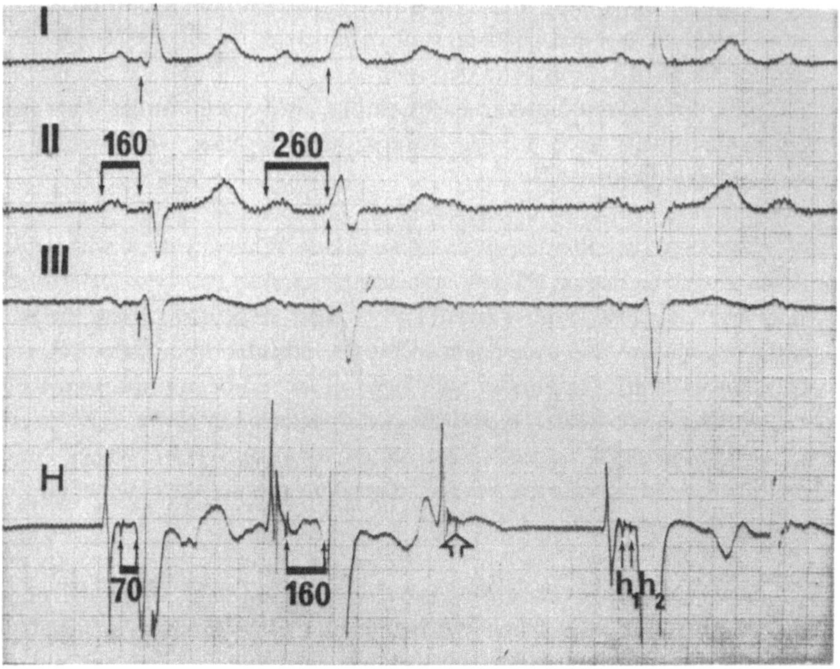

Figure 1. A rare exemple of infra-Hisian Wenckebach phenomenon. *Surface ECG:* Complex I: PR interval = 160 msec; QRS: extreme left axis deviation; Complex II: PR interval = 260 msec; QRS: complete left bundle branch block; Complex III: blocked P wave. *Bottom:* His bundle electrogram: lengthening of the HV interval from 70 to 160 msec between the first and second complex, block distal to the His after the third P wave (open arrow); A split His potential, h_1, h_2 is suggested on the next cycle (also probably present on the second cycle).

A paroxysmal conduction defect with a block limited to the main trunk of the His bundle should be suspected and endocavitary electrocardiography is mandatory (Figure 2). The technique is particularly delicate. A supple recording catheter is used and the longest HV interval is recorded during the progressive withdrawal from the ventricule to the atrium. The highest-amplitude His potential is searched for by gently rotating the catheter so as to demonstrate signs of a truncular block such as widening of the His potential greater than 20 msec, and above all splitting of the His potential into two separate electrical activities, h_1 and h_2. Care must be taken not to confuse h_1 with low atrial potentials. If need be, rapid atrial pacing must be performed to increase the nodal conduction time to separate them clearly (11).

– when the symptomatology is atypical and the atrioventricular block only partial (Wenckebach block, first-degree atrioventricular block, and various intraventricular blocks). The work-up should include continuous ambulatory electrocardiography (Holter monitoring). This may be informative if the malaises are fairly frequent; the times at which the malaises occur can be noted by

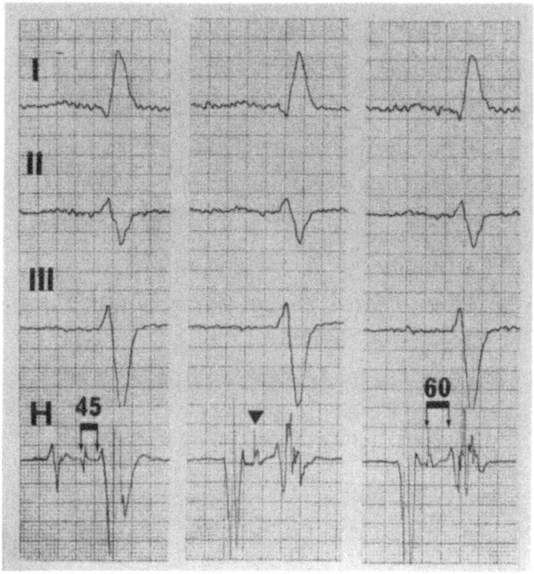

Figure 2. His-bundle electrophysiological study in a 55-year-old patient with typical attacks. ECG showed extreme left axis deviation. The recording catheter is gradually withdrawn from the ventricle to the atrium. The measurements are made from the first deflection of the His potential to the first deflection of the ventriculogram in all leads. *Left:* catheter in a distal position, HV interval normal at 45 msec; *centre:* catheter in an intermediary position – the His potential is widened and bifid; *right:* catheter in a proximal position, HV interval 60 msec – this suggests an *intra-Hisian* block (truncular block).

the patient in a diary or by a marker signal on the magnetic tape. Paroxysmal atrioventricular block and even unexpected arrhythmias such as sinus bradycardia or arrest or paroxysmal tachycardias (atrial fibrillation with rapid ventricular response) may be unmasked during rapid playback of the recording. Even in the absence of symptoms during the period of recording subclinical but significant abnormalities may be observed on the playback. However, these data, especially in youngsters, should be interpreted with caution (12).

Different techniques of electrophysiological investigation may be used (Figures 3, 4, 5, 6, 7 and 8). Atrial overdrive pacing (Figure 3) does not seem to be reliable in the detection of cases with atrioventricular conduction defects (13, 14) including long PR interval, a finding which has been sometimes observed before complete atrioventricular dissociation (15). In addition electrophysiological studies may show up latent atrioventricular conduction defects (normal PR interval on ECG may conceal an obvious conduction defect on His bundle

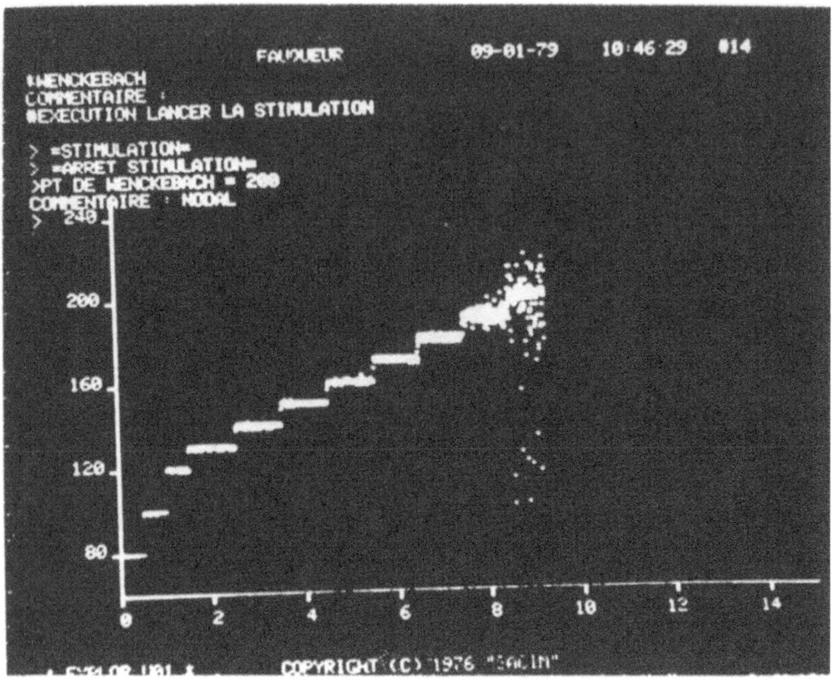

Figure 3. Measurement of the Wenckebach point: rapid atrial pacing at progressively faster rates for intervals of 30 seconds and then one minute until the appearance of second-degree atrioventricular block. The rate at which block occurs in known as the Wenckebach point. The graph drawn automatically on the computer console shows the time in minutes on the abscissa and the frequency of ventricular response to atrial pacing on the ordinate axis. The ventricular response in this case is regular up to 190/mn but at 200/mn the points of ventricular response are scattered because the recording intervals differ when second-degree block occurs.

electrocardiography) and also define the level of the block. When the AH interval is prolonged the block is supra-Hisian, situated inside the atrioventricular node, and when the HV interval is prolonged the block is situated in the trunk or the branches of the His bundle (16). This point is of particular importance. Infra-Hisian conduction defects are generally caused by degeneration of the His bundle or its branches and is often associated with a poorer prognosis. A retrospective study of the HV interval in patients presenting bundle branch block before developing complete atrioventricular block showed that most had long HV conduction times (17, 18, 19, 10). The question is now to determine the outcome of patients presenting a long HV interval, especially those with a typical symptomatology, as a history of malaises and dizzy spells is often found in elderly patients.

Several prospective studies are showing a clear difference between patients presenting a long HV interval who appear to go on to develop atrioventricular block and those with intraventricular or even atrioventricular blocks with a HV

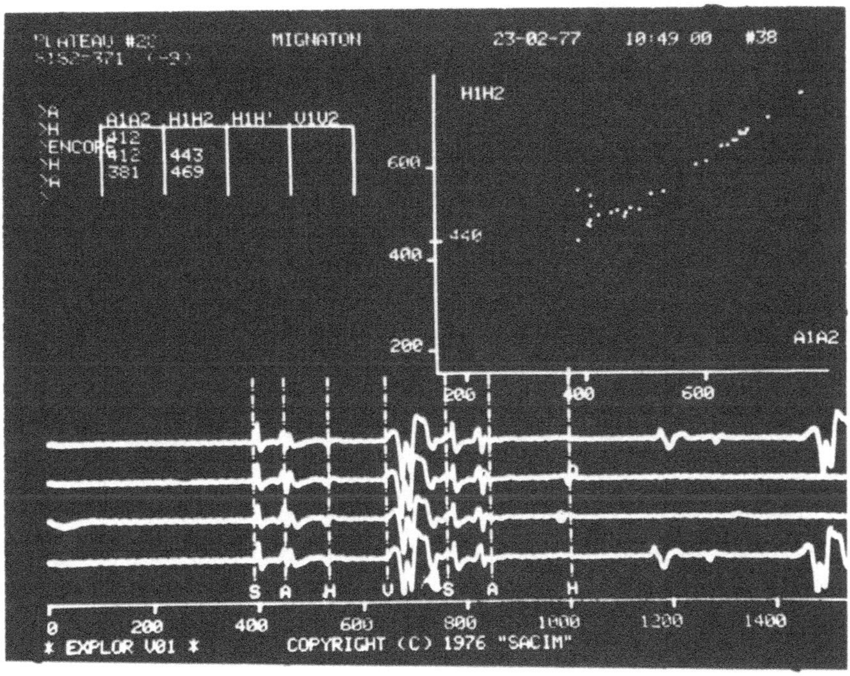

Figure 4. Premature extrastimulus technique in atrial pacing (programmed atrial pacing). The lower four recordings show the end of four successive series of pacing. The first cycle corresponds to the last basic cycle (frequency 80/mn) of atrial pacing; the second cycle is the response to the extrastimulus with a coupling interval of 381 msec. The bottom recording shows an auriculogram without a following His potential (nodal block); the recording just above shows the auriculogram followed by a His potential but no ventricular response. The same phenomenon is observed on the next tracing. The interval of 381 msec corresponds to the effective refractory period of the atrioventricular node in the bottom tracing and to that of the infra-Hisian conduction system in the second and third tracings. *Upper right:* the behaviour of nodal conduction with respect to the prematurity of the extra stimulus: on the abscissa the A1-A2 interval between two paced auriculograms, on the ordinate axis the H1-H2 interval, H1 being the last His potential of the basal cycle and H2 the His potential of the extra-stimulus response.

of 60 ms who seem to have a better prognosis.

This point has been contested by other investigators who have not found that patients with long HV intervals (21, 22, 23, 24) have a significantly worse prognosis and who suggest that the indication for permanent pacing should be its association with left bundle branch block or a documented complete atrio-ventricular block (21).

In fact it would seem that these differences may be explained by a difference in population of patients given their age, the low incidence of symptomatic patients in the series of the last-mentioned groups, the nature of the underlying disease process (cardiomyopathy), and the technique of measuring the HV interval (25).

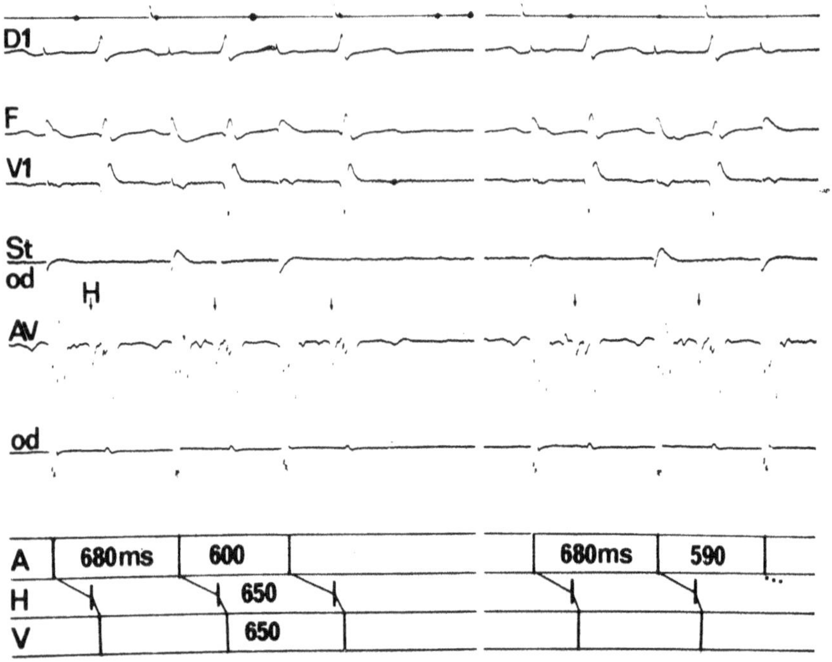

Figure 5. Electrophysiological investigation: the premature extrastimulus (A2) technique in atrial pacing (A1) demonstrates a latent nodal block: cycle A1-A1 of 680 msec on the left. The A2 atrial extrasystole with a coupling interval of 600 msec gives rise to physiological delay at the node. H1-H2 = 650 msec. *Right:* Increasing the prematurity of the extrastimulus by 10 msec (A1-A2 = 590 msec) gives rise to nodal block. The effective refractory period of the node is 590 msec (normal, less than 300 msec).

1.2. Asymptomatic patients

1.2.1. Intermittent (or permanent) slow pulse syndrome without symptoms due to complete atrioventricular block. Only a few years ago the limited life span of pulse generators justified an expectant attitude to avoid the risks of multiple operations. At that time the decision as to when to institute pacemaker therapy was based on:

- ECG features:
  - bradycardia less than 35 per minute with wide ventricular complexes,
  - ectopic pacemakers giving rise to double ventricular rhythms.
  - significant lengthening of the Q-U interval with giant T wave suggestive of severe desynchronization of repolarization which might lead to syncopal attacks by *torsades de pointes;*
- social or geographical factors:
  - living far away from a cardiological centre,

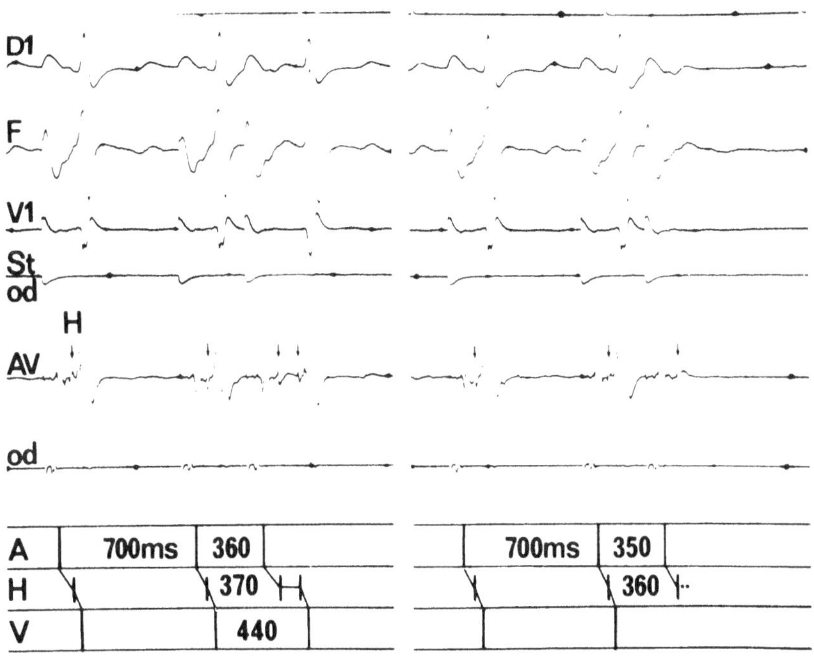

Figure 6. Extrastimulus technique: demonstration of latent intra-Hisian block: A1-A1 cycle of 700 msec. *Left:* atrial extrasystole with A2 coupled at 360 msec leads to prolongation of the nodal conduction time (H1-H2 = 370 msec) and an intra-Hisian block with split His potentials 50 msec apart. *Right:* shortening the coupling interval by 10 msec (A1-A2 = 360 msec) does not increase nodal delay (H1-H2 = 360 msec) but complete intra-Hisian block is observed after the first His potential.

– professions in which syncopal attacks could cause serious accidents,
– the need to drive a car.

Nowadays, the indications are less rigid especially since the appearance of long-life pulse generators and simpler techniques of implantation. This attitude is reinforced by the recognition of the long-term complications of permanent bradycardias:

– heart failure: left ventricular failure with dyspnoea of effort and at rest, right ventricular failure with severe dependent oedema and cardiomegaly which may eventually interfere with fixation of the pacing wire;
– cerebrovascular insufficiency which may markedly regress within days or weeks with pacing;
– essential hypertension aggravated by bradycardia or resulting from the slow ventricular rhythm which may regress soon after the re-establishment of a normal rhythm.

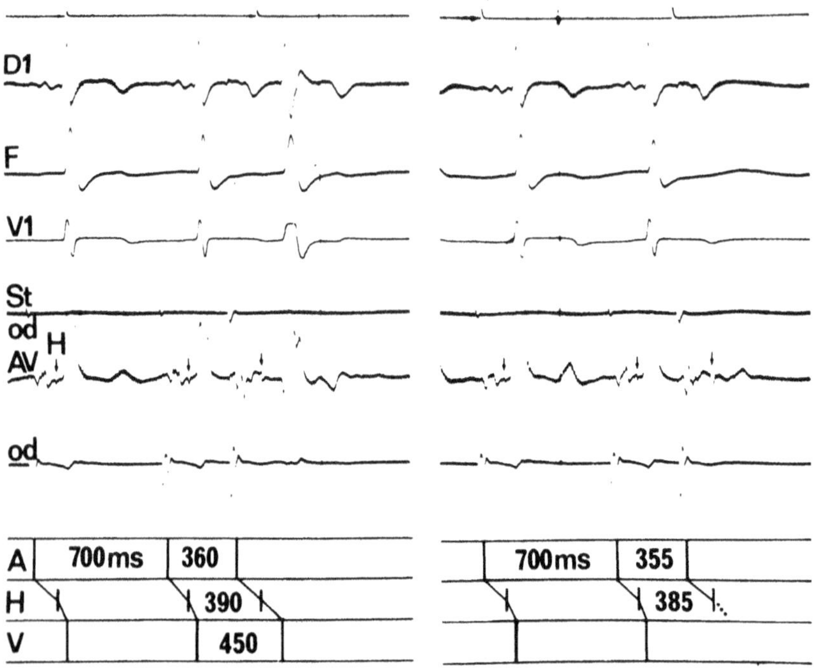

Figure 7. Extrastimulus techique: demonstration of a latent distal block, A1-A1 cycle: 700 msec. *Left:* a premature atrial extrasystole (A2) with a 360 msec coupling interval leads to lengthening of the nodal conduction time (H1-H2: 390 msec) and infra-Hisian block with lengthening of the HV interval from 40 (basal cycle) to 80 msec. *Right:* increasing the prematurity of A2 by 5 msec (A1-A2: 355 msec) does not increase the nodal delay (H1-H2: 385 msec) but complete block is observed after the Hisian potential: effective refractory period of the His-Purkinje system: 385 msec (normal, less than 250 msec).

Therefore, implantation of a pacemaker has become more or less systematic as soon as intermittent (or permanent) complete atrioventricular block is diagnosed. There is only one exception to this rule: congenital heart block when asymptomatic with a sufficiently rapid (50-60 per minutie) narrow-complex escape thythm and with adaptation to exercise.

1.2.2. Second-degree atrioventricular block. In these patients the analysis of the sequence of atrioventricular activation is of great importance in deciding whether or not to institute pacemaker therapy. The two sites of second-degree block have quite different prognoses. The type II (Mobitz) block on the one hand, where paroxysmal block is nearly always situated in the distal part of the His bundle as far as the origin of the main branches – infra-Hisian block (16) – seems to be associated with a definite risk. The 2/1 block with a normal PR interval comes into this group as the block is also nearly always infra-Hisian.

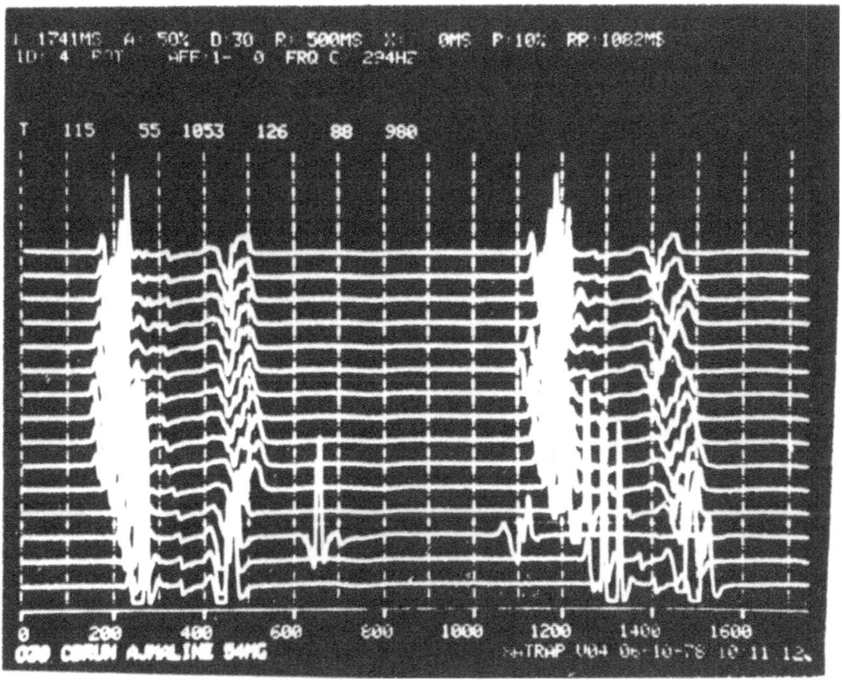

Figure 8. Study of effect of Ajmaline on the distal conduction (programmed endocavitary electrocardiography): the figure shows the His bundle recording during the injection of 1 mg/kg Ajmaline at the rate of 1 mg/sec. The recordings have been arranged side by side with the first ventricular complex always situated on the 400 msec line. The progressive lengthening of the HV interval from 55 to 88 msec in the three minutes following the start of the injection is shown on the sixth recording from the bottom. Lengthening of the HV interval by more than 100 percent or an HV interval of over 100 msec is considered diagnostic of severe infra-Hisian conduction defect.

The same attitude is adopted in patients with bundle branch block in whom it is thought that the preceding changes (Mobitz II, 2/1 block with normal PR interval) correspond either to a paroxysmal block of the permeable bundle branch or an infra-Hisian block associated with an intraventricular block. In all these cases the outcome is often complete atrioventricular block with the risks that it entails, and prophylactic implantation of a pacemaker is justified.

The type I (Wenckebach) block, on the other hand, whether the QRS complexes are narrow or widened by bundle branch block, in which the usual site of the atrioventricular block is in the atrioventricular node (16), is generally associated with a better prognosis and does not justify prophylactic pacemaker therapy. However, endocavitary electrocardiography is mandatory to determine the exact site of block as cases of infra-Hisian Wenckebach block, with only slight variation of the PR interval and cases of associated intranodal and infra-Hisian block are encountered.

1.2.3. First-degree atrioventricular block. Bundle branch or bifascicular block may be the first signs of localized disease of the intraventricular conduction system. Endocavitary electrocardiography is justified in these cases to determine the exact site of the block (26). In fact, the length of the PR interval is no guide. Although PR intervals greater than 0.2 sec usually correspond to the less severe intranodal block, they may be associated with relatively slight infra-Hisian lesions (truncular or on the permeable bundle) masked by the underlying delay of activation.

Conversely, and for reasons that are poorly understood, infra-Hisian block or a block on the permeable branch may very well be associated with only slight lengthening of the PR interval (26, 27).

– If the HV exceeds 55 msec or a truncular delay is associated with a split His potential or lengthening of the His bundle branch potential is observed prophylactic implantation of a pacemaker could be indicated.

– On the other hand, when lengthening of the PR interval is due to intranodal block alone only regular surveillance is required. Pacemaker therapy will only be undertaken when certain drugs which prolong the nodal conduction time (digitalis, beta-blockers, and so on) have to be used.

– Narrow QRS complexes or left axis deviation alone are strong argements against a degenerative disease at the origin of the intraventricular conduction system. In our opinion systematic endocavitary electrocardiography is not justified in these cases provided the patients are asymptomatic. As previously stated long PR intervals are nearly alsways due to intranodal block but nevertheless the possibility of a first-degree truncular block demands regular follow-up of these patients.

1.2.4. Absence of atrioventricular block on surface ECG. Permanent pacing may be indicated without further investigation when repeat ECG shows alternating bundle branch block with slight variations of the PR interval on the permeable bundle (28) or so-called 'trifascicular block' in its different commonest forms (29). On the other hand, asymptomatic patients with an isolated intraventricular block only require regular follow-up. This should be all in the more attentive in cases where one has reasons to fear rapid progression to complete atrioventricular block:

- rapidly progressive intraventricular block of recent onset, particularly right bundle branch block complicating known left anterior hemi-block;
- conversely a bifascicular block of over three years standing which may progress to complete atrioventricular block at short or medium term (15) – endocavitary electrocardiography may be perfectly justified for the safety of such patients when cardiological follow-up is difficult.

Therefore, the same problems are encountered here as in the symptomatic patients. Their solution is even more critical because the number of patients is that much greater. Although endocavitary investigation is very useful when the results are positive, a paroxysmal block cannot be formally excluded by a negative result. However, before significant prospective studies become available it would only seem justifiable to use prophylactic permanent pacing in patients with HV intervals, measured from the first deflection of the His potential and recorded with wide band-pass filters, greater than 75 msec.

In conclusion, in symptomatic patients the indication for permanent pacing may be posed from the analysis of the sequence of endocavitary atrioventricular activation under basal conditions. Pacing is indicated when the HV conduction time is clearly prolonged or a first-degree truncular block is observed with a split His potential of over 20 msec duration.

A similar indication in an asymptomatic patient implies a very careful recording of the His potential according to the techniques already described. In these cases, pharmacodynamic stress testing is most useful (30, 31). The most widely described test is the Ajmaline test where the variation of the HV interval after the intravenous injection of Ajmaline at 1 mg/kg/sec is measured. This test is not without danger and should not be used unless the HV interval is normal or less than 60 ms. It must not be used in cases with cardiomegaly or in the acute phase of myocardial infarction. A distal block or an increase of 100 percent in the HV interval or an HV conduction time greater than 100 msec are considered to be signs of severe distal conduction defects. Because of the risks involved this test has been criticized by some investigators (25).

Permanent pacing is not justified in cases of nodal block even when severe with AH intervals 300 msec (normal 50 to 150 msec).

1.3. Special cases

It has been seen that the indications for permanent pacing depend on symptoms suggestive of paroxysmal block in the absence of other pathology which could give rise to such symptoms, analysis of the surface ECG showing atrioventricular and intraventricular block associated, in some cases, with endocavitary electrocardiography to give the precise location of the block and therefore an indication of the prognosis. However, special cases are encountered which may influence the final decision.

1.3.1. Drug therapy. Cardiac glycosides and beta-blockers may aggravate previously well tolerated intranodal blocks (32). When such therapy is essential it is logical to implant a pacemaker prophylactically to avoid the consequences of complete block.

Certain antiarrhythmic agents increase the infra-Hisian conduction times. In such cases, a positive Ajmaline test in an asymptomatic patient or an HV interval at the upper limit of normal may justify permanent pacing if this type of drug is indispensable (33).

1.3.2. Anesthesia. It is quite common the find abnormal changes in routine preoperative ECGs. The same attitude is adopted as with asymptomatic patients with similar atrioventricular or intraventricular blocks. Temporary pacing is only needed when the patient has a clear indication for permanent pacing and has to be operated on as an emergency (34). A temporary pacing wire may also be indicated for intranodal blocks (long PR interval, Wenckebach block) likely to be aggravated by the anesthetic agents used for induction, but intravenous Atropine 1 mg is usually adequate in these cases. Nevertheless, the operation should be performed under continuous ECG monitoring. When there is a clear indication for permanent pacing, and it is possible to defer operation, it is preferable to implant a permanent pacemaker first, and perform the operation at a later date when the cardiac problem has been resolved. Asymptomatic patients with right bundle branch block, left axis deviation, and normal PR intervals generally do not require additional anesthetic precautions as the distal conduction system, unlike the atrioventricular node, is unaffected by anesthetic agents. However, a documented case of Mobitz II block has recently been reported (35). Therefore ECG monitoring is advisable.

1.3.3. Trauma to the right bundle. Complete atrioventricular block caused by trauma of the right bundle occurring during endocavitary electrocardiography in patients with existing complete left bundle branch block nearly always regresses a few hours or days and does not justify permanent pacing if the HV interval returns to normal, when right bundle branch block disappears (36, 37, 38).

1.3.4. Cardiac surgery. Atrioventricular block after cardiac surgery is a difficult problem. Permanent pacing is systematic in patients with complete or second-degree (especially type II Mobitz) atrioventricular block at the fifteenth post-operative day. In our opinion an endocardial study of conduction times is advisable even in cases where atrioventricular block regresses and in post-operative complete right bundle branch block to avoid missing a block situated in the bundle of His. This attitude is reinforced by reports of sudden death after complete repair of tetralogy of Fallot, closure of ventricular septal defect, and after aortic valve surgery (39). These blocks should however be preventable by preoperative electrophysiological localization of the His bundle.

If permanent pacing is required endocavitary pacing would appear to be the most appropriate technique as reoperation at a site already in the process of healing is avoided.

1.3.5. Calcified aortic stenosis. Patients with aortic stenosis and symptoms only of syncope should have endocavitary electrocardiography, especially in the presence of left bundle branch block, when external carotid pulse tracing does not suggest severe stenosis, and when syncope does not appear to be related to effort. When a distal or truncular block is found the pacemaker may be implanted preoperatively, should cardiac surgery be indicated.

1.3.6. Intraventricular block in the convalescent phase of anterior myocardial infarction. The mortality rate in the first month of acute anterior myocardial infarction complicated by intraventricular or atrioventricular block is very high. In the survivors the persistence of bifascicular block may justify endocavitary investigation of the conduction intervals. This attitude would seem to be all the more legitimate in that these patients are prone to ventricular arrhythmias requiring antiarrhythmic therapy likely to prolong the infra-Hisian conduction time and the mechanism of a certain number of sudden deaths in these patients is not always understood (40).

1.3.7. Atrial fibrillation. When drugs acting on the atrioventricular node, such as digitalis or beta-blockers, are not in use, patients in atrial fibrillation with slow ventricular rhythms are a difficult problem. Regular ventricular rhythm with wide QRS and bradycardia at 40 per min with normal QRS are signs of complete atrioventricular block and an indication for permanent pacing. On the other hand when the ventricular rhythm is *irregular* the investigation of choice is the RR interval histogram over a minimum period of half an hour. The statistical distribution of the ventricular QRS complexes transiting through the node-Hisian system may then be observed, and a shift to the right especially with diastolic periods exceeding 1.2 sec is abnormal. This is important because the information may be applied to the interpretation of large RR intervals found on conventional ECGs, so facilitating the decision as to the need for permanent pacing. The largest diastoles on the histogram are the result of concealed conduction accentuated by atrioventricular block, the level of which cannot be determined from the RR histogram. In patients with supra-Hisian block the indication for pacing is not formal unless the patient needs treatment with digitalis. However, experience has shown that the general condition and well-being of these patients improves with pacemaker therapy.

Cardioversion by electric shock may reveal latent blocks by showing lengthening of the PR interval. It is of course possible to perform endocavitary electrocardiography even in atrial fibrillation. However, the identification of the H-potential is sometimes difficult. It may be confused with the atrial fibrillation potentials making the measurement of the HV interval impossible.

In summary indications for permanent pacing in atrioventricular block are easy to identify in the context of documented complete atrioventricular block and documented symptomatic paroxysmal atrioventricular block. The diagnosis of the latter condition may be very difficult when the symptomatology is atypical and the surface ECG shows a 1/1 atrioventricular conduction. However the most

suggestive features for the diagnosis of paroxysmal block are:
- the rapidly progressive nature of the block;
- widespread disease of excitation and intracardiac conduction;
- alternating blocks on the left intraventricular bundles associated with a pattern of right bundle branch block.

Endocavitary electrocardiography, especially correct measurement of HV intervals, and to a lesser extent continuous ambulatory ECG and the technique of RR interval histograms are helpful in deciding on the indications for pacing. These investigations demand strict adherence to technique in order to avoid mistakes in their interpretation, to which end the experience and basic knowledge of the physician are of fundamental importance.

2. INDICATIONS OF PACEMAKER THERAPY BESIDES ATRIO-VENTRICULAR BLOCK

The success of cardiac pacing in the treatment of atrioventricular block in the prevention of syncope and side effects of bradycardia has led to its use in patients without atrioventricular block with dysfunction of the sinoatrial node or with disturbances of atrial activation.

2.1. Sinus node dysfunction and sinus bradycardia

Sinoatrial block is characterized by deficiency of sinus node activity or an abnormality in the conduction defects observed into type I and type II as in atrioventricular block.

Our concepts are hypothetical because the sinus node activation has not yet been recorded in the human with present-day investigatory techniques. Nevertheless, the results of these conduction defects are either abnormally long diastolic periods with absence of one or several sinus node depolarizations or slowing of the cardiac rhythm to the stage where differentiation from sinus bradycardia becomes very difficult. The symptoms experienced by these patients are of three types:

- true syncopes suggestive of the Stokes-Adams attacks of complete atrioventricular block (41);
- heart failure due to sinus bradycardia;
- angina pectoris also due to bradycardia.

Symptoms suggestive of low output state, with tiredness and anorexia, are also usually present. Although angina is quite easily controlled by simple drug regimes the other two categories of symptoms are usually resistant and only transient improvement with medical therapy is observed. Pacemaker therapy is therefore the treatment of choice and 30 percent of all pacemakers are implanted for this condition (42).

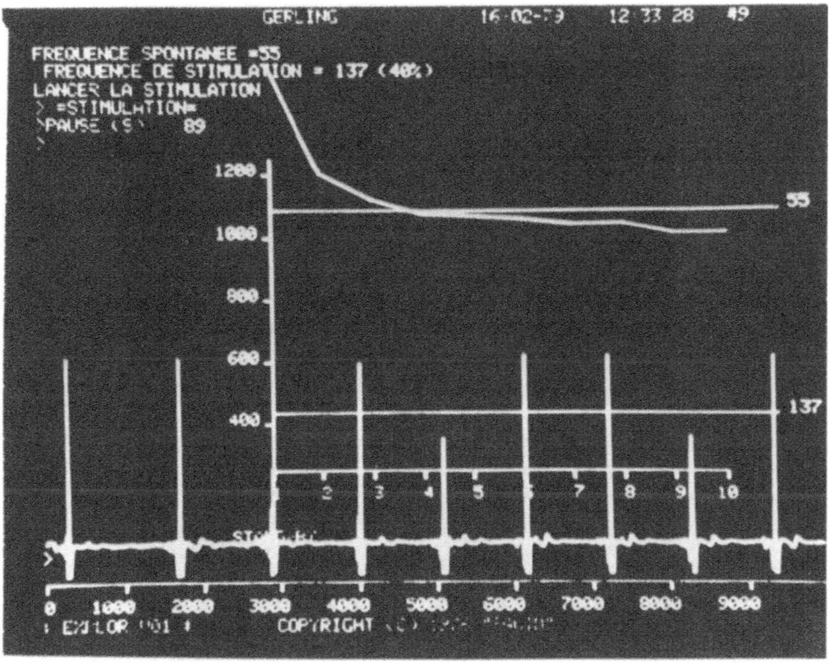

Figure 9. Study of sinus node by the measurement of the sinusal return cycle after atrial overdrive: at termination of overdrive and pacing at a fixed rate (137/min in this case) the corrected sinus node recovery time is obtained by the substraction of the basal cycle (55/min or 1090 msec) from the return cycle (1600 msec). The graph shows the behaviour of the periodicity of the 10 cycles following the termination of overdrive as well as the endocavitary Hisian recording. The normal value for the corrected sinus node recovery time is less than 500 msec.

The use of endocavitary electrocardiography in the assessment of sinus node function has been of much less practical value than in atrioventricular block as a significant number of false negative results are recorded. Two principal techniques are used: the first comprises the measurement of sinus node recovery time after overdrive pacing (Figure 9) and the second the assessment of sinoatrial conduction time by the extrastimulus technique (Figure 10). Prolongation of the sinus node recovery time is usually observed in patients with severe symptoms which require permanent pacing. The measurement of sinoatrial conduction times seems to be more useful in making the diagnosis of sinus node dysfunction than in the assessment of its severity (43).

When there is no associated atrioventricular block (atrioventricular conduction is investigated at the same time as the sinus node function) endocavitary atrial pacing with the pacing wire fixed in the right atrium or coronary sinus is the treatment of choice.

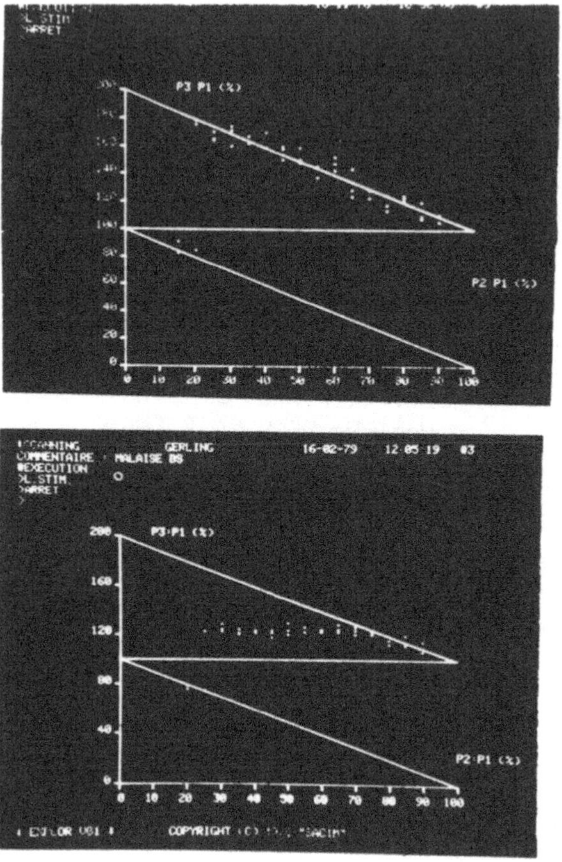

Figure 10. Study of sinus node function by the measurement of the sinusal return cycle after scanning the sinusal cycle with the premature extrastimulus technique (percentage of the cycle on abscissa; return cycle time as a percentage of the basal cycle on the ordinate). Normally the sinusal cycle remains initially unchanged as atrial depolarization conceals the sinus node activity (*bottom*), the return time is 'compensatory' and increases with the degree of prematurity of the extrastimulus. Beyond a certain prematurity (70%) the sinus node is *recycled* and the return time becomes constant, appearing on the graph as a plateau the height of which is related to the sinoatrial conduction time. In sinoatrial block (*top*) the extrastimulus cannot affect the sinus node whose cycle remains unaltered giving a constant aspect of 'compensatory pause'.

2.2. Bradycardia-tachycardia syndrome

This is a special form of sinus node dysfunction characterized by sinus arrest frequently occurring after rapid supraventricular tachycardia such as paroxysmal atrial tachycardia, flutter, or fibrillation (44). The duration of sinus arrest may be long enough to cause malaise or true syncope by cardiac standstill. This usually ends in a nodal escape rhythm or in the progressive reappearance of sinusal automatism. The symptoms experienced by the patients vary from palpitations to postcritical malaise. The extrastimulus technique often triggers atrial arrhythmias, especially when the prematurity coincides with the end of the atrial refractory period. The arrhythmias may be persistent and lead to the interruption of the investigation.

Pacemaker therapy is justified in these patients but it must be realized that it does not provide complete protection against rapid atrial arrhythmias and in many cases antiarrhythmic therapy has to be used. Besides the hemodynamic advantages atrial pacing may also prevent supraventricular arrhythmias by suppressing atrial extrasystoles and slow atrial rhythms. However, it is rarely employed in practice because many patients develop progressive disease of the conduction system leading to atrioventricular blocks. Therefore the pacing wire is positioned in the ventricle unless the technique of bifocal pacing is used (45).

An important clinical feature in these patients is the risk of systemic embolism and in general, anticoagulant therapy is advisable.

2.3. Pacemaker therapy in tachycardias

This question will be discussed in detail in chapter 4 and so we will confine ourselves to some general remarks, emphasizing from the outset that the indications for pacemaker therapy must be based on a rigorous electrophysiological study of the arrhythmia aimed at determining its mechnism and above all the efficacity of the pacing techniques to be used.

Permanent pacing may be considered as an intermediary technique to be employed when antiarrhythmic agents are either ineffective or give rise to unacceptable side effects, and when radical surgery on the arrhythmia is not clinically indicated. Pacing techniques in tachy-arrhythmias are principally directed to those probably arising from re-entry phenomena, the basic model of which is the reciprocating tachycardia observed in the Wolff-Parkinson-White syndrome (46). The presence of two different conduction pathways, the nodo-Hisian and the Kent, between the atria and the ventricles is a setup in which re-entry phenomena may arise. An appropriately timed electrical stimulus applied near enough to the pathway of the circus movement, either in the atrium or ventricle, may terminate this type of tachycardia. When the electrode is positioned at a distance from the pathway a single electrical stimulus may not be effective and doubled stimuli or a burst of rapid pacing may be required. To be safe, the electrode should be positioned in the atrium. It is important not to initiate atrial fibrillation or at least to be sure that if it does occur its transmission to the ventricles will not cause hemodynamic problems greater than that caused by the orthorhythmic tachycardia itself. Different methods of pacing are indicated in other supraventricular tachycardias not related to the WPW syndrome but probably caused by re-entry, such as paroxysmal atrial tachycardia, or reciprocating junctional rhythms (47).

Similar pacing techniques have been used in the treatment of ventricular tachycardia. In this condition the pacing wire must be positioned near to the re-entry pathway. The success of the method does not wholly depend on the physical distance but also on the electrophysiological properties of the muscle between the tip of the pacing wire and the zone of origin of the arrhythmia.

In adverse conditions, stimulation performed close to the pathway may not succeed in interrupting the arrhythmia. In other cases, under the same conditions, pacing at a distance from the re-entry pathway (even from the opposite ventricle) may be successful in initiating and terminating the arrhythmia.

In some exceptional cases patients have been provided with the means of triggering their pacemakers at rapid rhythms, either by a magnet or by a radio-frequency pacemaker (46, 48) so as to *terminate* attacks of tachycardia. In other cases, a permanent pacemaker is programmed to pace at a regular rhythm fast enough to *prevent* the tachycardia from occurring by changing the dynamic equilibrium of the ventricular depolarization.

3. CONCLUSION

The indications of permanent pacing are still expanding. In atrioventricular block the physician has to find a compromise between ignoring certain indications which may expose his patient to the risk of sudden death, and premature implantation, with the economic consequences this entails. This latter problem is felt to a variable degree in different countries. In the context of tachy-arrhythmias, the indications for pacing should be based on clinical and electrophysiological studies performed at specially equipped centres.

REFERENCES

1. Edhag O: Long-term follow-up of patients with implanted pacemakers. In: *Cardiac pacing*, Watanabe Y (ed), Amsterdam, Excerpta Medica, 1977, p 237.
2. Torresani J, Jouve J: Cardiac pacing for more than ten years. In: *Cardiac pacing*, Watanabe Y (ed), Amsterdam Excerpta Medica, 1977, p 245.
3. Johansson BW: Natural history of atrioventricular block. In: *Cardiac pacing*, Watanabe Y (ed), Amsterdam, Excerpta Medica, 1977.
4. Lenegre J: Etiology and pathology of bilateral bundle branch block in relation to complete heart block. *Prog Cardiovasc Dis* 6: 409, 1964.
5. Kulbertus HE: The magnitude of risk of developing complete heart block in patients with LAD RBBB. *Am Heart J* 86: 278, 1973.
6. Scherlag BJ, Lau SH, Helfant RH, Berkowitz WP, Stein E, Damato AN: Catheter technique for recording His bundle activity in man. *Circulation* 39: 13, 1969.
7. Lipski J, Cohen L, Espinoza J, Motro M, Dack S, Donoso E: Value of holter monitoring in assessing cardiac arrhythmias in symptomatic patients. *Am J Cardiol* 37: 102, 1976.

8. Slama R, Motte G, Grolleau R: Les Blocs atrioventriculaires paroxystiques: indications de l'exploration electrophysiologique et de l'implantation d'un stimulateur cardiaque chez un malade en rythme sinusal. In: *Les Troubles du rythme cardiaque*, Puech P, Slama R (eds), Nanterre, Corbière, 1978.
9. Krikler DM, Curry PVL: Torsade de pointes, an atypical ventricular tachycardia. *Brit Heart J* 38: 117, 1976.
10. Touboul P, Ibrahim H: Atrioventricular conduction defects in patients presenting with sy cope and normal P-R interval. *Brit Heart J* 34: 1005, 1972.
11. Narula OS: Validation of his bundle recordings: limitations of the catheter technique. In: *His bundle electrocardiography and clinical electrophysiology*, Narula OS (ed), Philadelphia, Davis, 1975, p 65.
12. Brodsky M, Wu D, Denes P, Kanakis C, Rosen KM: Arrhythmias documented by 24 hours continuous electrocardiographic monitoring in 50 male medical students without apparent heart disease. *Am J Cardiol* 39: 390, 1977.
13. Haft JI, Weinstock M, Deguia R, et al.: Assessment of atrioventricular conduction in left and right bundle branch block using His bundle electrograms and atrial pacing. *Am J Cardiol* 27: 474, 1971.
14. Gupta PK, Lichstein E, Chadda KD: Intraventricular conduction time (H-V interval) during aterograde conduction in patients with heart block *Am J Cardiol* 32: 27, 1973.
15. Zakaudin V, Mason DT, Fletcher RD, Awan NA, Massumi RA: Prolonged His-Q interval in chronic bifascicular block: relation to impending complete heart block. *Circulation* 53 (1): 46-55, 1976.
16. Puech P, Grolleau R, Guimond C: Incidence of different types of A-V block and their localisation by His bundle recordings. In: *The conduction system of the heart*, Wellens HJJ, Janse MJ, Lie KI (eds), Leiden Stenfert Kroese, 1976, p 467.
17. Narula OS, Gann D, Samet P: Prognostic value of H-V intervals. In: *His bundle electrocardiography and clinical electrophysiology*, Narula OS (ed), Philadelphia, Davis, 1975, p 437.
18. Gupta PK, Lichstein E, Chadda KD: Follow-up studies in patients with right bundle branch block and left anterior hemiblock: significance of H-V interval. *J Electrocardiol* 10: 221, 1977.
19. Scheinman MM, Peters RW, Modin G, Brennan M, Mies C, O'Young J: Prognostic value of infranodal conduction time in patients with chronic bundle branch block. *Circulation* 56: 240, 1977.
20. Altschuler H, Fisher JD, Furman S: Significance of isolated H-V interval prolongation in symptomatic patients without documented heart block. *Am Heart J* 97: 19, 1979.
21. Dhingra RC, Denes P, Wu D, Chuquimia R, Amat-Y-Leon F, Wyndham C, Rosen KM: Chronic right bundle branch block and left posterior hemi-block: clinical, electrophysiologic and prognostic studies. *Am J Cardiol* 36: 867, 1975.
22. Denes P, Dhingra RC, Wu D, Chuquimia R, Amat-y-Leon F, Wyndham CR, Rosen KM: H-V interval in patients with bifascicular block (right bundle branch block and left anterior hemiblock): Clinical, electrocardiographic and electrophysiologic correlations. *Am J Cardiol* 53: 600, 1976.
23. Dhingra RC, Denes P, Wu D, Wyndham CR, Amat-y-Leon R, Iowne WD, Rosen KM: Prospective observations in patients with chronic bundle branch block and marked H-V prolongation. *Circulation* 53: 600, 1976.
24. Seipel L, Breithardt G, Kuhn M: Significance of His bundle in bundle branch block. In: *To pace or not to pace*, Thalen HJTh, Harthorne JW (eds), The Hague, Martinus Nijhoff, 1978, p 33.
25. Fisher JD, Kulbertus HE, Narula OS: The prognostic value of the H-V interval PACE 1: 132, 1978.
26. Narula OS: Intraventricular conduction defects. In: *His bundle electrocardiography and clinical Electrophysiology*, Narula OS (ed), Philadelphia, Davis, 1975, p 177.
27. Narula OS: Evaluation of the cardiac conduction system by His bundle recordings. In: *To pace or not to pace*, Thalen HJTh, Harthorne JW (eds), The Hague, Martinus Nijhoff, 1978, p 16.
28. Wu D, Denes P, Dhingra RC, Amat-y-Leon F, Wyndham CR, Chuquimia R, Rosen KM: Electrophysiological and clinical observations in patients with alternating bundle branch block. *Circulation* 53: 586, 1976.

29. Wong BYS, Dunn M: Transient unifascicular-bifascicular block: electrophysiologic correlation in a patient with rate-dependant left bundle branch block and transient right bundle branch block. *Am J Cardiol* 39: 116, 1977.
30. Guérot C, Coste A, Valère PE, Tricot R: L'Épreuve à l'Ajmaline dans le diagnostic des blocs auriculo-ventriculaires paroxystiques. *Arch Mal Coeur* 66: 1241, 1973.
31. Motte G, Fournial C, Bodereau P, Kevorkian M, Welti JJ: Intérêt pronostic de l'intervalle H-V spontane et après ajmaline chez les patients ayant un bloc de branche. In: *Troubles du rythme et electrostimulation: symposium*, Toulouse, 1977.
32. Berkovitz WD, Wit AL, Lau SH, Sterner C, Damato AN: the effects of propranolol on cardiac conduction. *Circulation* 40: 885, 1969.
33. Gupta PK, Lichstein E, Chadda KD: Lidocaine-induced heart block in patients with bundle branch block. *Am J Cardiol* 33: 487, 1974.
34. Pirzada FA, Venkataraman K, Madias JE, Hood WB: Prophylactic preoperative pacing. In: *To pace or not to pace*, Thalen HJTh, Harthorne JW (eds), The Hague, Martinus Nijhoff, 1978, p 82.
35. Falkoff M, Stowe S, Ong LS, Heinle RA, Barold S: Unusual complication of bifascicular block during surgery under general anesthesia. PACE 1: 260, 1978.
36. Kimibiris D, Dreifus LS, Linhart JW: Complete heart block occurring during cardiac catheterization in patient with preexisting bundle branch block. *Chest* 65: 95, 1974.
37. Levites R, Toor M, Haft JI: Progressive improvement of His-Purkinje conduction during recovery from catheter-induced heart block. *Am Heart J* 91: 79, 1976.
38. Jacobson LB, Scheinman M: Catheter-induced intra-Hisian and intra-fascicular block during recording of His bundle electrogram. *Circulation* 49: 579, 1974.
39. Sung RJ, Iamer DM, Garcia OL, Castellanos Jr A, Myerburg RJ, Gelband H; Analysis of surgically-induced right bundle branch block pattern using intracardiac recording techniques *Circulation* 54 (3): 442-446, 1976.
40. Ritter WS, Atkins JM, Blomqvist CG, Mullins CB: Permanent pacing in patients with transient trifascicular block during acute myocardial infarction. *Am J Cardiol* 53: 205 1976.
41. Lister JE, Gosselin AJ, Swaye PS: Obscure syncope and the sick sinus syndrome. PACE 1: 68, 1978.
42. Jordan JL, Yamaguchi I, Mandel WJ: Function and dysfunction of the sinus node: clinical studies in the evaluation of sinus node function. In: *The sinus node: structure, function and clinical relevance*. Bonke FIM (ed), The Hague, Martinus Nijhoff, 1978, p 2.
43. Luderitz B, Steinbeck G, Naumann C, Rosenberger W: Relevance of diagnostic atrial stimulation for treatment in Sinoatrial disease. In: *The sinus node: structure, function and clinical relevance*. Bonke FIM (ed), The Hague, Martinus Nijhoff, 1978, p 77.
44. Short DS: The syndrome of alternate tachycardia and bradycardia. *Brit Heart J* 16: 208, 1954.
45. Dreifus LS, Berkovits BV, Kimibiris D, Moghadam K, Haupt G, Walinsky P, Thomas P, Brockman SK: Use of atrial and bifocal cardiac pacemakers for treating resistant dysrhythmias. *Eur J Cardiol* 3: 257, 1975.
46. Ryan GF, Easley RM, Zaroff LI: Paradoxical use of a demand pacemaker in the treatment of supraventricular tachycardia due to the WPW syndrome: observation of termination of reciprocal rhythm. *Circulation* 38: 1037, 1968.
47. Barold SS: Therapeutic uses of cardiac pacing in tachyarrhythmias. In: *His bundle electrocardiography and clinical electrophysiology*, Narula OS (ed), Philadelphia, Davis 1975, p 407.
48. Fontaine G, Frank R, Coutte R, Vachon JM, Laughlin LL, Grosgogeat Y: A new technique of radio-frequency pacing to interrupt the attacks of reciprocating tachycardia in the WPW syndrome. In: *Cardiac pacing*, Thalen HJTh (ed), Assen, Van Gorcum, 1973, p 389.

4. ELECTROPHYSIOLOGY RELATED TO CARDIAC PACING TECHNIQUES

BERNDT LÜDERITZ

1. GENESIS OF ARRHYTHMIAS

1.1. Bradycardias

Bradycardias originate either from a dysfunction of impulse formation in the sinoatrial node or from a disturbed conduction of the impulse. A decrease in the rate of the sinoatrial node automaticity may be caused by an increased duration of the action potential, an increase in the maximum diastolic potential (i.e. hyperpolarization which delays depolarization to the threshold potential) or a reduced rate of rise of diastolic depolarization. Conversely, changes of these variables in the opposite direction increase the trigger rate of the intrinsic cardiac pacemaker.

The conduction velocity is basically determined by the amplitude and maximum rate of rise of the action potential, by the threshold potential and by the intercalated discs. The conduction velocity increases with increasing amplitude and upstroke velocity of the action potential, with increasing negativity of the threshold potential, with an increasing number of intercalated discs and a decrease of their electric resistance. The maximum rate of rise and the amplitude of the action potential are determined by the fast influx of sodium ions. A depolarization of the membrane or a drug-induced inhibition of the sodium influx (e.g. by local anesthetics) lowers the conduction velocity by decreasing the rate of rise and amplitude of the action potential. Furthermore, an impaired functional connection of cardiac cells caused by necrosis, dehiscence or fibrosis may result in a decreased conduction velocity.

Conduction disturbances vary in their degrees: they range from a gradual delay to complete blockade of conduction. Clinically, disturbances of impulse formation and conduction are particularly relevant to the so-called sick sinus syndrome as well as in sinoatrial and atrioventricular blocks of different degrees.

1.2. Tachycardias

Two different pathogenetic mechnisms will be discussed as causes of tachycardias: focal automaticity and circus movement (re-entry). Circus movement is primarily caused by pathological changes in conduction and refractoriness (1). Ectopic focal impulse formation results from local disturbances of depolarization and repolarization of the cell membrane (2).

1.2.1. Focal impulse formation

Factors that enhance focal impulse formation include hypoxia, ischaemia, increased extracellular calcium levels, decreased intracellular potassium levels, and mechanical lesions of cardiac tissue. One has to differentiate between increased automaticity and so-called triggered activity. The former refers to a basically physiologic process which, however, is pathologically speeded up whereas the latter is understood as a disturbed process of repolarization of the cell membrane.

Increased automaticity. Ectopic impulse formation usually originates in the specific ventricular conduction system and only occassionally in the contractile system itself. The action potentials of the Purkinje fibres are initiated when, during the phase of diastolic depolarization, the efflux of potassium drops below the depolarizing influx of sodium, and the threshold potential of rapid sodium influx is reached. The velocity of diastolic depolarization as well as the levels of the threshold potential are particularly sensitive to electrolyte disturbances (3, 4, 5). In Purkinje fibres a fall of potassium concentration leads to an increased automaticity and spontaneous depolarization rate due to a decreased permeability of the cell membrane for potassium ions.

Triggered activity. A different mechanism of increased focal impulse formation underlies the phenomenon of 'triggered activity' (6). This involves a disturbance of the post-repolarization phase of the cell membrane. An intermittent lack of coordination between repolarizing and depolarizing ion shifts leads to alternating hyper- and depolarization. Accordingly the membrane potential oscillates around the resting potential and an action potential is triggered off whenever the threshold potential is reached. Cranefield et al. called this type of impulse formation 'triggered activity' (7).

1.2.2. Circus movement (re-entry).

The following conditions have to be fulfilled for a circus movement:
1. unidirectional block of an impulse in one or more than one region of the heart;
2. slow passage of an impulse via an alternative pathway;
3. delayed excitation of the tissue distal to the blocked site;
4. re-excitation of the tissue proximal to the site of block (8, 9).

The perpetuation of the tachycardia demands a refractory period shorter than the time needed for conduction of the activation wave around a loop. In mathematical terms: $RP < \oint \frac{1}{V}\, dl$. That is, the refractory period must be less than the circle integral 1 over V, (V = conduction velocity in the pathway) times the

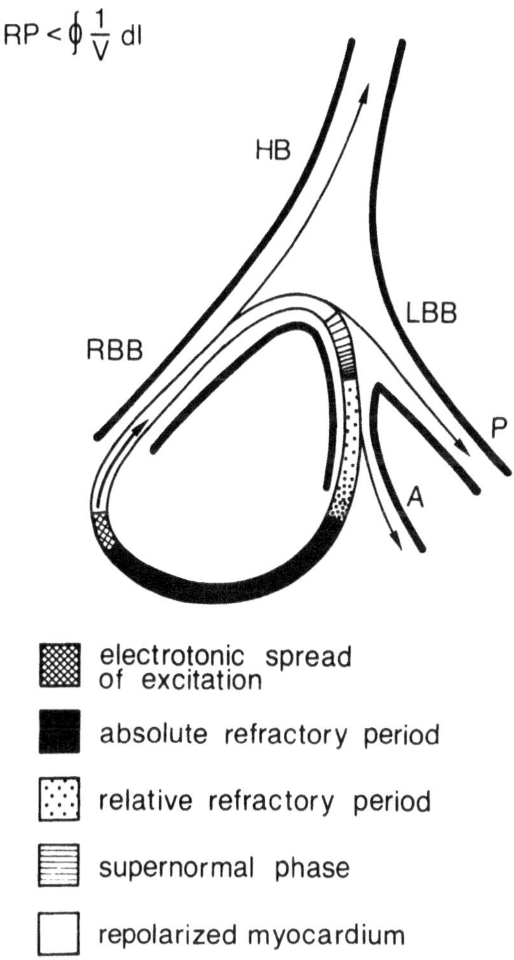

Figure 1. Complete right bundle branch block with bundle branch re-entry tachycardia: arrows indicate possible pathways for a re-entry ventricular tachycardia via the bundle brances. HB = His bundle, RBB = right bundle branch, LBB = left bundle branch, A = anterior fascicle, P = posterior fascicle, RP = refractory period, V = conduction velocity, dl = differential length of the pathway (11).

differential length of the pathway, (dl). The re-entrant tachycardia is terminated if the refractory period exceeds the conduction time around the loop (10). A schematic illustration is given in Figure 1 using the example of an antegrade right bundle branch block (11).

A re-entry tachycardia can be terminated by

1. a prolongation of the refractory period in the pathologic pathway (e.g. by drugs or appropriate electric stimulation);
2. an increased conduction velocity in the pathologic pathway;

3. a decreased radius of the pathologic circus;
4. external depolarization of the excitable gap ('window') by properly-timed electric stimulation.

Clinically, a sinus node re-entry has been discussed as the cause of supraventricular tachycardia and of atrial echo beats (12). Up to now, however, animal experiments have only been able to show that single-echo beats may be caused by a sinus node re-entry (13,14). On the other hand, it has been demonstrated that re-entry of the atria can cause tachycardia. For example, Lewis et al. showed in atrial flutter that the underlying excitations are impulses which circle around the entry of the superior and inferior vena cava into the right atrium (15). More recent investigations have shown atrial circus movement even without the existence of an anatomical obstacle around which the excitation circles (16, 17).

Atrial and ventricular echo beats and supraventricular tachycardia arising form the AV nodal area may be explained by the concept of functional longitudinal dissociation within the AV node (18). This theory suggests that the AV node contains two functionally separate pathways which differ in their duration of the refractory period and conduction velocity. Hence the conditions for a circus movement would be met. For example, a premature atrial impulse is blocked in one pathway but is conducted in the other one. By retrograde conduction it may then enter the first pathway which at that time is not refractory any more, leading to an atrial echo beat.

In the ventricles, re-entry has also been hypothesized as a cause of tachycardias, but this is far more difficult to prove than in the atria. Pathways may be the bundle branches, the Purkinje fibres with or without surrounding muscle cells, as well as infarcted or fibrotic muscle cells (9).

A relatively long duration of the action potential and refractory period in the ventricles may suggest a large re-entry circus – a 'marco re-entry'. It could be shown, on the other hand, that in case of block at the site of the transitions from Purkinje fibres to muscle cells a marked abbreviation of the action potential occurs in the Purkinje fibres (19, 20). This would favour a 'micro re-entry' at the peripheral transitions from the Purkinje fibres to the ventricular muscle cells. In addition a decrease in conduction velocity may play an important role in re-entry phenomena (21, 22).

2. DIAGNOSTIC PACING

2.1. *Atrial stimulation*

Recognition of the clinical importance of sinoatrial disease is growing. Impaired sinus node function in sinoatrial disease including sinus bradycardia, sinus arrest, sinoatrial block, and the bradycardia-tachycardia syndrome cannot easily be assessed, especially when rhythm disturbances are occurring intermittently, since the recording of the electric activity of sinus node pacemaker cells is not available in man. The analysis of atrial activity in the surface electrocardiogram permits only an overall estimation of sinus node function. This involves the ability to act as an impulse generator and includes the conduction of the impulse from the pacemaker site to the atrium. Therefore, methods of provocative atrial stimulation have been developed which are thought to allow indirect estimation of sinus node automaticity and sinoatrial conduction in man.

The method of rapid atrial stimulation was established to measure sinus node recovery time which is assumed to permit the evaluation of sinus node automaticity. When sinus node recovery time was prolonged in patients with sinoatrial disease this has been interpreted as a sign of disturbed sinus node automaticity (23, 24). In 1973 Strauss et al. described a way of determining sinoatrial conduction time in man by using the premature atrial stimulation technique. Thus, with both provocative atrial pacing methods a discrimination between sinus node automaticity and sinoatrial conduction seemed to be possible (26). In respect to the methodical limitations of each of these atrial stimulation procedures (27, 28, 29) we recommended the measurement of both sinoatrial conduction time and sinus node recovery time for the estimation of sinus node function in sinoatrial disease (26, 30). In a recent study we correlated the results of rapid atrial stimulation as well as premature atrial stimulation with clinical data in forty patients in whom sinoatrial disease was supposed to be present. The aim was to examine the diagnostic value of atrial stimulation in patients who may require pacemaker implantation (30). In our study a multipolar electrode catheter was inserted via the right basilic vein or the femoral vein, and the tip placed at the lateral wall of the right atrium. The caudal-distal pair of electrodes (interelectrode distance 8 mm) was always used for stimulation. From the proximal pair of electrodes, lying closer to the sinus node, a high right atrial electrogram was simultaneously recorded. An additional bipolar electrode catheter was passed percutaneously by way of the right femoral vein to the right atrium to lie across the tricuspid valve for the recording of a His-bundle electrogram by use of a previously described technique – see Figure 2 (31).

The sinus node recovery time is defined as the time interval between the last paced atrial activation and the first spontaneous beat of sinus origin after cessation of rapid atrial stimulation. Sinus node recovery time was measured after stimulation with rates slightly higher than sinus rhythm.

Applying the premature atrial stimulation technique, premature depolarizations are elicited after every eighth spontaneous activation of sinus origin by use of programmable stimulator. For that purpose, the bipolar atrial electrogram is used as trigger signal.

The post-extrasystolic cycle a_2-a_3 (see Figure 3) is plotted in a diagram as a function of curtailed cycle a_1-a_2, both values expressed as the percentage of the

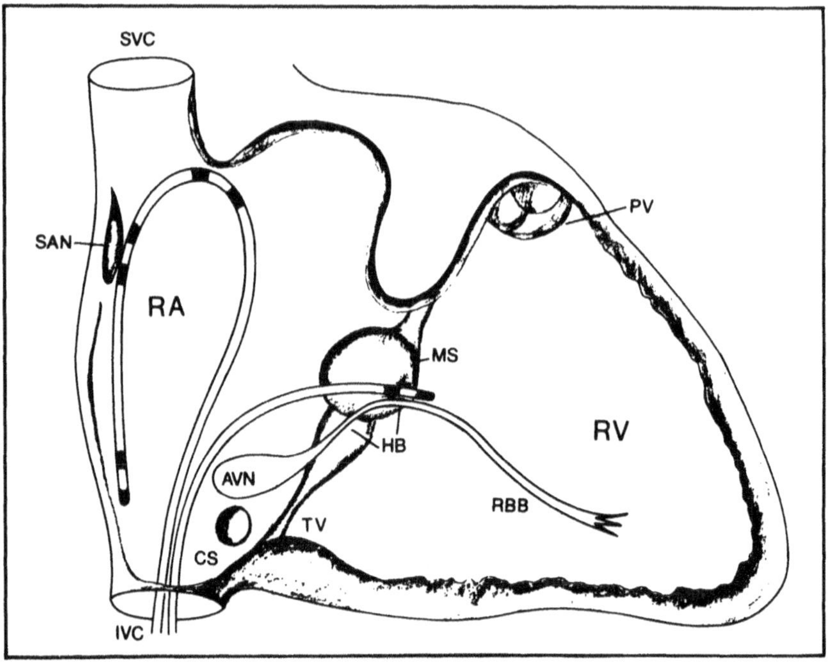

Figure 2. Diagnostic cardiac stimulation. Cutaway view of the heart demonstrating the electode catheter's postition. A multielectrode catheter is positioned in the right atrium, with another bipolar-electrode catheter lying across the tricuspid valve for the registration of His bundle potentials. SVC = superior vena cava, IVC = inferior vena cava, RA = right atrium, RV = right ventricle, TV = tricuspid valve, PV = pulmonic valve, SAN = sinoatrial node, AVN = atrioventriculat node, HB = His bundle, CS = orifice of the coronary sinus, MS = membranous septum, RBB = right bundle branch.

spontaneous atrial cycle a_1-a_1. For calculation of sinoatrial conduction time, the post-extrasystolic cycle just after the longest curtailed cycle which was followed by a non-compensatory pause is taken (see Figure 3). Hence we used the transition from the compensatory to the non-compensatory pause. This method has been further discussed elsewhere (29).

In single cases a changed configuration of a_3 as expression of a premature beat-followed pacemaker shift was observed (see Figure 4). This electrophysiologic event consists of a concomitant change in shape of high right atrial electrogram and an increase of atrial cycle length. Simultaneous alteration of P-waves was also observed. Assuming that the pacemaker shift indicates the arrivial of ectopic activation in the sinus node, capture of the sinus node by the premature beat could be distinguished from failure to capture. Thus, a pacemaker shift can be used for estimating sinoatrial conduction time in addition to the conventional methods of measuring the post-extrasystolic atrial interval (32).

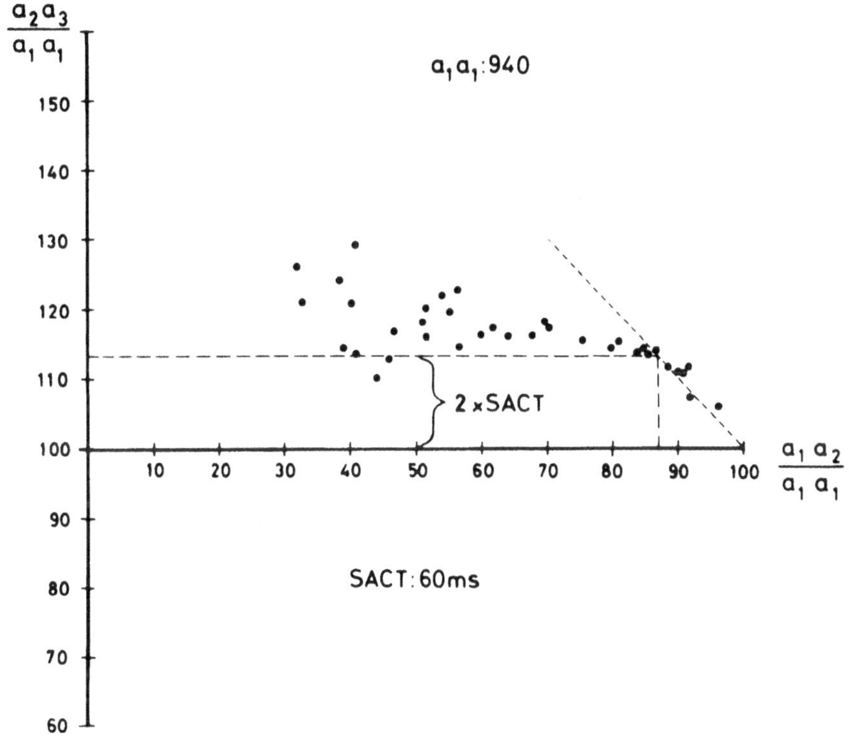

Figure 3. Post-extrasystolic cycle a_2-a_3 as a function of the curtailed cycle a_1-a_2. Both values are related to the precedinga_1-a_1 interval; a_1-a_1 interval=960 ± 55 msec (± SD), n=36. Transition from compensatory to non-compensatory a_2-a_3 interval occurs at a curtailed cycle of 87 percent of the a_1-a_2 interval. The post-extrasystolic interval a_2-a_3 at this borderline (113%) minus the spontaneous atrial cycle a_1-a_1 (=100%) represents conduction time into and out of the sinus node, i.e., the sum of the conduction time from the atrium to the sinus node plus from the sinus node to the atrium. Half of the total sum of conduction time results in the sinoatrial conduction time; in this case, 60 msec.

2.1.1. Controls. In 13 patients without sinus node dysfunction sinus node recovery time (SNRT) was 1172 msec ± 200 (± SD), and sinoatrial conduction time (SACT) was 66 msec ± 17 (± SD). Concerning SACT our normal values ranged between 40 and 95 msec which is understood as half of the conduction time into and out of the sinus node. With respect to SNRT we obtained results similar to other authors (see Table 1). Concerning SACT, different values were reported by other investigators (Table 2) since these authors used the non-compensatory pause for indirect calculation of SACT (see 29). In contrast, experimentally determined SACT was found to be much shorter in animal studies (43).

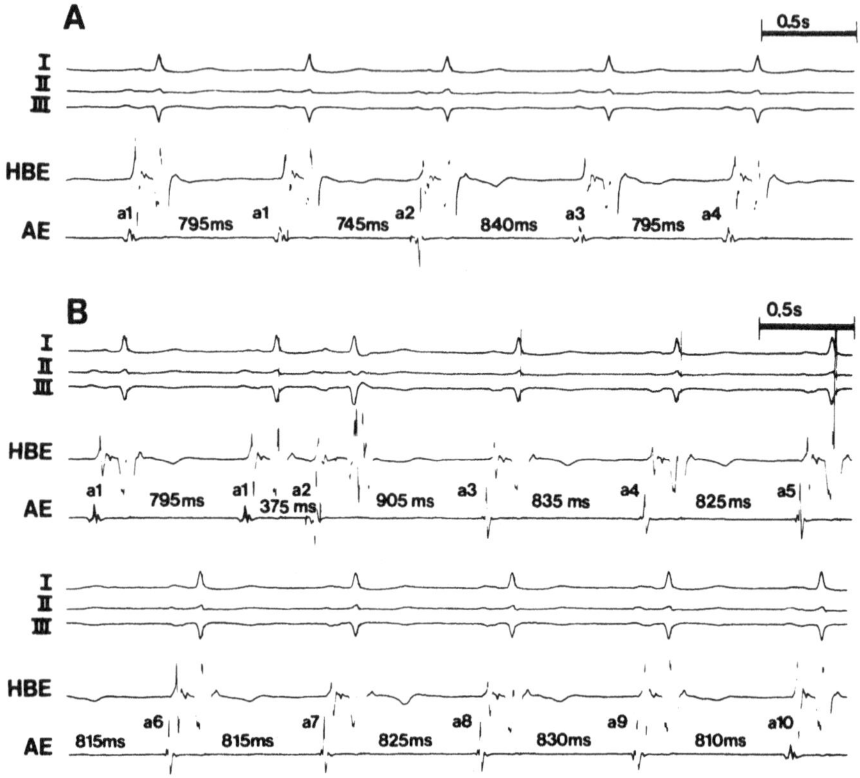

Figure 4. Lead I, II, III, His bundle (HBE), and atrial electrogram (AE) during premature atrial stimulation. A: After the second spontaneous atrial activation of sinus origin a late premature beat is followed by a compensatory pause (745 msec + 840 msec ≤ 2 × 795 msec). Five spontaneous cycles preceding a_2 ranged from 785 msec to 795 msec. B: Two continuous tracings are shown: a curtailed cycle of 375 msec followed by a non-compensatory pause (375 msec + 905 msec < 2 × 795 msec). Three cycles preceding a_2 with complexes identical to a_1 ranged from 795 msec to 800 msec. Alteration of activation pattern is apparent in the atrial electrogram as well as in the surface leads (the P-waves corresponding to a_3 and a_4 being negative in III, and isoelectric in II), whereas changes are not apparent in the HBE; a_5 to a_8 represent an intermediate activation pattern with return of small postive P-waves in II, but P remaining negative in III. With reappearance of an initial negative vector in AE in a_9 and more clearly in a_{10}, the P-waves have become normal (positive in II, biphasic in III). Cycle length up to a_8-a_9 is increased following one premature beat; a_9-a_{10} tends to become normal (From Steinbeck and Lüderitz [32], *Circulation* 56 (3), 1977, by permission of the American Heart Association, Inc).

2.1.2. Sinoatrial disease. In a total of 40 patients with clinical and electrocardiophic evidence of sinoatrial disease values of SNRT and SACT are both increased (Tables 1 and 2). The maximum sinus node recovery time was 1895 msec ± 1068 (± SD) and SACT ranged from 45 to 165 with a mean of 110 msec ± 31 (± SD) (n=34). The results of SNRT agree with those of other authors

Table 1. Sinus node recovery time (SNRT) in patients with and without sinoatrial disease (mean ± SD).

Author	Control	Sinoatrial disease
Breithardt et al. (33)	1044 msec ± 216 (n=20)	2110 msec ± 1269 (n=41)
Delius et al. (34)		2925 msec ± 331 (n=21)
Kulbertus et al. (35)	1100 msec ± 190 (n=30	
Mandel et al. (24, 36)	1041 msec ± 56 (n=43)	3087 msec ± 464 (n=31)
Rostock et al. (37)	1153 msec ± 122 (n=15)	
Lüderitz et al. (30)	1172 msec ± 200 (n=13)	1859 msec ± 1068 (n=40)

Table 2. Sinoatrial conduction time (SACT) in patients with and without sinoatrial disease (mean ± SD).

Author	Control	Sinoatrial disease
Breithardt et al. (33)	82 msec ± 19 (n=20)	126 msec ± 47 (n=41)
Crook et al. (39)	112 msec ± 30 (n=11)	128 msec ± 27 (n=14)
Dhingra et al. (40)	92 msec ± 30 (n=36)	
Masini et al. (41)	70 msec ± 15 (n=18)	127 msec ± 24 (n= 7)
Rostock et al. (37)	98 msec ± 11 (n=15)	
Strauss et al. (42)		103 msec ± 55 (n=16)
Luderitz et al. (30)	66 msec ± 17 (n=13)	110 msec ± 31 (n=34)

(Table 1). The agreement concerning SACT values depends on the calculation method used, i.e. the non-compensatory pause or the transition from the compensatory to the non-compensatory pause (see 29).

Patients with sinoatrial disease were clinically divided into two groups. 20 patients (group A) were kept on conventional drug therapy whereas 20 patients (group B) required pacemaker implantation. 13 patients without clinical or electrocardiographic evidence of sinoatrial disease represented the control group (group C).

The electrophysiological data of the no-pacemaker (A) and the pacemaker group (B) were compared with those of the control group (Figure 5). The sinus rate was markedly decreased in patients who required pacemaker implantation. However, no significant changes were observed between the control and the no-pacemaker group. A similar pattern was observed for the maximal sinus node recovery time. SNRT is conspicuously prolonged in patients requiring pacemaker therapy. Patients without pacemaker requirement revealed no prolongation of SNRT when compared with the control group. The feature of calculated sinoatrial conduction time was completely different. Patients with sinoatrial disease showed significantly prolonged SACT values in comparison to the con-

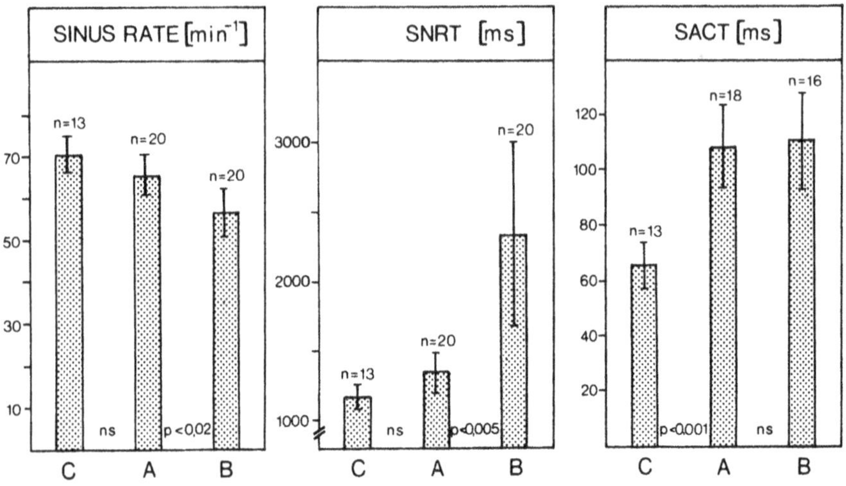

Figure 5. Electrophysiological data of sinus node function for the patients studied by diagnostic atrial stimulation. Control group (C), and patients with sinoatrial disease; A = no pace-maker requirement, B = pacemaker requirement (*ns* = no significant difference).

trol group. However, there was no difference between the no-pacemaker and the pacemaker group.

In conclusion, in cases of moderate sinoatrial disease SNRT was nog significantly different from the control values. While determination of SNRT seems to be useful for the additional differentiation between severe and mild cases of sinoatrial disease, calculation of SACT fails in this respect. Sinoatrial conduction time is conspicuously prolonged in the whole group of patients with sinoatrial disease; however, no difference between severe and mild forms could be detected (Figure 5). A patient follow-up over a period of 18-24 months with regular visits of the patient revealed a marked improvement of all patients in group B (pacemaker implantation). So far no patient has died. The persisting severe symptoms in patients of group A were not related to sinoatrial disease.

Hence, the decision for pacemaker treatment in sinoatrial disease is largely determined by the particular symptoms which are troublesome to the patient and which correlate with electrocardiographic and electrophysiological abnormalities. Prolonged SNRT is associated with a high incidence of clinically severe sinoatrial disease in patients requiring pacemaker therapy. The calculation of SACT seems to be helpful for the diagnosis rather than for the estimation of the severity in sinoatrial disease. In our opinion moderate prolongation of SNRT or SACT in the absence of clinical symptoms is not an indication for (prophylactic) pacemaker implantation.

2.2. His-bundle electrography

In 1957 Giraud, Puech et al. first succeeded recording His-bundle potentials in man. The registration was obtained during a catheterization in a patient with Fallot's tetralogy (44). After extensive animal studies His-bundle electrography HBE) was introduced to clinical medicine by Scherlag in 1969 (32).

The present routine technique of HBE requires an electrode to be inserted via the right femoral vein. It is placed in a way such that the elctrodes touch the septum of the right ventricle shortly below the septal cusp (Figure 2). When using catheters with four or six electrodes it is possible, using switching techniques, to select two adjacent electrodes which deliver the optimal His-bundle potential. In most cases HBE is used in connection with atrial stimulation. A transvenous catheter inserted into the right atrium via the right or left arm allows stimulation at chosen rates.

His-Bundle electrograms are recorded simultaneously with conventional leads. Right atrial potential close to the electrodes show as a group of spikes which lie within the P-wave of the ECG. After 80-100 msec these potentials are followed by a single spike of about 15 msec duration which represents the His-bundle potential. After a gap of another 40-60 msec a second group of potentials is recorded and indicates depolarization of the septum near to the electrodes.

HBE is best suited for the diagnosis of conduction defects of the specific conduction system which cannot be identified by conventional leads. In addition, some information can be obtained with regard to orthograde conduction or retrograde conduction disturbances. First-degree AV blocks are primarily localized above the bundle of His. Therefore a PQ-prolongation in the conventional ECG is mostly based on an increased AH interval. A second degree AV block is also localized above the bundle in most cases of blockade of the Wenckebach type. In Mobitz type II second-degree AV block, however, the site of the block is primarily distal to the bundle of His. In third-degree AV block the site of the block can be either proximal or distal to the bundle of His.

Using HBE it has been shown that supraventricular rhythms, previously regarded as junctional (nodal) rhythms, arise from the bundle of His. Furthermore, the HBE allows differentiation between ventricular ectopic beats and aberrant conduction in atrial fibrillation. Ventricular ectopic beats have no preceding H-potential. Supraventricular tachycardia which functional bundle branch block can also be identified.

His-bundle elctrography has become particularly important for the diagnosis of paranodal atrioventricular junctions. In the LGL syndrome[1] often a shortened AH and HV interval is present. The Wolff-Parkinson-White(WPW) syndrome is typically indicated by the His bundle spike lying inside the delta

[1] Lown-Ganong-Levine syndrome: short P-R interval and normal QRS complex.

wave, i.e. inside the excitation of the ventricles. This finding confirmed the hypothesis of atrioventricular conduction via an accessory pathway.

Pharamacological studies which included HBE have become important for differential therapeutic decisions in the treatment of various cardiac arrhythmias. For example, the AH interval is shortened by atropine, isoprenaline, and diphenylhydantoin but prolonged by verapamil, digitalis, and propranolol (see also 45).

Finally, HBE has proven useful for the interpretation of various patterns of bundle branch block. A separate analysis of the conduction within the AV node and the intraventricular conduction system has become possible. By additional rapid atrial stimulation latent intraventricular conduction defects may be detected. Thus, an HBE may provide further information for the decision as to whether the implantation of an external pacemaker is inducted or not.

These fields of application have made the HBE a useful tool in cardiac research as well as in special clinical investigation – particularly for a detailed analysis of atrioventricular conduction defects. However, the catalogue of absolute indications for the registration of the HBE is very small. This is because diagnostic problems necessitating HBE are rare and rather special. In AV blocks the result can be predicted in most cases. Therefore the decision for pacemaker therapy can primarily be made without invasive diagnostics purely on the basis of clinical symptoms and the surface ECG. In intraventricular block an HBE is only necessary if the clinical symptoms remain unclear.

The prognostic relevance of a prolonged HV interval is of particular importance. The definition of prolongation, however, has not yet been ultimately established (46, 47).

3. THERAPEUTIC PACING

3.1. Pacing in bradycardias

Symtomatic bradycardias represent the standard indication for cardiac pacing particularly with implantable pacemakers. Based on clinical electrophysiology various types of pacemakers are available at present (Figure 6). The variety of implantable pacemakers can be devided into five cathegories:

3.1.1. Atrial triggered pacemakers. Atrial triggered pacemakers (VAT) are controlled by an atrial electrode which picks up the depolarization of the atrium and initiates ventricular excitation after a delay comparable to the normal PQ interval. In case of normal atrioventricular conduction atrial pacemakers of the fixed rate or demand type are used.

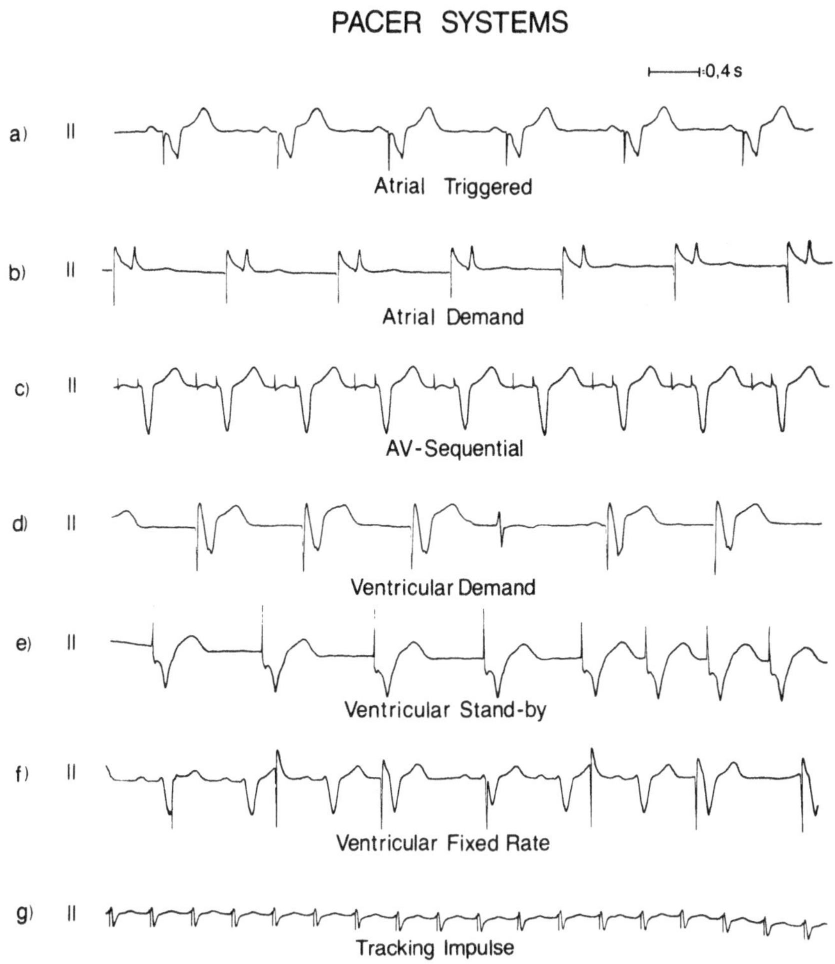

Figure 6. ECGs after pacemaker implantation: the atrial triggered pacemaker (a) detects the P-wave and initiates ventricular depolarization after a physiological interval. The atrial pacemaker (*b*) may be a demand, a triggered, or a fixed rate device. Normal AV conduction provided, it guarantees a more or less physiological order of contraction and rate control, the latter if the sinus node is still eleciting spontaneous impulses. In sequential pacemakers (*c*) ventricular stimulation follows the atrial one after an interval comparable to the PQ-interval. There have to be detection units for the atrial as well as for the ventricular actions. The demand-inhibited pacemaker (*d*) is reset after spontaneous beats whereas the fixed rate pacemaker (*f*) leads to parasystole if there are spontaneous actions. Demand-triggered pacemakers (e) pace at a basic rate and discharge additional impulses in response to spontaneous beats or even external signals (e.g. chest-wall stimulation as the figure). Tracking impulse pacemakers (*g*) discharge a short impulse below the threshold into the QRS-complex of every spontaneous beat. This allows the detection of spontaneous beats by telephonic control.

3.1.2. AV-sequential pacemakers. AV-sequential pacemakers (DOO) first stimulate the atrium and then the ventricles after a defined interval. This type of stimulation preserves the physiological sequence of contraction of the atria and ventricles except for premature contraction of the right ventricle. In addition an atrial triggered pacemaker allows the preservation of autonomic rate control, normal sinus node function provided. Newly-developed 'optimated sequential pacemakers' (DDI) prevent supraventricular as well as ventricular parasystole by working as demand pacemakers at both levels (48).

3.1.3. Demand pacemakers. In demand pacemakers (VVI) an impulse is only triggered off if no electric activity has been registered during an interval between 400 msec (refractory period of the device) and 800 msec (basic pacemaker rate) after the preceding depolarization. In demand pacemakers with positive hysteresis the duration of the first stimulation interval is extended to 1000 msec. Impulse suppression by external electric impulses – in some models even by magnetic fields – is possible. Therefore clinically relevant parameters such as the post-stimulation pause, the intrinsic heart rate, an ECG free of artefacts or the refractory period of the pacemaker can be checked. Thus, if there is a sufficient intrinsic heart rate an intermittent pacemaker suppression can be effected in

- stimulation or sensing defects,
- pacemaker racing with preserved sensing function,
- 'runaway pacemakers' (uncontrolled rate increase in battery failure),
- pacemaker-induced skeletal or diaphragmatic contractions.

In some pacemaker models of Edwards Laboratories or Telectronics a tracking impulse within the QRS complex is triggered off. It lies below the threshold but allows one to differentiate between spontaneous and pacemaker-induced impulses by telephonic control.

3.1.4. Stand-by pacemakers. Stand-by pacemakers (VVT) discharge impulses into the QRS complexes up to an upper limit. Effective stimulation only results if the intrinsic heart rate drops below a preset basic pacemaker rate. Stand-by pacemakers allow positive control by an external impulse generator. In this way, for example, a test rate can be effected or if required special stimulation via chestwall electrodes can be obtained.

3.1.5. Fixed rate pacemakers. Fixed rate pacemakers (VOO) permanently discharge impulses at a defined stimulation interval. This type, as well as the stand-by pacemaker, has recently regained importance for the treatment of tachycardias.

3.2. Tachycardias

Clinically significant tachycardias necessitate immediate therapy in most cases.

Besides the conventional drug treatment electrotherapeutic means have gained a place particularly in emergencies. This applies to defibrillation in ventricular fibrillation as well as to electrostimulation in certain types of recurrent supraventricular and ventricular tachycardias (Table 3).

Table 3. Cardiac pacing in tachy-arrythmias.

Indication	Method
DC shock	
Atrial Fibrillation	Defibrillation
Atrial flutter	Cardioversion
Supraventricular tachycardia	
Ventricular tachycardia	
Ventricular fibrillation	
Pacemaker stimulation	
Atrial flutter	Rapid atrial and ventricular stimulation
Supraventricular tachycardia	Overdrive pacing
(pre-excitation syndromes)	Coupled stimulation
Ventricular extrasystoles	Programmed stimulation:
Ventricular tachycardia	1. Fixed rate stimulation
	2. Stimulation with progressive coupling intervals
	3. Simultaneous atrial and ventricular stimulation
	4. Rate related interval stimulation

3.2.1. DC shock. The termination of tachycardias by electric shock applied through the chest wall is called electroconversion. In atrial or ventricular fibrillation it is named defibrillation. It has been used worldwide for more than 15 years now. The clinical application is based on the work of Lown et al. (51, 52), who could show experimentally as well as clinically that atrial and ventricular tachycardias can be terminated without serious complications by short but intensive DC shocks. In a rhythmically beating heart a DC impulse falling into the repolarization period may trigger off ventricular fibrillation. Therefore Lown developed an R-wave-triggered defibrillator which guarantees that the application of the shock occurs outside the vulnerable period of ventricular repolarization.

According to investigations by Antoni the mechanism of action of electric defibrillation is assumed to be a synchronous depolarization of all non-refractory myocardial areas. Synchronous depolarization is essential and this demands a sufficiently strong electric charge to all areas: new excitations are evoked in non-refractory areas of the myocardium which, however, cannot spread out through the rest of the heart. Therefore fibrillation stops and sinus rhythm can regain control over the heart. The electric suppression of focal automaticity is probably of minor importance. Electric defibrillation is more likely to be successful the more homogenous the electric current (53).

3.2.2. Cardiac pacing. In some cases electrical pacing offers advantages over standard DC cardioversion for the termination of tachycardias because:
1. no general anesthesia is required;
2. digitalis-induced arrhythmias may be abolished – a condition in which DC cardioversion is dangerous and usually ineffective; and
3. pacing can be effected rapidly, simply, and repeatedly, leaving the pacing catheter in place (54).

3.2.3. Mechnisms of cardiac pacing in tachycardias. Termination of tachycardias by properly-timed premature stimulation has been regarded as being indicative of the existence of a re-entry mechanism (9). For the explanation of this termination of a tachycardia one assumes that the artificial additional impulse depolarizes an excitable gap of the pathologic re-entry pathway which in return becomes refractory to the circling excitation. On the bais of some theoretical considerations as well as more recent findings in animal experiments, however, it has become doubtful again whether success or failure of electric stimulation can serve as a differential diagnostic criterion to distinguish between focal or re-entry tachycardia. One could, for instance, argue that the artificial impulse might perhaps not reach the circus if the distance between the electrode and the site of the circus movement is too long or if the conduction velocity is too slow. Furthermore, the chances of terminating the circus movement by an additional impulse become less promising if an anatomically very small circus pathway is present. Ultimately the circus could be just as short as the wavelength of the excitation itself. Thus, there would be no excitable gap for an additional artificial stimulus between the beginning and the end of the excitation wave. This leads to the conclusion that a failure of pacemaker therapy does not exclude a re-entry mechanism just as much as a success does not necessarily contradict focal impulse formation. This point results from animal experiments which contradicted the general view that focal impulse formation can be triggered off as well as interrupted by artificial electric stimulation (6, 55; see also 50).

Several different modes of cardiac pacing are now used to suppress supraventricular, junctional, and ventricular tachycardias.

3.2.4. Types of pacing modes in tachycardia.

a) Rapid intra-atrial stimulation. Rapid intra-atrial stimulation is an effective electrotherapeutic tool in atrial flutter, atrial and junctional (nodal) tachycardias. Regardless of the underlying condition atrial flutter with fast conduction can lead to dangerous situations because of the risk of 1:1 conduction to the ventricles. The conventional therapy involves administration of digitalis substances with the aim of converting the flutter into sinus rhythm or into atrial fibrillation with slow ventricular rate. If digitalis is contraindicated or if cardioversion is out of the question (e.g. in case of overdigitalization), rapid atrial stimulation (56) is an alternative method. Unlike cardioversion it can be performed without general anesthesia. This is an advantage in the elderly or in patients with a poor general condition. Treatment with digitalis does not have to be interrrupted.

A bipolar stimulation catheter is transvenously inserted into the right atrium under X-ray control and put against the atrial wall. Ventricular stimulation (e.g., caused by a shifting electrode) must be avoided. Short-term (seconds to minutes) rapid stimulation is effected by an impulse generator. The effective rate normally ranges from 150 to 600 per minute. In rare cases rates up to 2000/min have been applied (57). The procedure may be repeated several times. An ECG registered simultaneously allows one to recognize, for instance, the conversion of atrial flutter into fibrillation, which often spontaneously converts into sinus rhythm within a short time. Rapid atrial stimulation by no means alsways has to last for minutes. In our experience stimulation with a salvo of a few rapid impulses can be effective. Figure 7 shows the conversion of a supraventrivular tachycardia via atrial fibrillation into sinus rhythm following stimulation with five impulses at an interval of 30 msec (representing a rate of 2000/min).

The rate of success of rapid atrial stimulation – success defined as a conversion into sinus rhythm or atrial fibrillation – reaches 70 percent. Reversion into sinus rhythm within seconds or minutes is achieved in approximately 50 percent of the patients treated successfully. Sometimes the conversion is delayed by hours or even days although conversion into sinus rhythm is usually observed within 48 hours (57).

In atrial fibrillation intra-atrial stimulation is inefficient. Supraventricular tachycardia (except atrial fibrillation) can also be treated successfully with programmed single stimulation or with stimulation at a rate below the rate of the tachycardia.

Also the so-called radio-frequency pacemaker seems to be promising. Kahn and Citron reported a patient-controlled implantable pacemaker system for the suppression of supraventricular tachycardia. The system is based on externally triggered intermittent rapid atrial stimulation. The system includes an implantable receiver connected to a bipolar atrial electrode and an external battery-powered transmitter which is to be handled by the patient (58). Successful application demands an exact diagnosis of the tachycardia by previous stimulation, and a normal atrioventricular conduction, as well as considerable cooperation by the patient: he has to be able to recognize the bouts of tachycardia. The authors observed successful conversion of drug-resistant supraventricular tachycardia in 15 out of 18 patients. The new stimulation system was used by the patients approximately 10,000 times (58).

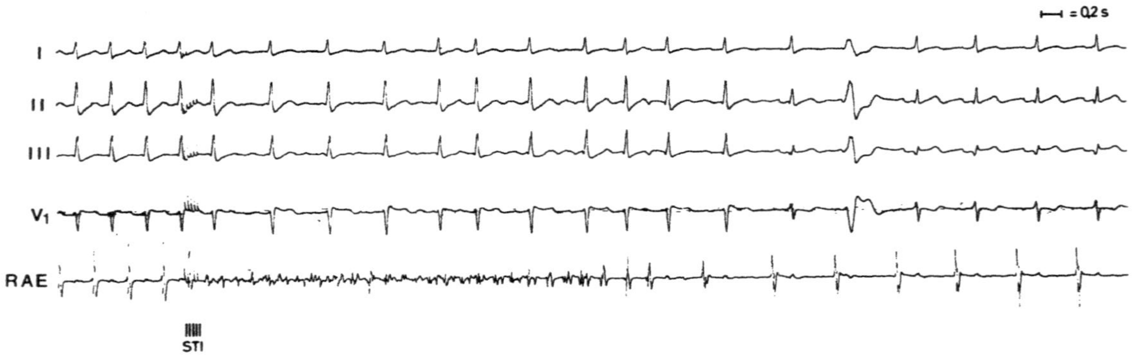

Figure 7. Conversion of supraventricular tachycardia into normal sinus rhythm in a 44-year-old patient. A burst of five electrical impulses (stimulation intervals 30 msec) leads to atrial fibrillation which is followed by normal sinus rhythm. I, II, III: standard ECG leads; V_1: precordial lead; RAE: right atrial electrogram, STI = stimulation (50).

There is only limited experience about trans-oesophageal atrial stimulation. First reports, however, sound encouraging, The advantage of this method lies in its simple noninvasive application. Moreover, an X-ray check of the position of the electrode can be omitted in emergencies (59).

The mechanism of the reversion into sinus rhythm by rapid atrial stimulation has not yet been elucidated. In may cases a re-entry tachycardia might be interrupted. But the suppression of an automatic focus also seems to be plausible. The initiation of atrial fibrillation by rapid stimulation can be explained by impulses falling into the vulnerable period of the atria.

b) Rapid ventricular stimulation. Supraventrivular re-entry tachycardias can also be terminated by short-term rapid intraventricular stimulation provided there is sufficient retrograde conduction.

In ventricular tachycardias rapid stimulation has so far only been used in special cases. Occasionally, the time necessary for effective ventricular stimulation can be very short and may only consist of a singly series of external impulses (Figure 8). Furman et al. have already described an implantable pacemaker system which can terminate ventricular tachycardia by rapid ventricular stimulation (60). They used a special QRS-inhibited pacemaker at a rate of 80/min. The rate can be increased up to 295/min or 300/min respectively by a magnetic relay. The rapid stimulation is automatically stopped after 2.5 sec. Ventricular fibrillation has so far never been observed.

c) Overdrive pacing. Increasing the rate in order to suppress ventricular or supraventricular ectopic activity is called 'overdrive pacing' (61). The stimulation rate has to be higher than the spontaneous rate, but it can be markedly lower than the ectopic rate to be suppressed. Often a rate just slightly above the spontaneous one suffices. This type of stimulation is particularly successful in extrasystoles. Overdrive pacing can be used in emergencies for hours or even days and is particularly suitable for cardio-surgical patients or patients with myocardial infarction suffering from drug-resistant extrasystoles. Epicardial application of the electrodes is to be preferred.

The electrophysiologic mechanism of overdrive suppression is still unclear. For example, the ventricular fibrillation threshold could be set to a higher level by the higher stimulation rate, or the spontaneous rate might be increased above the rate of the focus, or a re-entry circus could be interrupted by a change in myocardial conduction. In this context, not only the rate but also the site of stimulation are decisive (57).

d) Coupled stimulation. The frequency of drug-resistant tachycardias may also be reduced in some cases by coupled stimulation providing a prolongation of the electric refractory period. Closely following the last QRS complex, a second electric depolarization is prevented by the artificially-induced refractory period. Thus, by lengthening the period of inexcitability, the heart rate is significantly reduced.

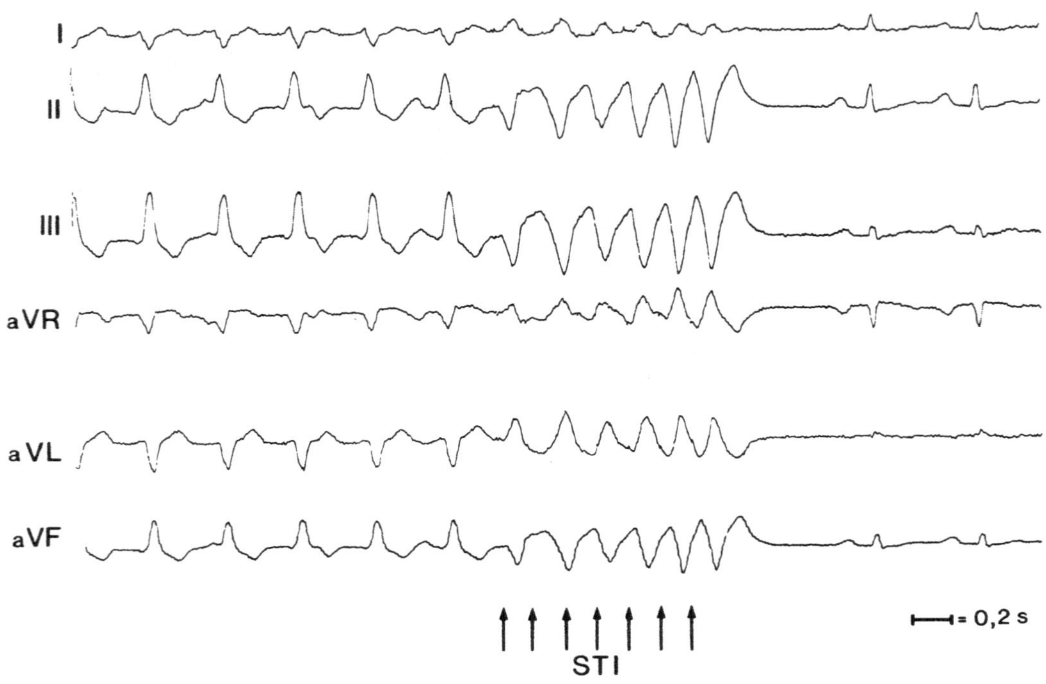

Figure 8. Termination of a sustained ventricular tachycardia (163/min) by rapid ventricular stimulation applied to the right ventricule. Seven impulses were elicited at a rate of 400/min according to a stimulation interval of 150 msec. Following pacemaker intervention a normal sinus rhythm is reestablished.

e) Fixed-rate pacemaker stimulation. The switching of the ventricular demand pacemaker to fixed-rate stimulation by a magnetic relay is called a paradoxic application of a demand pacemaker. Ryan et al. succeeded in interrupting rapid supraventricular re-entry tachycardias in WPW syndrome using this method (62; see 63). A randomized depolarization of the excitable gap of a re-entry circus is hypothesized as the underlying mechanism.

The application of programmed intermittent fixed-rate stimulation is not only limited to supraventricular tachycardias in patients with pre-excitation syndromes. For example, supraventricular tachycardia in myocarditis can also be terminated by this type of stimulation.

f) Stimulation with progressive coupling intervals. Spurrell described a so-called 'scanning pacemaker' which works by ventricular stimulation in supraventricular re-entry tachycardias (64). This system allows the variation of the optimal time of stimulation – which can vary by up to 30 msec. The scanning system automatically starts when a supraventricular tachycardia arises and it discharges single or double impulses after certain intervals: the first stimulation falls into the refractory period of the stimulated ventricle. One second later, a second impulse is given with 5 msec delay. Every following second another impulse is discharged, every one being delayed by another 5 msec until the overall delay has reached 400 msec. The stimulation stops as soon as the tachycardia is terminated (64).

g) Simultaneous atrial and ventricular stimulation. Coumel et al. developed a pacemaker system by which a certain type of supraventricular tachycardia (caused by a uniderectional block in the presence of two functionally different pathways) can be controlled by simultaneous atrial and ventricular stimulation. The pacemaker intervenes after the P-wave at the beginning of the tachycardia and, at the same time, stimulates the ventricles without delay like an artificial pre-excitation. The re-entry tachycardia is interrupted by concealed backwards conduction into the two atrioventricular pathways of the circus (65).

h) Programmed rate-related stimulation. The principle of precisely timed premature stimulation can be realized by programmed rate-related interval stimulation (orthorhythmic pacing) (66, 67). The delivery of an electric impulse is determined by the preceding interval of atrial or ventricular depolarization. Therefore this pacing mode is automatically rate-dependent (see Figure 9). Rate-related pacing is characterized by programmable demand pacing with escape intervals related to the length of the preceding cardiac cycle. Whereas conventional demand pacemakers operate at a fixed escape interval, the so-called orthorhythmic system possesses a variable hysterisis: the pacemaker takes into consideration the exact time of the extrasystole and produces a response delay which automatically varies as a function of the premature beat interval. The variable response delay (stimulation interval) may be identical to the premature beat interval. The ratio of these two intervals can, however, be modified. The

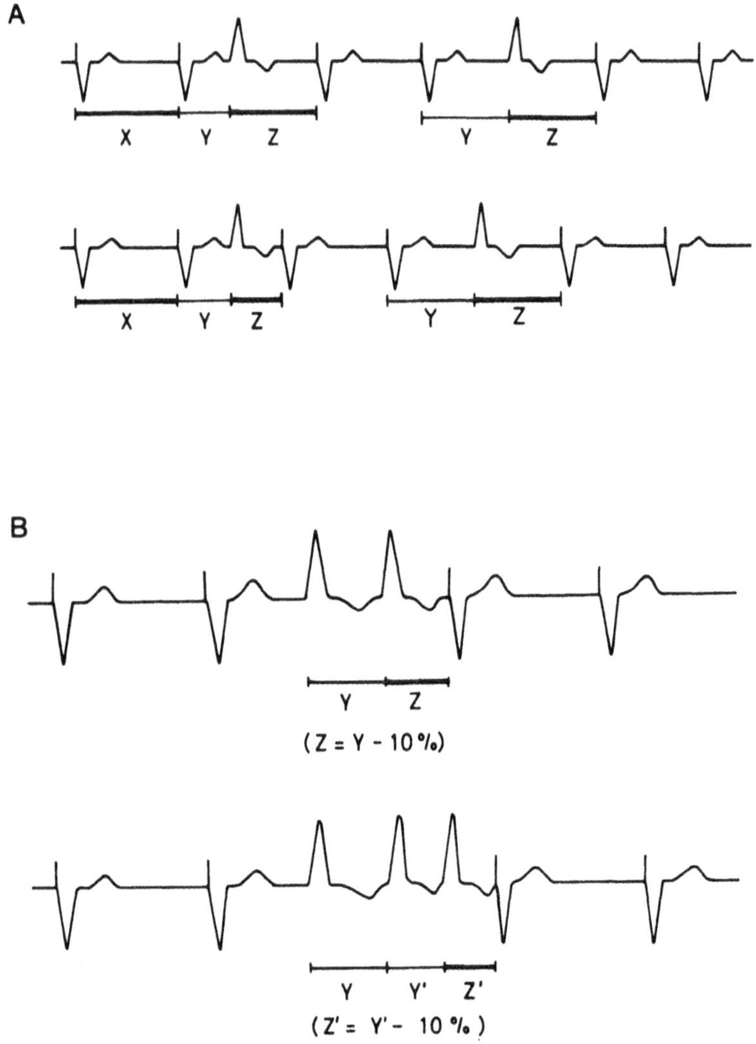

Figure 9. Operation mode of conventional demand pacing and programmed rate-related pacing following premature beat. X=basic cycle, Y=pre-extrasystolic interval, Z=post-extrasystolic interval. A: *Upper trace*: following extrasystroles with varying prematurity demand pacemakers will keep the same fixed delay (Z) before delivering the next impulse; *Lower trace:* applying rate-related stimulation, the moment of delivery of the impulse following the extrasystole can be modified as a function of Y: $Z = (f)\ Y$. B: rate-related pacing at repetitive extrasystoles. *Upper trace:* in two consecutively-occurring extrasystoles the stimulation interval Z is determined by the time Y between these two extrasystoles. In this case Z is 10 percent shorter than Y. The electrically-induced premature beat anticipates a possibly emerging third extrasystole. *Lower trace*: if consecutive extrasystoles occur with increasing prematurity rate-related pacing automatically processes the shorter interval (Y') between the last two extrasystoles.

orthorhythmic system consists of an external pacemaker which is connected to temporary endocardial electrodes. Temporary epicardial electrodes after open-heart surgery may also be used. The power source consists of two 9-volt alkaline batteries. Orthorhythmic pacing can be applied to the atrium or to the ventricle. It can be performed with single or repeated stimulations delivered according to an adjustable program which takes into account the spontaneous or stimulated heart rate. This kind of stimulation – controlled by sensing of the local intracardiac potentials either in the atrium or in the ventricle – provides the possibility of consecutive stimulation such as paired, tripled, or quadrupled impulses in very rapid coupled salvos. This on-demand stimulation coupled to the preceding cardiac depolarizations can be applied in bradycardias as well as in various types of tachycardia (68, 69).

When applied in drug-resistant spontaneously occurring bursts of ventricular extrasystoles or recurrent tachycardias in 56 patients programmed rate-related stimulation either by single or multiple impulses was effective in interrupting the tachycardia in 54 percent of cases (Table 4). In most cases the ventricular tachyarrhythmias were terminated after several attempts with rate-related stimulation using different rate-dependent stimulation intervals.

One of the side effects of injecting radiocontrast material into the coronary system as well as into the ventricle is the occurrence of ectopic beats, and sometimes ventricular flutter or even ventricular fibrillation – either by mechanical irritation of the ventricular wall or as a consequence of sinus slowing (70).

Table 4. Success of rate-related stimulation in ventricular tachycardias

	%	No. of patients
Spontaneous	54	56
During cardiac catheterization	21	20

In order to control ventricular tachycardia rate-related stimulation was therefore applied in patients with tachy-arrhythmias occurring during diagnostic right and left heart catheterization and angiocardiography. The overall success of rate-related interval stimulation is shown in Table 4. The suppression of ventricular arrhythmias occurring in diagnostic heart catheterization was about half as successful (21%) as in spontaneously–arising drug-resistant tachyarrhythmias (54%). As a complication the initiation of vertricular tachycardias due to the stimulation procedure was observed in three cases. It has been shown experimentally that stretching of the Purkinje fibres leads to an increase in the rate of depolarization. Single fibres of the myocardium may gain transient pacemaker properties as well (71). These effects are completely reversible within a few seconds after such stretching. A similar mechnism can be assumed during cardiac catheterization.

In some cases of tachy-arrhythmias two or even three coupled rate-related premature stimuli have to be delivered in close succession to terminate the tachycardia, especially if the rate is high. Ventricular tachycardias which could not be terminated by one or two stimuli were occasionally suppressed by sequential RR-related multiple stimulation.

Rate-related stimulation may not only be useful in ventricular tachycardias but also in supraventricular arrhythmias. Atrial flutter was converted via atrial fibrillation into sinus rhythm by interval-related multiple stimulation produced by an atrial electrode catheter. Junctional tachycardias can sometimes be suppressed by ventricular stimulation due to retrograde penetration of the ventricular impulse and interruption of the re-entry circuit.

Programmed rate-related stimulation was also applied in ventricular extrasystoles or recurrent tachycardias in 74 patients suffering from chronic coronary heart disease. Rate-related stimulation was effective in 40 patients by terminating the tachycardia. In four patients the tachycardia occurred within 24 hours after admission to the coronary care unit for acute myocardial infarction. In three of them the tachycardia could not be teminated by programmed stimulation – Table 5 (72).

Table 5. Efficiency of rate-related stimulation in ventricular tachyarrhythmias.

Condition	Total no. of patients	Termination achieved
Chronic coronary heart disease	74	40
Acute myocardial infarction	4	1

The rate-related stimulation technique was effective only in one case which was impressive from the clinical point of view: a 66-year-old patient with acute myocardial infarction developed a mural aneurysm, drug-resistant congestive heart failure and ventricular tachycardia (Figure 10). Programmed stimulation was effective in repeatedly terminating ventricular tachycardias as well as ventricular extrasystoles. In this case the pacing catheter was left in place for permanent use while an aneurysmectomy was performed.

While programmed rate-related stimulation is effective in dysrhythmias due to chronic coronary heart disease, this mode of pacing usually fails in ventricular tachy-arrhythmias following acute myocardial infarction. This finding suggests that the mechanism of ventricular tachycardias during acute myocardial infarction differs from the chronic recurrent type of tachycardia.

In conclusion, at the present time different modes of cardiac pacing techniques are in use in order to suppress supraventricular, junctional, and ventricular

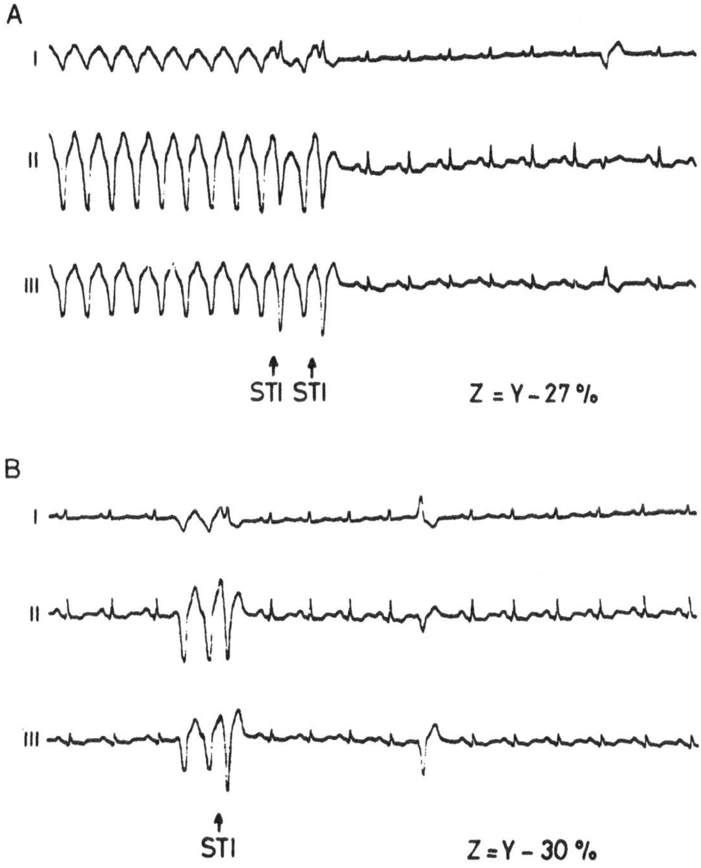

Figure 10. Suppression of ventricular dysrhythmias by programmed stimulation. A: ventricular tachycardia is terminated by the second electrical intervention according to the program $Z = Y - 27\%$. B: two ventricular premature beats which may indicate the beginning of a ventricular tachycardia. One properly-timed impulse elicited by the program $Z = Y - 30\%$ immediately terminates the arising tachycardia (73).

tachycardias. These are: rapid atrial stimulation; overdrive pacing; coupled stimulation; patient-initiated atrial pacing; precisely-timed single or multiple premature stimulation, and programmed rate-related stimulation. The termination of ectopic tachycardias by premature stimulation is easily understood if a re-entry mechanism is held responsible. The theory postulates that the premature electrical impulse creates refractoriness in a part of the re-entry pathway so that the next circulating impulse dies out in the refractory area. Thus, the tachycardia is terminated. The perpetuation of the tachycardia demands a refractory period shorter than the time needed for conduction of the activation wave around a loop; and the re-entrant tachycardia is terminated if the refractory period exceeds the conduction time around the pathologic pathway. Necessary conditions for a re-entrant tachycardia are unidirectional block in one or more regions of the heart; slow passage of the impulse along an alternative pathway; delayed excitation of the tissue distal to the blocked site; and re-excitation of the tissue proximal to the site of block. However, a distinct differentiation between focal automaticity and re-entry tachycardia has not yet become possible by clinical means.

REFERENCES

1. Mines GR: On circulating excitations in heart muscles and their possible relation to tachycardia and fibrillation. *Trans Roy Soc Can* 3 (4. 8): 43, 1914.
2. Aronson RS, Cranefield PF: The effect of resting potential on the electrical activity of canine cardiac Purkinje fibers exposed to Na-free solution or to ouabain. *Pflügers Arch* 347: 101, 1974.
3. Dominguez G, Fozzard HA: Influence of extracellular K^+- concentration on cable properties and excitability of sheep cardiaç Purkinje fibers. *Circ Res* 26: 565, 1970.
4. Weidmann S: Effects of calcium ions and local anesthetics on electrical properties of Purkinje fibres. *J Physiol* 129: 568, 1955.
5. Hoffman BF, Suckling EE: Effect of several cations on transmembrane potentials of cardiac muscle. *Am J Physiol* 186: 317, 1956.
6. Wit AL, Cranefield PF: Triggered activity in cardiac muscle fibres of the simian mitral valve. *Circ Res* 38: 85, 1976.
7. Cranefield PF, Aronson RS: Initiation of sustained rhythmic activity by single propagated action potentials in canine cardiac Purkinje fibres exposed to sodium-free solution of ouabain. *Circ Res* 34: 477, 1974.
8. Wellens HJJ: *Electrical stimulation of the heart in the study and treatment of tachycardias*, Leiden, Stenfert Kroese, 1971.
9. Wellens HJJ, Schuilenburg RM, Durrer D: Electrical stimulation in patients with ventricular tachycardia. *Circulation* 46: 216, 1972.
10. Lüderitz B, Steinbeck G: The pacemaker for managing tachy-arrhythmias. *Comprehensive Ther* 3: 46, 1977.
11. Naumann d'Alnoncourt C, Lüderitz B: Therapie tachykarder Rhythmusstörungen mit implantierten Schrittmachern. *Dtsch med Wschr* 1979 (in press).
12. Narula OS: Sinus node reentry: a mechnism for supraventricular tachycardia. *Circulation* 50: 1974.
13. Allessie MA, Bonke FIM: Is sustained circus movement into the sinus node possible? In: *The sinus node: structure function and clinical relevance*, Bonke FIM (ed), The Hague, Martinus Nijhoff, 1978.
14. Han J, Malozzi AM, Moe GK: Sino-atrial reciprocation in the isolated rabbit heart. *Circ Res* 22: 355, 1968.
15. Lewis T, Feil HS, Stroud WD: Observations upon flutter and fibrillation: nature of auricular flutter. *Heart* 7: 191, 1920.
16. Allessie MA, Bonke FIM, Schopman FJG: Circus movement in rabit atrial muscle as a mechanism of tachycardia. *Circ Res* 33; 54, 1973.
17. Allessie MA, Bonke FIM, Schopman FJG: Circus movement in rabbit atrial muscle as a mechnism of tachycardia III: 'the leading circle' concept: a new model of circus movement in cardiac tissue without the involvement of an anatomical obstacle. *Circ Res* 41: 9, 1977.
18. Moe GK, Preston JB, Burlinton H: Physiologic evidence for a dual AV transmission system. *Circ Res* 4: 357, 1956.
19. Mendez C, Mueller WJ, Meredith J, Moe GK: Interaction of transmembrane potentials in canine Purkinje fibers and of Purkinje-fiber muscle junctions. *Circ Res* 24: 361, 1969.

20. Sasyniuk BI, Mendez C: A mechanism for re-entry in canine ventricular tissue. *Circ Res* 28: 3, 1971.
21. Cranefield PF, Klein HO, Hoffman BF: Conduction of the cardiac impulse I: delay, block, and one-way block in depressed Purkinje fibers. *Circ Res* 28: 199, 1971.
22. Wit AL, Cranefield PF, Hoffman BF: Slow conduction and re-entry in the ventricular conduction system II: single and sustained circus movement in networks of canine and bovine Purkinje fibers. *Circ Res* 30: 11, 1972.
23. Narula OS, Samet P, Javier RP: Significance of the sinus node recovery time. *Circulation* 45: 140, 1972.
24. Mandel WJ, Hayakwa H, Allen HN, Danzig R, Kermaier AI: Assessment of sinus node function in patients with the sick sinus syndrome. *Circulation* 46: 76, 1972.
25. Strauss HC, Saroff AL, Bigger JT, Giardina EGV: Premature atrial stimulation as a key to the understanding of sinoatrial conduction in man. *Circulation* 47: 88, 1973.
26. Steinbeck G, Lüderitz B: Comparative study of sinoatrial conduction time and sinus node recovery time. *Br Heart J* 37: 956, 1975.
27. Miller HC, Strauss HC: Measurement of sinoatrial conduction time by premature atrial stimulation in the rabbit. *Circ Res* 35: 935, 1974.
28. Seipel L, Breihardt G, Both A, Loogen F: Diagnostische Probleme beim Sinusknoten-Syndrom *Z Kardiol* 64: 1, 1975.
29. Steinbeck G, Lüderitz B: Sinus node recovery time and sinoatrial conduction time. In: *Cardiac pacing: diagnostic and therapeutic tools.* Lüderitz B (ed), Berlin, Springer, 1976.
30. Lüderitz B, Steinbeck G, Naumann d'Alnoncourt C, Rosenberger W: Relevance of diagnostic atrial stimulation for pacemaker treatment in sinoatrial disease. In: *The sinus node; structure, function and clinical relevance.* Bonke FIM (ed), The Hague, Martinus Nijhoff, 1978.
31. Scherlag BJ, Samet P, Helfant H: His-bundle electrogram. Circulation 46: 601, 1972.
32. Steinbeck G, Lüderitz B: Sinoatrial pacemaker shift following atrial stimulation in man. *Circulation* 56 (3): 402, 1977.
33. Breithardt G, Seipel L, Loogen F: Sinus node recovery time and calculated sinoatrial conduction time in normal subjects and patients with sinus node dysfunction. *Circulation* 56: 43, 1977.
34. Delius W, Wirtzfeld A: The significance of the sinus node recovery time in the sick sinus syndrome. In: *Cardiac pacing: diagnostic and therapeutic tools.* Lüderitz B (ed), Berlin, Springer, 1976.
35. Kulbertus HE, de Leval-Rutten F, Mary L, Casters P: Sinus node recovery time in the elderly. *Br Heart J* 37: 420, 1975.
36. Mandel WJ, Hayakawa H, Danzig R, Marcus HS: Evaluation of sinoatrial node function in man by overdrive suppression. *Circulation* 44: 59, 1971.
37. Rostock KJ, van Knorre GH: Zur Analyse der nomotopen Reizbildung des menschlichen Herzens. *Dtsch Gesundh Wes* 31: 304, 1976.
38. Steinbeck G, Lüderitz B: Sinuatriale Funktionsstörungen. In: *Elektrische Stimulation des Herzens,* Lüderitz B (ed), Berlin, Springer 1979.
39. Crook B, Kitson D, McComish M, Jewitt D: Indirect measurement of sinoatrial conduction time in patients with sinoatrial disease and in controls *Br Heart J* 39: 771, 1977.
40. Dhingra RC, Wyndham C, Amat-y-Leon F, Denes P, Wu D, Rosen KM: Sinus nodal responses to atrial extrastimuli in patients without apparent sinus node disease. *Am J Cardiol* 36: 445, 1975.
41. Masini G, Dianda R, Graziina A: Analysis of sinoatrial conduction in man using premature atrial stimulation. *Cardiovasc Res* 9: 498, 1975.
42. Strauss HC, Bigger JT, Saroff AL, Giardina FGV: Electrophysiologic evaluation of sinus node function in patients with sinus node dysfunction. *Circulation* 53: 763, 1976.
43. Sano T, Yamagishi S: Spread of excitation from the sinus node. *Circ Res* 16: 423, 1965.
44. Giraud G, Puech P, Latour H, Hertault I: Variations de potentiel liées à l'activité du système auriculoventriculaire chez l'homme (enregistrement électrocardiographique endocavitaire). *Arch Mal Coeur* 53: 757, 1960.
45. Neuss H, Schaumann H-J, Stegaru B: Drug effects on AV-conduction. In: *Cardiac pacing: diagnostic and therapeutic tools,* Lüderitz B (ed), Berlin, Springer, 1976.
46. Narula OS: Evaluation of the conduction system of the heart by His-bundle recordings. In: *To pace or not to pace,* Thalen HJTh, Harthorne JW (ed), The Hague, Martinus Nijhoff, 1978.

47. Seipel L: Atrioventrikuläre und intraventrikuläre Leitungsstörungen. In: *Elektrische Stimulation des Herzens*, Lüderitz B (ed), Berlin, Springer, 1979.
48. Funke H: Die optimierte sequentielle Stimulation von Vorhof und Kammer: ein neuartiges Therapiekonzept zur Behandlung bradykarder Dysrhythmien. *Herz/Kreisl* 10: 479, 1978.
49. Naumann d'Alnoncourt C, Lüderitz B: Grundlagen der Elektrostimulation. In: *Elektrische Stimulation des Herzens*, Lüderitz B (ed), Berlin, Springer, 1979.
50. Lüderitz B (ed): *Elektrische Stimulation des Herzens*, Berlin, Springer, 1979.
51. Lown B, Amarasingham R, Neumann J: New method for terminating cardiac arrhythmias: use of synchronized capacitor discharge. *J Am Med Ass* 182: 548, 1962.
52 Lown B, Perlroth MG, Kaidberg S, Abe T, Harken DE: 'Cardioversion' of atrial fibrillation: a report of the treatment of 65 episodes in 50 patients. *New Engl J Med* 269: 325, 1963.
53. Antoni H: Physiologische Grundlagen der Elektrostimulation und der Elektrokonversion des Herzens. *Intensivmedizin* 9: 166, 1972.
54. Barold SS, Linhart JW: Recent advances in the treatment of ectopic tachycardias by electrical pacing. *Am J Cardiol* 25: 698 1970.
55. Cranefield PF, Aronson RS: Initiation of sustained rhythmic activity by single propagated action potentials in canine cardiac Purkinje fibres exposed to sodium-free solution or ouabain *Circ Res* 34: 477, 1974.
56. Massumi RA, Kistin AD, Tawakkol AA: Termination of reciprocating tachycardia by atrial stimulation. *Circulation* 36: 637, 1967.
57. Barold, SS: Therapeutic use of cardiac pacing in tachyarrhythmias. In: *His bundle electrocardiography and clinical electrophysiology*, Narula OS (ed), Philadelphia, Davis, 1975, p 407.
58. Kahn AR, Citron P: Patient initiated rapid atrial pacing to manage supraventricular tachycardia. In: *Cardiac pacing: diagnostic and therapeutic tools*, Lüderitz B (ed), Berlin, Springer, 1976.
59. Montoyo JV, Angel J, Valle V, Gausi C: Cardioversion of tachycardias by transesophageal atrial pacing. *Am J Cardiol* 32: 85, 1973.
60. Furman S, Fisher J, Mehra R: Ectopic ventricular tachycardia treated with bursts of ventricular pacing at 300 per minute. In: *Cardiac pacing*, Watanebe Y (ed), Amsterdam, Excerpta Medica, 1977.
61. Sowton E, Leatham A, Carson P: The suppression of arrhythmia by artificial pacing. *Lancet* 1098 (2), 1964.
62. Ryan GF, Easley RM, Zaroff LI, Goldstein S: Paradoxical use of a demand pacemaker in the treatment of supraventricular tachycardia due to the Wolff-Parkison-White syndrome: observation of termination of reciprocal rhythm. *Circulation* 38: 1037, 1968.
63. Krikler DM, Curry P, Buffet J: Dual-demand pacing for reciprocating atrioventricular tachycardia. *Br Med J* 1: 1114, 1976.
64. Spurrell RAJ: Future aspects of cardiac pacing. In: *Cardiac pacing: diagnostic and therapeutic tools*, Lüderitz B (ed), Berlin, Springer, 1976.
65. Coumel P: Management of paroxysmal tachycardia. In: *Symposium on cardiac arrhythmias*. Sandoe E, Flensted-Jensen E, Olesen KH (eds), Melsingör, AB Astra, 1970, p 783.
66. Guize L, Zacouto F, Lenègre J: Un nouveau stimulateur du coeur: Le pacemaker orthorythmique. *Presse Méd* 79: 2071, 1971.
67. Zacouto F, Guize L: Fundamentals of orthorythmic pacing. In: *Cardiac pacing: diagnostic and therapeutic tools*, Lüderitz B (ed), Berlin, Springer, 1976.
68. Lüderitz B, Steinbeck G, Zacouto F: Significant reduction of recurrent tachycardias by programmed rate-related premature Stimulation. In: *Cardiac pacing*, Watanabe Y (ed), Amsterdam, Excerpta Medica, 1977.
69. Lüderitz B (ed): *Cardiac pacing: diagnostic and therapeutic tools*, Berlin, Springer, 1976.
70. Benchimol A, McNally EM: Atrial pacing during selective coronary angiography. *Br Heart J* 29: 767, 1967.
71. Kaufmann R, Theophile K: Automatiefördernde Dehnungseffekte an Purkinje-Fäden, Papillarmuskeln und Vorhoftrabekeln von Rhesus-Affen. *Pflügers Arch* 297: 174, 1967.
72. Lüderitz B: Programmed electrostimulation. In: *The first 24 hours in myocardial infarction*, Kaindl F, Pachinger O, Probst P (eds), Baden-Baden, Witzstrock, 1977.

73. Lüderitz B, Steinbeck G, Guize L, Zacouto F: Schrittmachertherapie tachykarder Rhythmusstörungen durch frequenzbezogene Intervallstimulation. *Dtsch med Wschr* 14: 730, 1975.
74. Wellens HJJ: Cardiac pacing in the study and treatment of arrhythmias, tachycardias. In: *Cardiac pacing: proceedings of the fourth international symposium*, Thalen HJTh (ed), Van Gorcum, Assen, 1973.

5. PACING MODES AND RELATED HAEMODYNAMICS

ANTHONY F. RICKARDS

A trained athlete, under conditions of maximal exercise, is able to increase his cardiac output by a factor of about 9. These changes are brought about in approximately equal measure by increasing cardiac frequency and stroke volume, and the control mechanisms which regulate the resultant changes are complex.

A patient who suffers from a disorder which requires cardiac pacing is usually unable to maintain a cardiac output appropriate to his physiological requirements, and although cardiac pacing is highly successful in providing a safety mechanism preventing symptomatic or dangerous bradycardias, only a minority of paced patients continue to have physiological and appropriate control of their cardiac output. This article reviews some of the haemodynamic consequences of heart block and disorders of physiological rate control, and describes the effects of various modes of cardiac pacing.

There are three main results of A-V dissociation with the slow idioventricular rhythm which will be considered in some detail:

Loss of physiological rate control,
Loss of synchronised atrial contraction, and
Abnormal ventricular activation.

1. LOSS OF PHYSIOLOGICAL RATE CONTROL

Figure 1 indicates the relationship between heart rate and cardiac output in a resting subject. The schematic indicates that at any given rate the end-systolic volume remains constant, and changes in stroke volume are the result of changes in end-diastolic volume. The control mechanism responsible for maintaining the constancy of end-systolic volume is that underlying the Frank-Starling law, where increasing cardiac muscle fibre stretch produces an increase in the extent of fibre shortening, resulting in the same contracted fibre length, providing the load against which the muscle is contracting remains unchanged. In the schematic shown in Figure 1, no changes in the duration of systole or the volume of venous return are implied to explain the relationship between cardiac output and

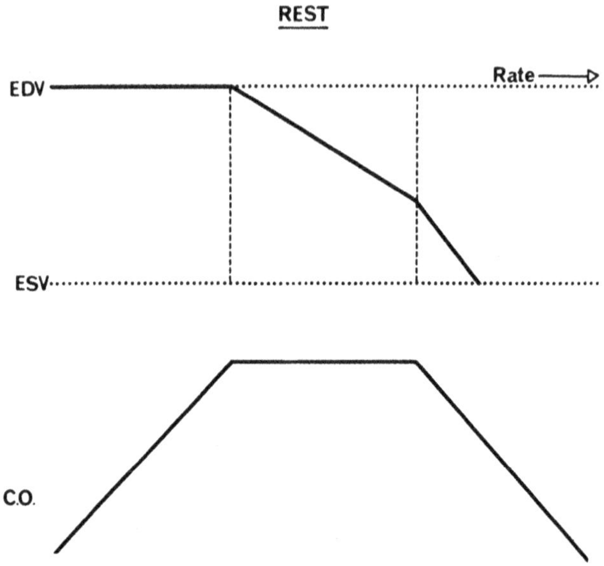

Figure 1. Indicates a theoretical relationship between end-diastolic volume, end-systolic volume and heart rate. The upper dotted line represents the maximum end-diastolic volume, the lower dotted line the minimum end-systolic volume. The change in end-diastolic volume with increasing rate is shown by the solid upper line. The lower vertical bound represents the rate at which the low end-diastolic volume can increase no further, and the upper vertical bound represents the rate beyond which diastolic filling is impeded. The lower line (CO) indicates the expected theoretical change in cardiac output with increasing rate.

rate in the resting patient.

The two vertical lines indicate the lower and upper bounds, above and below which cardiac output remains constant with increasing rates. Between these bounds an increase in rate produces a linear fall in stroke volume which results in an unchanged cardiac output. Thus as rate increases, end-diastolic volume falls progressively. The optimum cardiac output is therefore achieved over a wide range of heart rates.

Below the lower of the two bounds, end-diastolic volume can increase no further, and therefore stroke volume remains constant. Any reduction in rate will therefore produce a proportional reduction in cardiac output. The only method of adaptation possible to a chronic bradycardia is to increase the maximum possible end-diastolic volume, and therefore move the lower boundary to the left. Any increase in end-diastolic volume must be accompanied by an increase in ventricular wall thickness, if myocardial wall stress is to be kept constant during isovolumic systole, and this form of adaptation manifests as ventricular hypertrophy which is often seen in patients with a chronic bradycardia. However, the interpretation of electrocardiographic voltage changes of hypertrophy must be cautious in patients with a bradycardia, as an increase in ventricular size alone will produce a larger electrical moment of the QRS complex when viewed from surface recordings. Above the upper bound, cardiac output will fall as the rate increases, due to an increasing reduction in stroke volume. In the normal patient this fall in cardiac output is not achieved until rates of around 150 or 160 are reached, and occurs because diastolic filling time becomes too short to allow adequate ventricular filling. As will be seen later, this upper bound is moved to the right in the exercising patient, as sympathetic stimulation shortens the duration of systole allowing a longer filling time at high rates.

1.1. Effects of heart failure

Probably the best general purpose definition of heart failure is an inappropriately large end-systolic volume for any given end-diastolic volume. This allows us to construct a second schematic (Figure 2), which would indicate the effects of changes in rate on cardiac output in a subject with a small potential stroke volume. In Figure 2 the lower bound again delineates the level below which the end-diastolic volume cannot increase any further, and therefore stroke volume becomes fixed. As it is fixed at a lower level than that of a normal patient, the cardiac output itself is proportionally lower and decreases in rate produce decreases in cardiac output. In the centre section of the schematic, stroke volume as in the normal patient continues to fall with increasing rate, but as the stroke volume starts off at a lower value, then the optimum cardiac output is itself

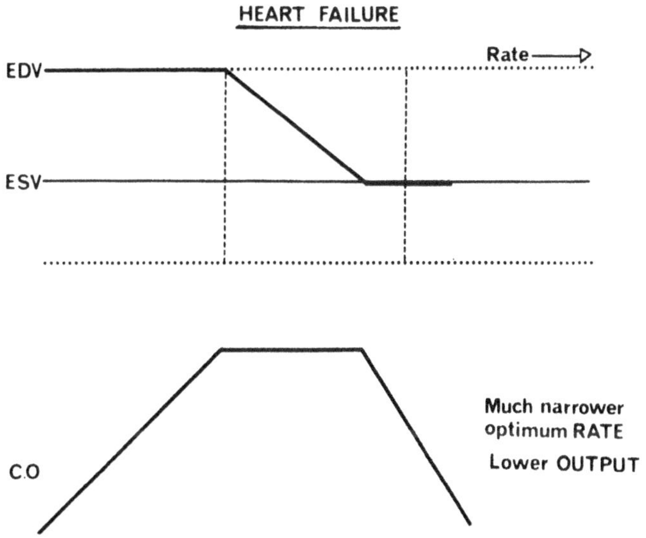

Figure 2. Indicates a similar schematic to that shown in Figure 1. Note that heart failure is here defined as a decrease in end-systolic volume relative to end-diastolic volume.

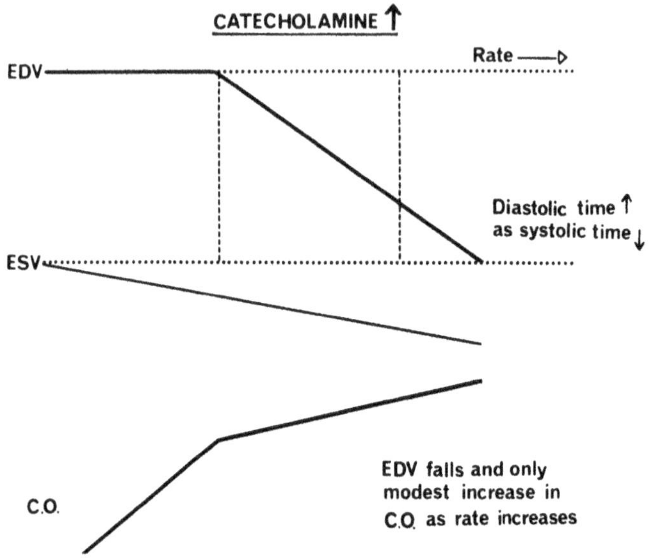

Figure 3. The effect of catecholamines on the relationship between cardiac output and rate. Legend as in Figure 1.

lower, and the point at which stroke volume can no longer be maintained, is reached at a lower rate. The effect, therefore, of heart failure is to reduce the maximum cardiac output, and to produce a narrower range over which the cardiac output is optimal.

1.2. Effect of increasing sympathetic drive

The effect of increasing sympathetic drive and circulating catecholamines is to reduce end-systolic volume (by improving myocardial contractility) and to shorten the duration of systole. Both these effects occur progressively, as the level of sympathetic stimulation increases, and the schematic shown in Figure 3 depicts effects on cardiac output in a subject in whom heart rate and sympathetic stimulation are increasing progressively. Again to the left of the lower rate bound, the end-diastolic volume is fixed as its maximum value, but as sympathetic stimulation increases towards the lower bound, end-systolic volume will fall, and therefore cardiac output will rise more steeply than in the normal subject, as stroke volume is capable of a small increase by virtue of the decrease in end-systolic volume. The same effect continues in the middle section where stroke volume is able to increase at a rate progressively greater than that seen in the resting patient, producing a larger increase in cardiac output as rate increases. The upper bound depicts the level at which diastolic filling becomes impeded in the normal patient, but as one of the prime effects of catecholamine drive is to shorten the duration of systole, this upper bound is not reached under conditions of sympathetic drive. The effects, therefore, on cardiac output of combined rate increase and sympathetic drive, are of a steep rise in cardiac output until the lower bound is reached at which end-diastolic volume starts falling, followed by a progressive rise in cardiac output until diastolic filling becomes impeded at very high rates.

1.3. Effect of increasing venous return

Physiological exercise is accompanied by improved venous return mainly due to the effects of muscular action on peripheral veins. Figure 4 depicts the schematic during which venous return is increased as heart rate is increased, but without concomitant sympathetic stimulation. The effect of this increased venous return is to maintain end-diastolic volume at its maximum levels over a much wider rate range, and this can be seen as a progressive rise in cardiac output, proportional to rate well beyond the point of the lower bound. Stroke volume will remain constant until the point at which end-diastolic volume can no longer be maintained at its maximum level, and then as end-diastolic volume falls, cardiac output will stabilise as heart rate increases.

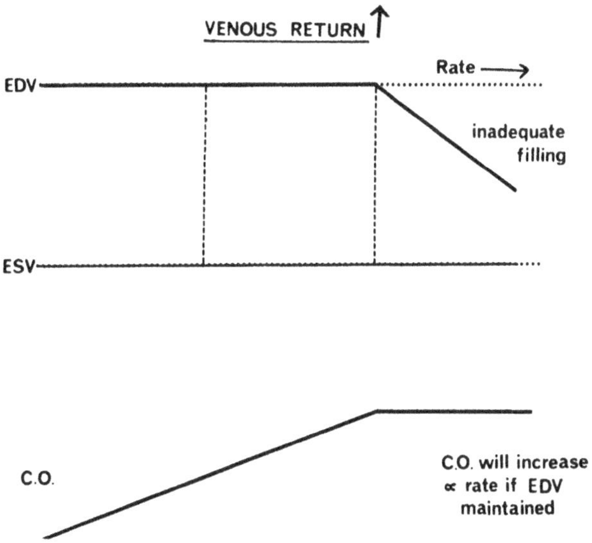

Figure 4. Effect of increasing venous return on the relationship between cardiac output and rate. Legend as in Figure 1.

1.4. Effects of exercise

The effects of physiological exercise can be depicted by combining the effects of increasing venous return with those of a sympathetic stimulation. The schematic depicting these effects is shown in Figure 5, and it will be seen firstly that end-diastolic volume remains constant over a wide rate range, and only starts to fall when the heart rate is at a high enough level to impede diastolic filling. Concomitant with the stabilisation of end-diastolic volume, end-systolic volume falls progressively due to sympathetic stimulation, and therefore over the whole rate range under conditions of physiological exercise, both stroke volume and heart rate are increasing, resulting in an additive effect, producing a steep rise in cardiac output. In the highly trained athlete the rise in venous return during exercise is responsible for a threefold increase in stroke volume, and therefore a rise in frequency of the same magnitude will produce a ninefold increase in cardiac output.

A patient who therefore has a chronic bradycardia which will not respond to the normal physiological mechanisms to increase heart rate, has two discrete and well defined disadvantages, resulting from this condition. The first is that at low heart rates cardiac output becomes critically dependant upon the rate itself as stroke volume is fixed and therefore it is easy to envisage a situation where output is insufficient for the basic physiological needs, and symptoms result. The second is that the ability to improve cardiac output by changing cardiac frequency is denied to the patient, and therefore at best the maximum improvement in cardiac output must occur as a direct result of increasing end-diastolic volume

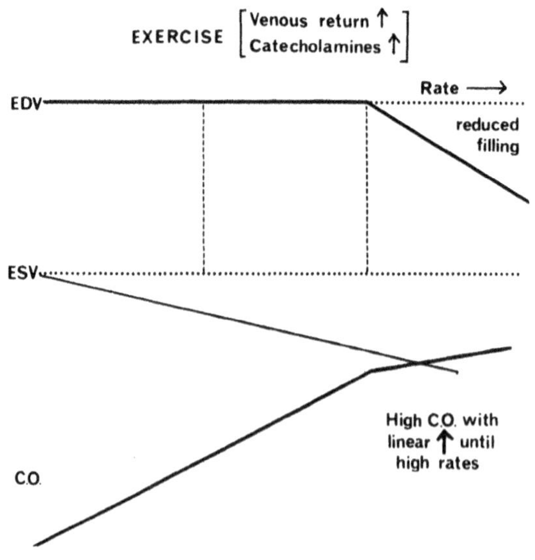

Figure 5. Effect of exercise on the relationship between cardiac output and increasing rate. Legend as in Figure 1.

by improved venous return. In a patient with a bradycardia where the end-diastolic volume is already at its maximum level, this may not be possible, and only in the patient who is operating at rest below the maximum end-diastolic volume, would an improvement in cardiac output be expected, due to increasing venous return. The patient, however, does have the ability to produce a decrease in end-systolic volume due to circulating catecholamine stimulation, and it is this effect which is largely responsible for the increases in the cardiac output seen in exercising patients with low heart rates. The exercising patient whose end-diastolic volume is not at a maximum at rest, will have a slightly greater improvement in cardiac output as venous return increases, and catecholamine stimulation occurs during exercise. Only a limited amount of adaptation is possible for the patient with a chronic bradycardia, and this occurs by increasing end-diastolic volume, but at the expense of generating ventricular hypertrophy.

2. LOSS OF SYNCHRONISED ATRIAL CONTRACTION

Although during physiological exercise the main function of the atrium is to increase ventricular rate by virtue of the sensitivity of the sinus node to physiological conditions, the atria themselves have important mechanical functions. The atria act as reservoirs within which blood is stored prior to ventricular filling, and ventricular filling is improved by the booster pump effects of synchronised atrial contraction. Finally, the effect of increasing blood velocity across the atrio-ventricular valves by atrial contraction aids the closure of the atrio-ventricular valves prior to ventricular systole, but is not essential to that function.

Figure 6 demonstrates the immediate change in aortic pressure when synchronous atrial contraction is abruptly withdrawn. Very large changes in aortic pressure have been demonstrated by experiments of this type, and occur presumably due to the reduced end diastolic volume following the abrupt withdrawal of atrial systole. However, in the normal subject where baroreceptor reflexes are intact, the systemic pressure is reset close to its original values within 20-30 seconds follwing withdrawal of synchronised atrial systole.

Figure 7 demonstrates that in subjects in whom aortic pressure is compared in the steady state period following 2 minutes of continuous ventricular or A-V sequential pacing, the changes seen in aortic pressure are only small. This demonstrates that in the subject in whom ventricular filling is unobstructed, the effect of loss of atrial systole on ventricular filling and aortic pressure, is not as great as would be imagined from looking at the effects of acute withdrawal of atrial systole. During ventricular filling, the majority of the stroke volume moves from atrium to ventricule during the rapid filling phase, both due to the active relaxation of the ventricle, and due to the pressure difference which has

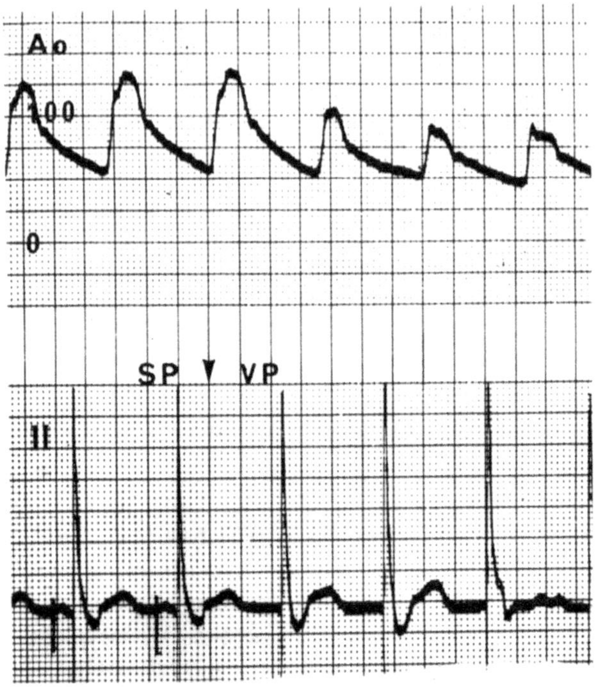

Figure 6. The effect of acute withdrawal of atrial transport. The upper tracing (AO) shows an arterial pressure tracing. The lower tracing (II) shows lead II of the electrocardiogram. The first two beats show atrioventricular synchrone, achieved by sequential pacing (SP) and the last three beats show ventricular pacing alone, with no atrial activity. Note the decrease in aortic pressure.

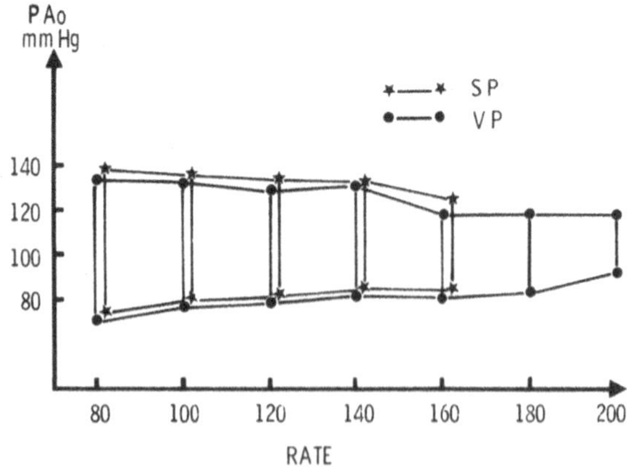

Figure 7. Relationship between increasing rate during sequential pacing (SP) and ventricular pacing (VP) on aortic pressure. Both systolic and diastolic pressures are shown.

accumulated between atrium and ventricle during systole. The loss of synchronised atrial contraction can be minimised by a rise in atrial pressure, and the consequent increase in filling, both during the early diastolic rapid filling phase, and extending ventricular filling into the period of ventricular diastasis. In a patient, however, in whom it is impossible to increase the transfer of blood from atrium to ventricle during early ventricular filling, such as mitral stenosis, the loss of synchronised atrial systole might be expected to produce a fairly dramatic reduction in aortic pressure and cardiac output, and indeed, in clinical practice, this is what is observed in such individuals. Figure 8 shows recordings of pulmonary artery pressure in the same experiments as depicted in Figure 7, where ventricular pacing was compared against A-V sequential pacing while measurements of pulmonary artery pressure were made. The rise in left sided filling pressures is shown by the higher pulmonary artery pressure present at all heart rates, and this increased left sided filling pressure is responsible for an increased

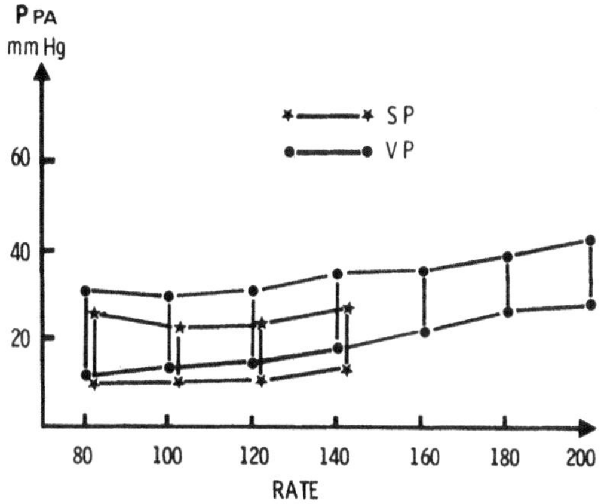

Figure 8. Relationship between increasing heart rate showing sequential pacing (SP) and ventricular pacing (VP) on pulmonary artery pressure. Both systolic and diastolic pressures are shown.

blood flow across the mitral valve during diastole, and therefore the maintenance of end diastolic volume and consequent aortic pressure. In the subject with heart failure manifesting as a high initial left atrial pressure, then the withdrawal of synchronised atrial contraction may result in a rise in atrial pressure to levels at which pulmonary oedema may occur, but in the normal subject, the rise in atrial pressure itself would not be expected to have any important consequences. It has been shown by a number of investigations that the apparent improvement in cardiac output afforded by synchronised atrial contraction is greater as heart rate increases. Figure 9 demonstrates a series of experiments where cardiac output was measured during A-V sequential

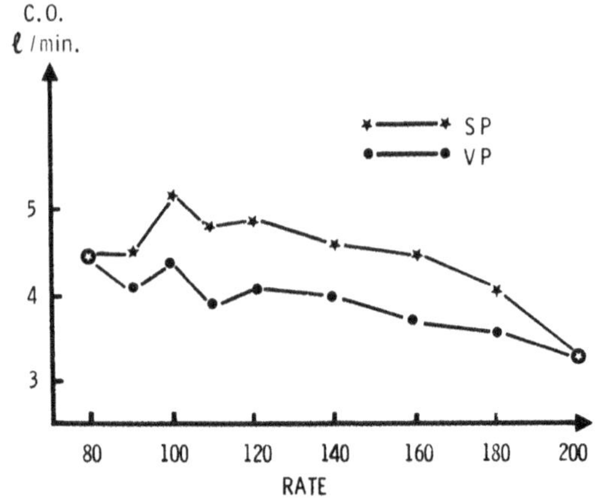

Figure 9. The change in cardiac output as measured between sequential pacing (SP) and ventricular pacing (VP) with increasing heart rate. Note that at low heart rate there is very little increasing in cardiac output afforded by synchronised atrial contraction, but beyond the heart rate of 100, a consistent 15-20% improvement is seen in cardiac output when assessed after two minutes of pacing.

and ventricular pacing, and show that at the lower rate chosen (80 b.p.m.) little difference occurred in the cardiac output. As heart rate increased, and as therefore the available diastolic filling time decreased, a small but significant improvement of around 15-20% could be consistently demonstrated between the two modes of pacing. This effect is somewhat surprising in view of the fact that at the intermediate values of these heart rates, diastolic filling time should be adequate to allow complete diastolic filling, albeit at the expense of a raised atrial pressure.

However, the effects of the loss of synchronised atrial contraction are not only those of withdrawing atrial systole just prior to ventricular systole, but also those of randomly distributing atrial systole throughout the cardiac cycle. It has been well documented that the timing of atrial systole is of critical importance to ventricular filling in the single beat situation, and that if atrial systole occurs against closed atrioventricular valves, the large rise in atrial pressure resulting from atrial contraction will impede venous return. This situation may consistently occur in patients who have intact retrograde conduction. Apart from the clinically observed discomfort of pulsation in the peripheral veins, the synchronous contraction of the atrium against the closed A-V valve will have a positive deleterious effect, which cannot be offset by the mechanism of a passive increase in the atrial volume at the onset of ventricular diastole.

The long-term effects of A-V dissociation and loss of correctly timed atrial systole are more difficult to evaluate. The patient in whom atrial systole is occurring at random throughout the cardiac cycle will experience some subjective discomfort, both because of atrial contraction against closed atrioventricular valves, resulting in high venous pressure, and also because of large and random

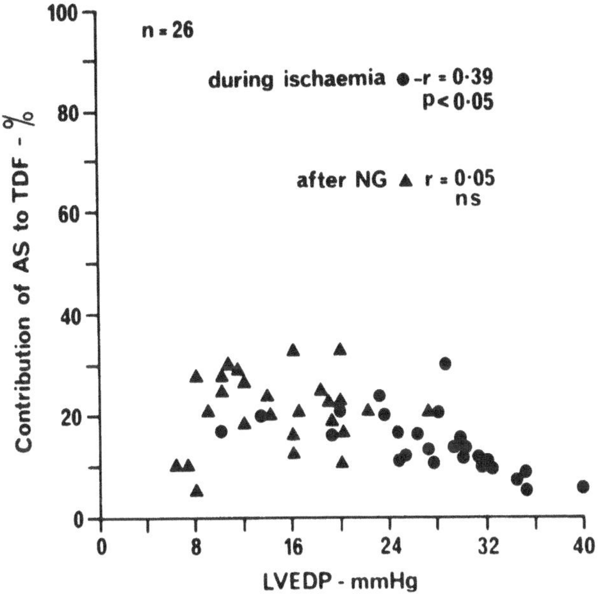

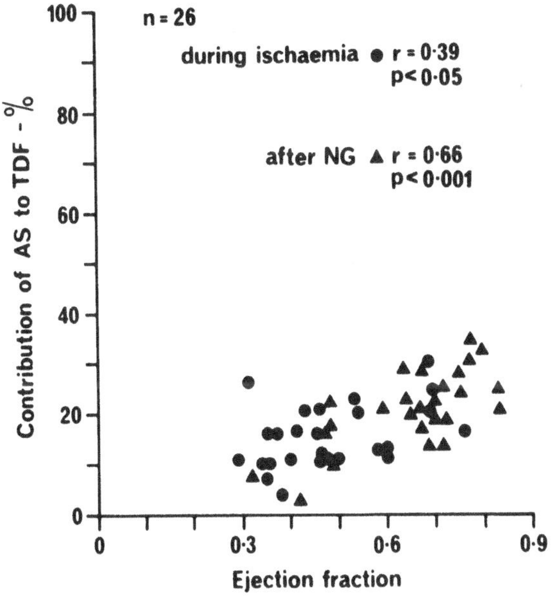

Figures 10 and 11. The relationship between the contribution of the atrial systole (AS) calculated as fraction of total diastolic filling (TDF), and the end-diastolic pressure (LVEDP) and the ejection fraction in a variety of subjects with coronary artery disease.

These figures indicate that at high levels of end-diastolic pressure the atrium is unable to deliver a large quantity of blood across the mitral valve.

fluctuations in aortic pressure. However, in the subject with normal ventricular function, and in whom there is no mechanical obstruction to diastolic filling, one would not expect a large impairment of resting cardiac output, and indeed, this has been demonstrated. Indeed, in this situation, a chronically paced patient with A-V dissociation and active atria would probably be better off from the subjective point of view by having concomitant atrial fibrillation.

In the patient with heart failure however, the situation may be different. The rise in atrial pressure which is necessary to overcome the effect of synchronised atrial contraction may produce left- and right-sided failure, as ventricular diastolic pressures are already elevated as part of the mechanism of cardiac failure. In such subjects it might be anticipated that the mechanical effects of loss of atrial systole, as distinct from the resultant rise in atrial pressure, might be more important. However, this is not the case, and as shown in Figures 10 and 11, in which the volume of blood crossing the mitral valve during atrial systole was calculated as a fraction of total diastolic filling in a variety of subjects with coronary artery disease. It appeared that in those subjects with the most important ventricular abnormality manifested by high end-diastolic pressure and low ejection fractions the contribution to end-diastolic volume produced by atrial systole was lower. This indicated that at high levels of end-diastolic pressure, which are achieved as the left ventricle fills, the atrium is unable to deliver a large quantity of blood across the mitral valve, as its ability to contract against

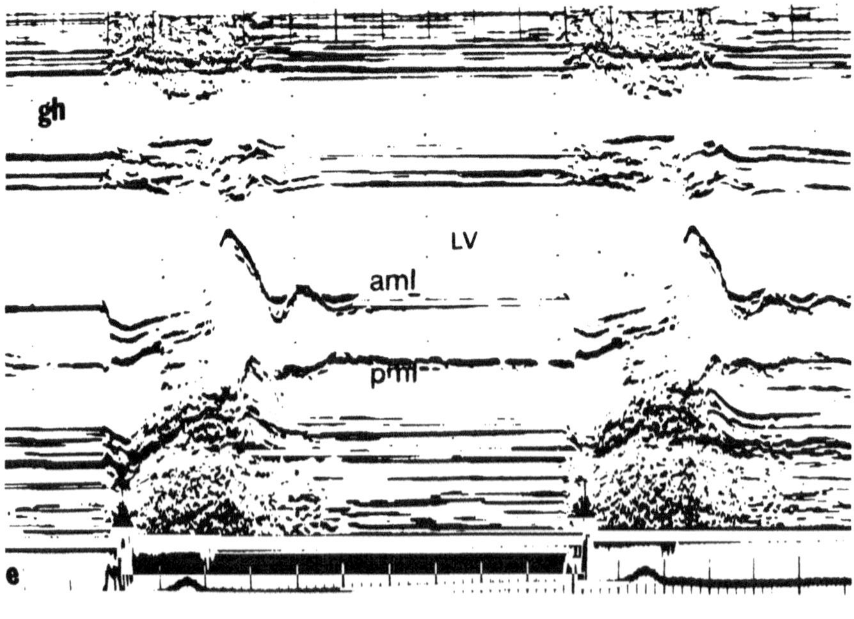

Figure 12. This echocardiogram shows that the normale features of the mitral valve echogram, including the mitral 'a' movement, occur even in the absence of atrial contraction.

such a large load is not surprisingly difficult for such a thin wall structure. This fits well with subjective observations in clinical practice, where contrastingly, patients with pure mitral stenosis, small left ventricles, and normal ventricular function appear to suffer quite markedly with the onset of atrial fibrillation, whereas individuals who have large ventricles with high pressures and low ejection fractions appear to suffer remarkably little with the onset of atrial fibrillation.

Finally, there is no doubt that theoretically at least, atrial contraction and the resultant pulsatile flow across the mitral valve in late diastole appears to create pressure differentials inside the ventricle, which aid atrioventricular valve closure. Figure 12 demonstrates an echocardiographic examination of a subject in whom the atria were electrically and mechanically silent, and shows that the normal features of the mitral echogram, including the mitral 'a' movement, occur even in the absence of atrial contraction. However, on theoretical grounds, at least, it is likely that the atrioventricular valves are not fully closed at the end of diastole when synchronisational contraction has not occurred, and that a slight degree of A-V valve regurgitation may occur. However, clinically this does not appear to be an important problem as demonstrated by the relative paucity of systolic murmurs heard in the ventricular paced patient.

MODES OF PACING

(Heart Block)

	RATE CONTROL	A-V SYNC	ABNORMAL DEPOLARISATION	ECTOPIC SENSING A	ECTOPIC SENSING V
VOO	-	-	+	-	-
VVI	-	-	+	-	+
VVT	-	-	+	-	+
VAT	+	+	+	-	-
VDTI	+	+	+	-	+
DVI	-	+	+	-	+
DDD	+	+	+	+	+

Figure 13. Advantages and disadvantages of various pacing modes in patients with AV dissociation and apparently normal atrial function.

3. ABNORMAL VENTRICULAR ACTIVATION

The final and probably least important effect of atrioventricular dissociation with an idioventricular or paced rhythm, is that the contraction sequence of left and right ventricles is abnormal. While this can be demonstrated electrocardiographically, and angiographically, it appears that in studies performed where synchronous activation versus asynchronous activation has been examined, the resultant decline in ventricular performance is only marginal. One would expect to see the greatest effects on the determinants of isovolumic systole whereas the ejection phase indices of ventricular performance, including cardiac output, are largely unchanged.

However, in certain circumstances, it does seem that the abnormal activation of the ventricle produces a disturbance in the organisation of the atrioventricular valve, and that A-V valve regurgitation may occur, solely because of abnormal ventricular activation. This effect is unusual, but may occasionally occur in clinical practice.

Asynchronous ventricular activation is followed by asynchronous relaxation and the consequent loss of the 'ventricular sucking' effect which normally aids ventricular filling by lowering cavity pressure at the onset of diastole. The paced patient would therefore be expected to have a higher ventricular pressure throughout diastole and this diastolic pressure increase does not occur with increased diastolic volume or reduced compliance. This is therefore the third discrete mechanism which raises filling pressure in the paced patient with A-V dissociation (random atrial systole, A-V valve regurgitation and asynchronous relaxation).

4. PACING MODES IN ATRIOVENTRICULAR DISSOCIATION

Figure 13 documents a table indicating the advantages and disadvantages of various pacing modes which are likely to be used in patients with atrioventricular dissociation and apparently normal atrial function.

From the physiological point of view the ideal pacemaker is obviously that which reproduces as closely as possible the normal contraction sequence of atrium and ventricle and is responsive to the changes in sinus node frequency and therefore to the physiological demands of the body. Both these requirements are met almost completely by atrial synchronous units with or without atrial and/or ventricular sensing functions. For a patient with intact sino-atrial function and A-V dissociation the atrial synchronous unit is, apart from the minor disadvantage of causing asynchronous ventricular contraction, the ideal pacemaker. However, there still remain technical problems in establishing reliable long-term atrial sensing and atrial synchronous units still offer significant shorter life expectancy than ventricular units. In practical terms the majority of patients who would benefit from an atrial synchronous unit are paced by ventricular pacemakers because of the practical difficulties. The loss to the patient who receives a ventricular unit is not so much the absence of synchronised atrial contraction, but as can be seen from the earlier remarks on the haemodynamics of heart block, mainly the loss of physiological control of heart rate. Some of these disadvantages may be partially overcome by rate programmable systems.

If a decision is made to employ a ventricular pacemaker there are two main considerations from the haemodynamic point of view in the selection of the pacemaker. The first is whether the escape interval of the pacemaker is the same as the pacing rate: that is whether the unit demonstrates negative hysteresis. In the patient with established complete heart block in whom there is no competitive rhythm, the use of a negative hysteresis unit is not necessary as a competitive rhythm does not occur. Indeed, such patients are probably best treated with a fixed rate unit. However, the use of a non hysteresis pacemaker in a patient whose pacing rate is set close to the rate at which a competitive rhythm would frequently occur results in 'hunting' between the pacemaker and the natural heart rate which may be uncomfortable for the patient especially in the early weeks after pacemaker implantation. In this context it appears more sensible to use a pacemaker with a wide negative hysteresis so that in the event of a natural competetive rhythm occurring the pacemaker does not take over until the natural rate drops below say 50 beats per minute. This has the advantage that normal physiological contraction will occur until the sinus rate has dropped below 50 beats per minute but then the pacemaker takes over at a pre-set ventricular rate (say 70 beats per minute) with consequent abolition of the 'hunting' syndrome with its haemodynamic disadvantages. The use of negative hysteresis pacemakers will however, produce an effective bradycardia in patients who develop coupled ectopic rhythms: an arrhythmia which may well be controlled by using positive hysteresis. The ideal solution would appear to be the use of units which allow independent programming of both the escape interval and pacing rate.

The second consideration is the selection of the heart rate to be employed when using a ventricular unit. As has been discussed in the previous part of this article, patients with normal ventricular function at rest have a wide band of rates over which a small change in rate makes little difference to cardiac output. The selection of an average rate of around 70 beats per minute is therefore entirely appropriate for such individuals. However, such an individual when exercising is unable to increase his ventricular rate and it has been shown that below paced rates of about 110 beats per minute the exercising patient does not approach his optimal cardiac output.

In the patient with heart failure selection of an appropriate rate may be more difficult. Many studies have been reported documenting the effects of varying rate on cardiac output in such individuals and it is common practice to perform measurements of cardiac output on the patient at various rates under resting conditions to determine which rate to choose and indeed to determine whether atrial synchronous pacing is of value. It should be pointed out that if a patient has a *normal* cardiac output under conditions of ventricular pacing when at rest and a slightly increased cardiac output during short-term atrial synchronous pacing, this does not imply a beneficial effect of atrial synchronous versus ventricular pacing, as reflex control of output and pressure will reset output to values appropriate at that moment. However, in the patient with heart failure and a low resting output, such measurements of the contribution of heart rate and atrial contraction may be of more benefit even though they are performed at rest.

A fairly simple technique in the presence of normal sino-atrial function is to assess the patient by varying the ventricular paced rate over a wide range and plotting the resultant PP interval against the ventricular rate. At the extreme ends of the rate range the PP interval will be short reflecting a high sympathetic drive to the patient because aortic pressure and cardiac output are reduced resulting in baroreceptor reflex stimulation. However the PP interval will be at its longest (that is the atrial rate at its slowest) where the cardiac output and aortic pressure are optimal and an elegant inverted bell shaped curve can be plotted by examining these relationships. Such an examination is simple to perform and requires no special apparatus other than the ability to vary the rate of the ventricular pacemaker and it is quite appropriate to perform such investigations both at rest and during exercise to determine the ventricular rate at which the atrial rate is slowest and therefore presumably the sympathetic drive induced by baroreceptor reflexes at a minimum.

5. PACING MODES IN SICK SINUS SYNDROME

Figure 14 documents details of pacemakers which may be used to pace those patients who have sino-atrial abnormalities. These patients can broadly be broken down into two groups – those with intact atrioventricular conduction and those who have abnormal atrioventricular conduction who need additional ventricular pacing.

The former group from the physiological point of view are adequately treated by an atrial pacing system which will allow normal sinus rhythm to occur but which will provide atrial pacing if the sinus rate drops below a pre-set limit. The use of a negative hysteresis function in this context is less appropriate as the oscillation between atrial sensing and atrial pacing will not cause subjective discomfort to the patient or random large changes in arterial pressure.

In those patients who have impairment of atrioventricular conduction and in whom a ventricular pacing system is necessary then the only current solution is to

MODES OF PACING

(SSS)

	RATE CONTROL	A-V SYNC	ABNORMAL DEPOLARISATION	ECTOPIC SENSING	
VOO	-	-	+	-	-
VVI	-	-	+	-	+
VVT	-	-	+	-	+
AOO	-	+	-	-	-
AAI	+	+	-	+	-
AAT	+	+	-	+	-
VAT	+	+	+	-	-
VDTI	+	+	+	-	+
DVI	-	+	+	-	+
DDD	+	+	+	+	+

Figure 14. Advantages and disadvantages of various pacing modes in patients with SSS.

use a pacemaker which is capable of providing atrial synchronous pacing when the sinus rate is above a pre-set limit and if the sinus rate falls below a pre-set limit then provides atrioventricular sequential pacing with or without a ventricular demand function. Such pacemakers are in the process of development but the haemodynamic developments offered by such a pacing system are only marginal as the patient with sick sinus syndrome is by definition denied the advantage of increased heart rate which is probably the single most important function of the atria in the physiological control of cardiac output. The potential problems produced by the universal (DDD type pacemaker) would therefore seem, in the patient with sinoatrial disease, to outweigh the haemodynamic disadvantages and in practice such patients would not be expected to suffer from the use of a conventional ventricular pacing system or an atrial synchronous system with a hysteresis function.

6. THE IDEAL PACEMAKER

The ideal pacemaker has not yet been conceived. The disadvantages exemplified in the use of a DDD system in a patient with sinoatrial and AV conduction disease exemplify that further input to the pacemaker is needed which enables the pacemaker to decide on the physiological requirements of the body independent of the sinus rate. Some remarkable achievements have been made with pH triggered pacemakers and investigations have been performed with pacemakers sensitive to changes in body temperature and respiration rate.

All of these possibilities open important new avenues for future research which should now concentrate on the creation of the intelligent pacemaker which is able to decide on appropriate atrial and ventricular rates by using more direct information concerning the physiological requirements of the body.

6. SURGICAL TECHNIQUES IN CARDIAC PACING

CLAUDE MEERE and JACQUES LESPÉRANCE

Since the first implantation of a cardiac pacemaker in 1958, the pacing systems have changed continuously. These changes have influenced the surgical techniques. With the development of the transvenous stimulating catheter, the transthoracic implantation of the electrode has decreased to under ten per cent of the overall implantations. New transvenous electrodes have changed the implantation site and in temporary pacing also the procedure.

This survey tries to outline the surgical techniques as they have been used with an emphasis on the techniques most applied today.

To this purpose this chapter is divided into techniques with temporary pacing and techniques with long-term pacing, both of them in turn are split into the transvenous and transthoracic methods of approach.

1. TEMPORARY PACING

If in the cardiac dysrhythmic patient the bradycardia or cardiac arrest cannot be controlled by pharmacological treatment (e.g. isoprenaline), or if in the tachycardias or brady-tachysyndrome pharmacological treatment is ineffective, temporary pacing is indicated.

Temporary pacing is also used in diagnostic procedures or as a preventive measure with certain (cardiac) interventions (1, 2, 3).

1.1. Facility for implantation

The implantation of a temporary pacemaker lead should be performed in a room with fluoroscopy facilities under sterile conditions. A catheterization laboratory or operating theatre with radiological facilities seems most suited. These precautions have to be taken into account, as infection and electrode displacement are the most frequently met complications of temporary pacing. The infection will complicate and most probably delay the implantation of a permanent pacing system and the electrode displacement may be dangerous for the patient. Sometimes the emergency situation may indicate implantation of the electrode at the bedside. In these cases usually the subclavian approach is chosen.

1.2. Selection of pacing system

Besides for the operating facilities, the pacing system also is very important, especially the electrode. As the application of an indifferent electrode can cause problems with an extracorporal pacemaker, in temporary pacing usually a bipolar catheter electrode is applied. Originally somewhat rigid electrodes were used, but lately the semifloating catheters are becoming more popular, especially for the subclavian approach, to be described later.

The external pacemaker is in principle identical to the implantable pacemaker, but it enables variation of parameters such as impulse frequency, impulse duration, output voltage c.q. current and sensitivity. The energy for the external pacemaker is supplied by disposable standard batteries.

External pacemakers can be fixed to the chest or the arm of the patient, preventing complete immobilization.

With postoperative stimulation in cardiac surgery, usually peroperative fixed epicardial or intramural electrodes are used, connected with an extension lead through the skin to the external pacemaker as will be explained later.

1.3. Placement of temporary electrode

1.3.1. Transvenous approach. Any vein suitable for introduction of a catheter electrode may be selected. Three main sites of introduction are the femoral vein, the brachial veins, and the subclavian vein. The jugular vein is seldom used for temporary stimulation.

The veins of the upper extremities may be entered with more ease than the femoral vein. They enable also some mobilization of the patient. The subclavian vein is used especially in emergencies and more and more has replaced the brachial approach, which has a higher incidence of dislocations.

The approach through the femoral vein is the choice in arrhythmia studies, especially for His bundle recordings. For all three approaches the patient is placed on a fluoroscopy table, the skin near the entrance route is desinfected, locally anesthetized and draped. In some cases, especially with the femoral approach, the area may have to be shaved first.

Femoral vein. Mostly the right side is chosen. This approach is transcutaneous. First the inguinal ligament and the femoral artery are located. The femoral vein is situated just medially from the femoral artery.

After local anesthetics are applied, a stab wound is made over the femoral vein, 3-4 fingers below the ligament. A needle on a saline-filled 20 ec syringe is advanced towards the vein under a 45° angle. As the dark venous blood usually does not spontaneously enter the syringe, the syringe has to be aspirated gently. When the venous blood appears and the vein is located, the syringe is disconnected and a guide wire is introduced into the vein through the needle, whereupon the latter is replaced by an introducer through which the catheter can be introduced and guided to the right ventricle. Puncture of the vein is also possible with a special teflon coated needle set, where after withdrawal of the needles, the teflon coating functions as an introducer. This system functions without a metallic guide wire.

The risks of extended tearing of the vein wall are increased by a more tangential introduction of long-bevelled needles. The tangential puncture may also enhance the risk of entering more proximally, into the iliac vein. Hemorrhage at this point of entry is less controllable and may infiltrate the retroperitoneal space and the abdominal wall. The obese patient is at greater risk in this respect; A-V fistulas, false aneurysms, transsections of the femoral profunda artery and damages to inguinal nerves are well documented complications of this approach.

The fluoroscopic guidance and positioning of the catheter in the right ventricle is easily performed since it bends naturally in the upper atrium towards the anterior leaflet of the tricuspid valve. Wedging or perforation of the right auricular appendage is avoided if resistance to progression is sensed and corrected by retraction. Risks of entering the coronary sinus are higher if the catheter is introduced via the superior vena cava.

Brachial veins. This approach, mostly from the right arm, can be performed by percutaneous puncture, that to some extent limits the choice of the electrode, but is mostly used with a veinal section. The cephalic vein located laterally should be avoided, because of the angle it makes in the deltopectoral triangle to reach the axillary vein.

Preferable are the median antecubital and the basilic vein, the same veins that are used for diagnostic right-heart catheterization.

The veins can be localized by pressing the upper arm to produce veinal congestion. After the usual preparations, a percutaneous puncture or a routine veinal section is performed, and the stimulating catheter electrode is guided towards the right ventricle.

Instability of the electrode in the right ventricle is one of the disadvantages of this site of introduction. To minimize this complication the arm should be moved around under fluoroscopic control. The electrode should allow these movements which usually result in a small curve of the lead in the right atrium to allow a certain flexibility, before the electrode is fixed in the antecubital fossa.

The atrial curve, however, entails also the risk of movement of the electrode towards the right ventricular outflow tract or pulmonary artery and myocardial perforation. Because of these complications the subclavian approach has become more popular.

Subclavian vein. The subclavian vein is situated under the clavicle as the name indicates and has to be located with the help of other anatomical landmarks. The patient is placed recumbent with his head turned away from the side to be used. After the usual preparations, a needle with syringe, as with the femoral approach, or a special needle set for the semifloating catheter is used. The needle is inserted at the junction of the middle and inner thirds of the clavicle under the clavicle and guided gently medially. The needle should be directed slightly above and behind the suprasternal notch. In some clinics the attachment of the sternocleidomastoid on the clavicle is used as reference point or the tip of the chin as the head is turned far away from the introduction side. The needle will enter the subclavian vein under the inner third of the clavicle as can be diagnosed with gentle aspiration of the syringe, whereupon the usual previously described regimen is followed and the catheter is positioned in the right ventricle under fluoroscopy (see Figure 4).

The technique is quick and the catheter tip position is usually stable. Trendelenburg's position will help to distend the subclavian vein, making the puncturing of the vein easier.

A complication with this method, unlike the other two approaches, is that sometimes the pleural cavity may be punctured and a pneumothorax may result. In these cases the femoral or brachial approach should be used or the opposite side approached.

Postimplantation protocol. Before the electrodes are fixed, the anatomical position should be checked carefully by fluoroscopy and the electrophysiological data such as stimulation threshold and R-wave signal should be determined. If inacceptable data are found, repositioning of the electrode in the right ventricle is indicated. Following the implantation the electrophysiological data should be checked at regular intervals, e.g. every 8-12 hours to diagnose early dislocations, perforations etc. Anticoagulants are not indicated by the stimulating catheter per se, nor is the catheter a contraindication for anticoagulants if this indication exists for other reasons.

Antibiotic prophylaxis may prove useful if temporary pacing is planned for more than 48 hours or if the general status of the patient is poor. Local antiseptics may prevent superficial infection at the entrance site of the catheter-electrode. Right ventricular perforation should be suspected if diaphragmatic stimulation occurs. Pulmonary embolism is probably caused more often by immobilization of the patient than by the presence of the catheter.

1.3.2. Transthoracic approach. In the early days of cardiac stimulation transthoracic puncture in the apex of the left ventricle has been applied for temporary pacing (5). Especially the subclavian puncture has replaced the complicated and rather dangerous transthoracic puncture techniques that will be mentioned here for the sake of completeness.

Two options are available: intramyocardial hooking or endocardial positioning (Figure 1).

In the first case, the electrode wire is placed in the needle prior to puncturing. One centimeter of its denuded part is bent over the proximal part of the needle's bevel. The needle is then advanced into the apex or septum. Pulsating contact without bleeding signifies adequate positioning. Withdrawal of the needle is performed gently while pushing slightly on the wire.

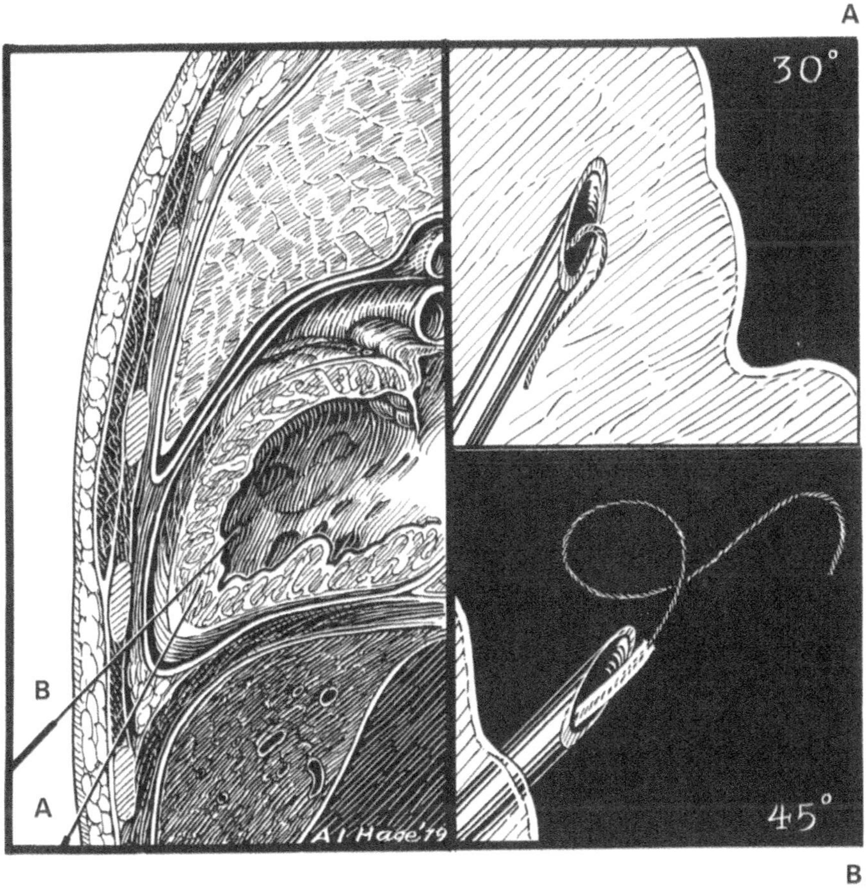

Figure 1. Transthoracic puncture for temporary pacing. Apical axial needle puncture avoids tearing of the superficially located vessels.

A – Intramyocardial hooking is technically more difficult.

B – Left ventricular endocardial pacing with an extended denudation of the temporary wire is quickly performed. Embolization of an apical thrombus is a major risk factor. (Use a 17-18 gauge needle, 12-15 cm long.)

In the second alternative, the left ventricular cavity is first punctured. After withdrawal of the mandrel, the wire is introduced in the cavity. The denuded part of the wire should be 3 to 4 cm long to ensure a constant contact with the endocardium.

In a normal chest configuration, the apex may be reached by puncturing halfway between the anterior axillary line and the mammary line in the sixth or seventh intercostal space. (Figure 2). The needle is introduced at a 45 degree angle to reach the left ventricular cavity and somewhat more tangentially for the muscular wall. The needle is directed towards the second right intercostal space.

Emphysematous thoraces, enlarged hearts may add difficulties and alter these approximate guidelines.

It is probably better to risk a puncture of the lung by a more lateral approach, than a coronary artery puncture by an anterior approach. A fibrotic apex may

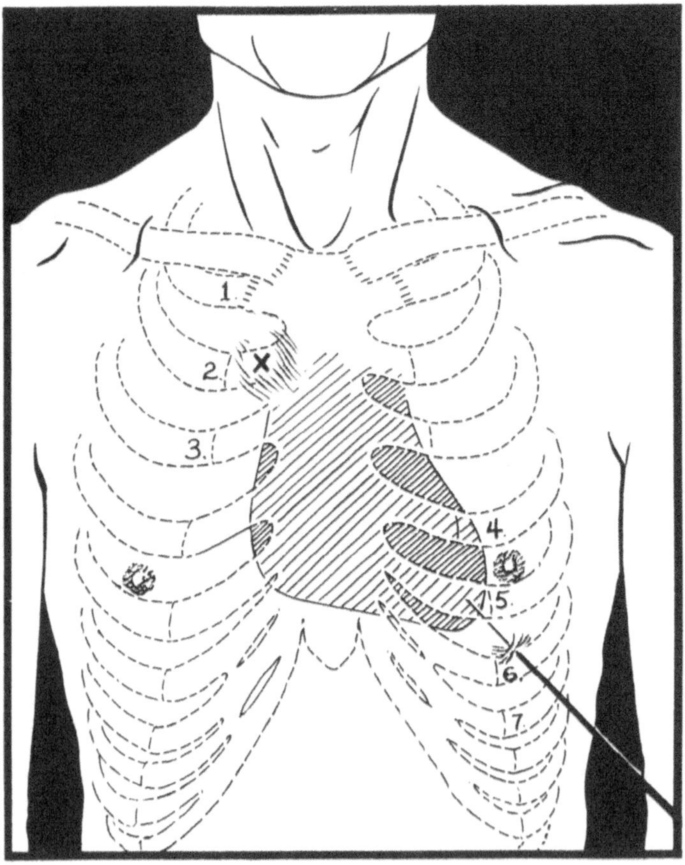

Figure 2. Landmarks for left apical puncture. The long axis of the L.V. points to the right second interspace. Apex location is best palpated but previous x-rays may give more accurate information.

be responsible for high thresholds. Aneurysmal apices should be avoided, for threshold problems, hemorrhage and left ventricular thrombus mobilization.

The postimplantation management with the transthoracic approach is the same as for the transvenous approach, but anticoagulants should be prevented because of the changes for cardiac tamponade.

In general the method can entail many complications and therefore is almost completely replaced by the transvenous approaches.

1.3.3. Temporary pacing following heart surgery. A special form of temporary pacing is cardiac stimulation following heart surgery. In many instances the cardiac surgeon feels it necessary to leave temporary epicardial electrodes after corrective heart surgery (6, 7, 8, 9).

Intramyocardial fixation is usually performed on the fat-free surface of the anterior right ventricle, if necessary, on the diaphragmatic side of the right ventricle. The electrode wire should enter the myocardium in an opposite direction to the postoperative withdrawal direction in order to avoid tearing of the epicardium.

Specific pacing modes such as sequential pacing may be useful in the postoperative period. Electrodes are therefore often secured to the right atrial wall (Figure 3) by means of mattress stitches leaving one or two electrodes embedded in atrial grooves parallel to the withdrawal direction.

Attempts to remove temporary epicardial electrodes should be abandoned if resistance is great, rather than risking acute tamponade.

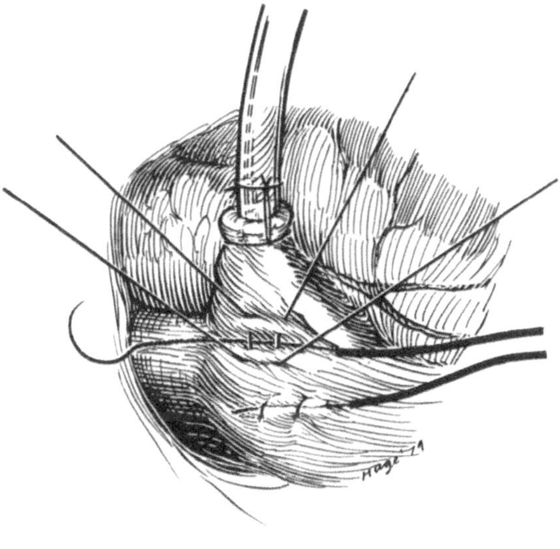

Figure 3. View of canulated right atrium. Technique for preoperative temporary atrial lead fixation allowing atraumatic closed-chest removal.

2. PERMANENT PACING

Initially permanent pacing was only used with electrodes positioned on the left ventricular myocardium by thoracotomy, later followed by the transvenous technique, whereas some centers also used the endoscopic technique for the placement of epicardial electrodes.

Of these three approaches the transvenous technique is most widely used by far for permanent cardiac pacing nowadays.

2.1. Transvenous technique

The transvenous technique was introduced in 1958, by Furman and others (12).

2.1.1. Sites of introduction. Initially the external jugular vein was used. Skin erosion over the implantation site and electrode displacements due to movements of the neck made the cephalic vein more popular. Recently the direct subclavian approach, as used for temporary pacing, has been used also for long-term pacing. With the last two sites, as a rule a single skin incision should be used for both vein dissection and pacemaker implantation (Figure 4).

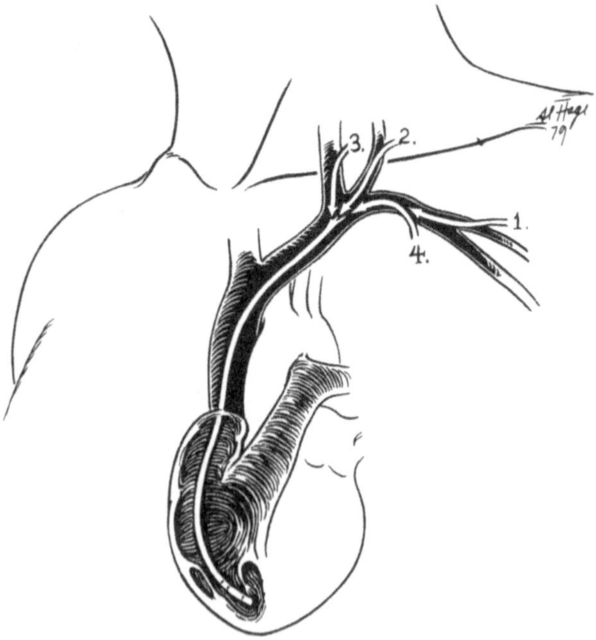

Figure 4. View of the various ways to enter the upper caval venous system including the direct puncture of the subclavian vein, the contra-lateral approach being identical.
1 – Cephalic vein; 2 – External jugular vein; 3 – Internal jugular vein; 4 – Subclavian vein.

Adequate fluoroscopic equipment in a sterile environment is needed for the three approaches that will be discussed.

Cephalic vein. The cephalic vein runs in a sulcus between the lower edge of the deltoid muscle and the most lateral fibers of the pectoralis major (Figure 5). Its size is often adequate. The skin incision is made above the projected vein's course and should not exceed the width of the powerpack to be implanted. After subcutaneous fat transsection, both muscle limits are found. The deltoid and pectoralis major are separated by a fatty sulcus which is covered by a thin fibrotic layer. The cephalic vein lays in this fatty sulcus or immediately under-

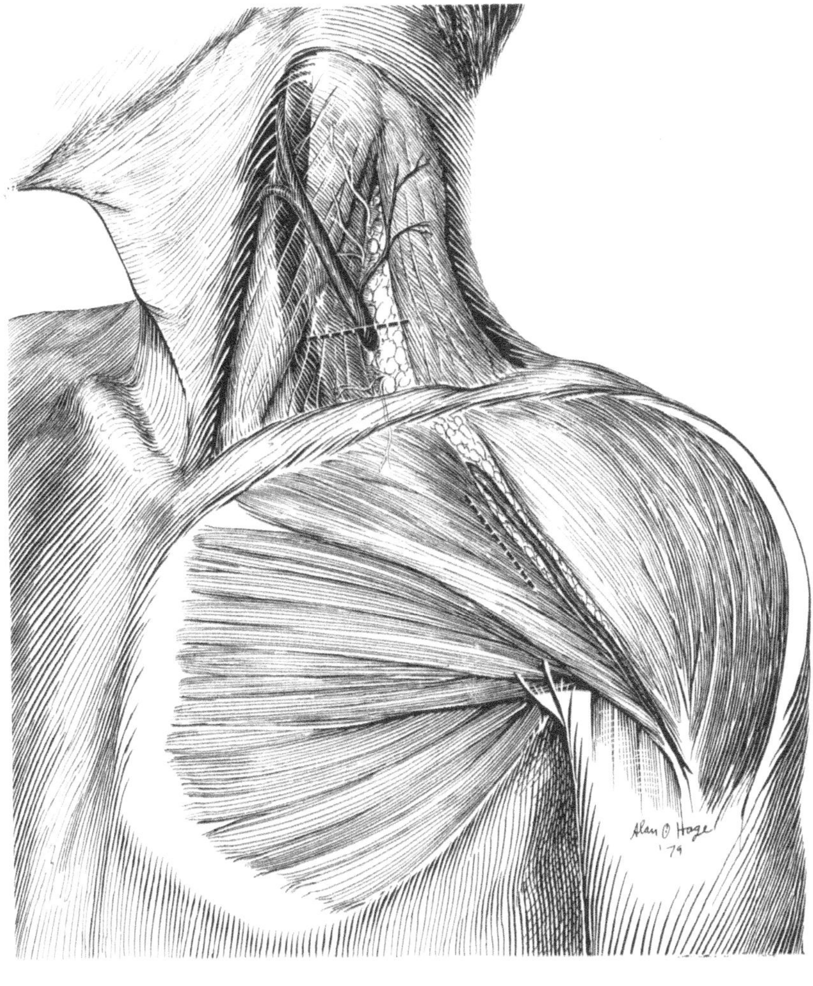

Figure 5. Antero-lateral view of external jugular and cephalic veins in relation to sterno-cleido-mastoid, pectoralis major, deltoid muscles and clavicle.

neath the edge of the pectoralis major muscle. If several smaller veins are found, occasionally with an accompanying artery, the larger cephalic vein may be absent and another approach is preferred. Otherwise, the lead is introduced into the cephalic vein about 5 cm beneath the clavicula. Vein dissection should not exceed 3 cm in length. A double-looped thread prevents proximal hemorrhage at the lead introduction, while distally, the vein is ligated and pulled outwards by the weight of a hemostat.

If the lead blocks shortly after its entrance point, further dissection is carried on along the vein. Usually, a venous Y bifurcation is found with the lead in a wedged position in a muscular branch running retrograde. (Figure 6)

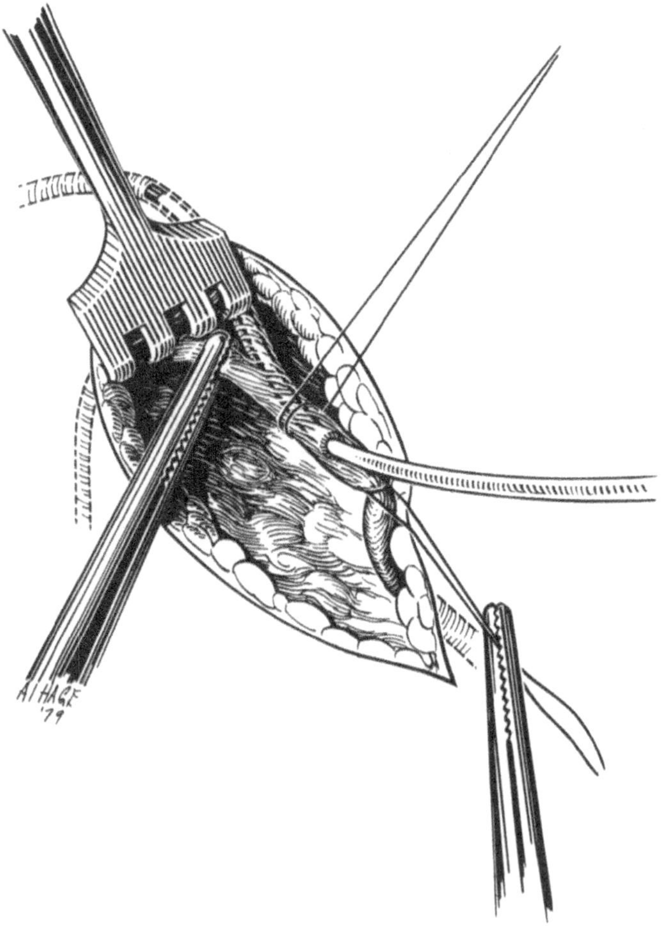

Figure 6. Cephalic vein approach. Extended subclavicular dissection towards clavicle demonstrating a temporarily clamped muscular vein, preventing the catheter-electrode from wedging in the shoulder muscles.

After slight withdrawal and temporary clamping of this upper medial vein, the lead may be guided into the upper lateral branch leading towards the subclavian vein.

Jugular veins. The patient should always be prepared and draped to allow access both to the neck and the cephalic vein. In case of unsuccessful catheterization of the cephalic vein, dissection of the ipsilateral jugular venous system can be performed (Figure 5 and Figure 7).

The external jugular is easily found behind the platysma. Its size is usually adequate but sharp angulation of its junction with the subclavian vein may sometimes direct the lead continuously upstream to the arm.

Thrombosis or hypogenesis of the external jugular vein are other reasons for extending the skin incision medially in search for the internal jugular vein (Figure 8).

The omohyoid muscle is transected, as well as its downward investing fascia and the clavicular fibers of the sternocleido mastoid muscle.

A purse-string suture can be placed in this large vein, while the patient's head is turned in the opposite direction and the remaining part of the sternocleido mastoid muscle is gently retracted. (Figure 9) The catheter is then introduced through a stab wound inside the purse-string and the latter tightened gently to control bleeding.

Subclavian vein. In case of failure to enter the cephalic vein, the surgeon may elect to dissect the subclavian vein through the same extended subclavicular incision rather than approach the jugular veins. A large muscular transection close to the clavicular insertion of the pectoralis is therefore needed.

More recently, direct subclavian puncture has been advocated (13) and may well become the method of choice after unsuccessful attempts at cephalic vein catheterization. This technique has been discussed in the subclavian vein section on temporary pacing (1.3.1.).

Inferior vena cava (Figure 10). Problems may arise if all superior veins are judged inadequate. (Previous usage, thrombosis, contiguous tissue infection, other skin conditions.)

The epicardial approach may also be contraindicated by pericardial conditions.

In such extremely rare cases a lumbotomy, as used for a right lumbar sympathectomy, will allow an adequate approach to the inferior vena cava after reclining the peritoneum anteriorly.

Entrance through a lumbar vein or through a purse-string suture in the inferior vena cava is easily performed.

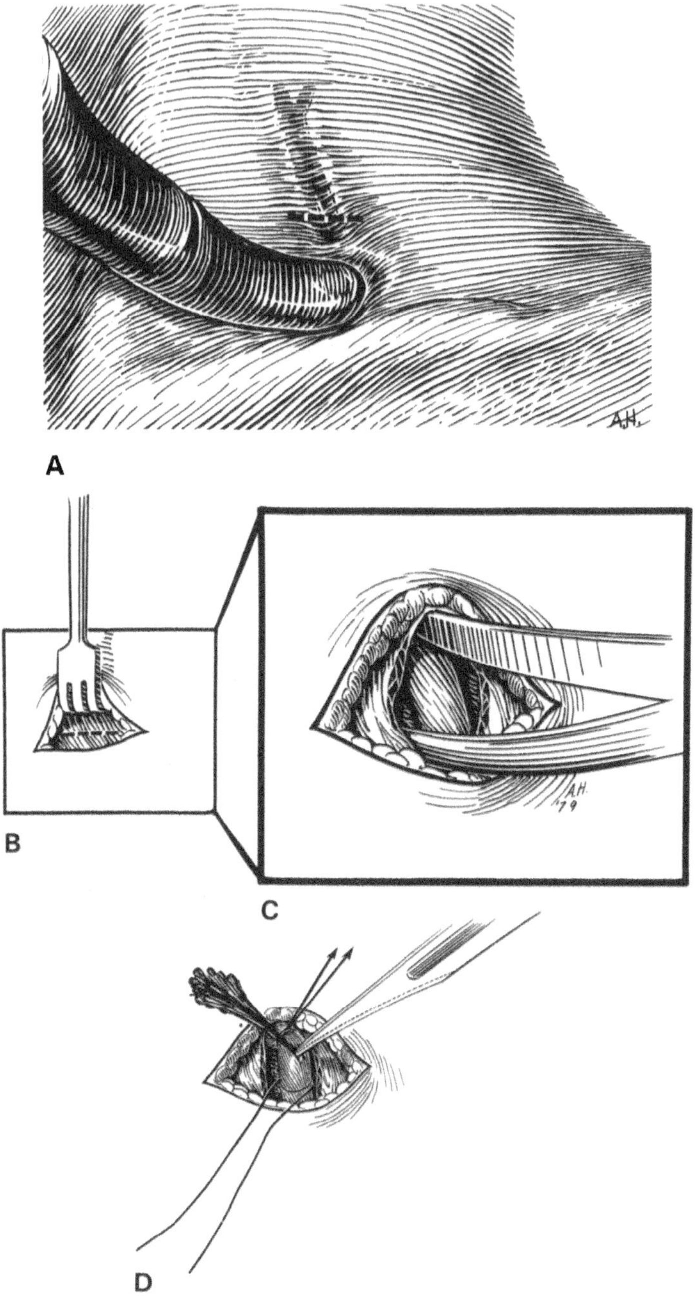

Figure 7. A – External jugular vein detection by supraclavicular finger pressure.
B – 1.5 cm horizontal skin incision and opening of platysma.
C – Axial vein dissection.
D – Caudal ligation allows some exteriorization of the vein while control of hemorrhage is performed by a proximal looping thread.

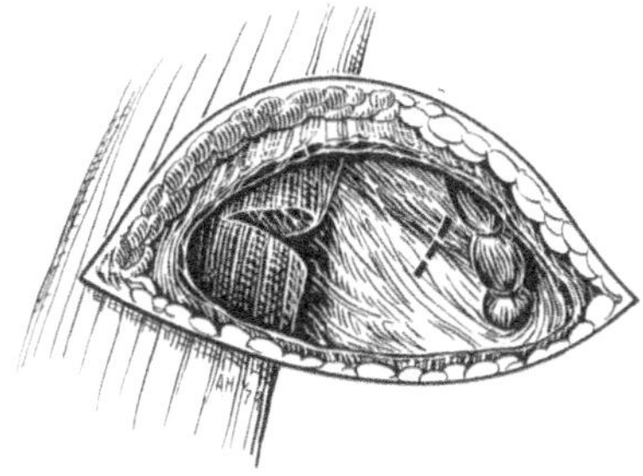

A

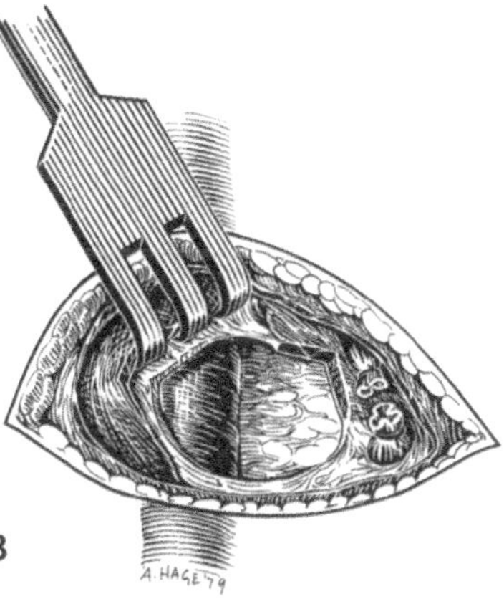

B

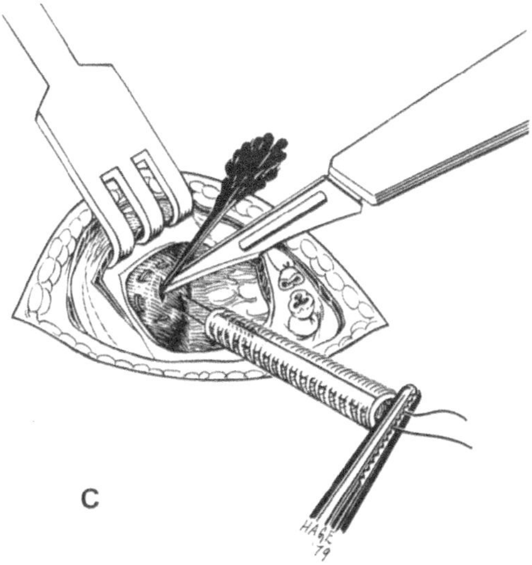

C

Figure 8. Internal jugular vein approach. Failure of external jugular catheterization and medial extension towards internal jugular vein. Opening of fascia, (A) transection of omohyoid and external incision of sterno-cleido-mastoid muscle uncovering the internal jugular vein. (B) Purse-string and tourniquet control for catheter introduction (C).

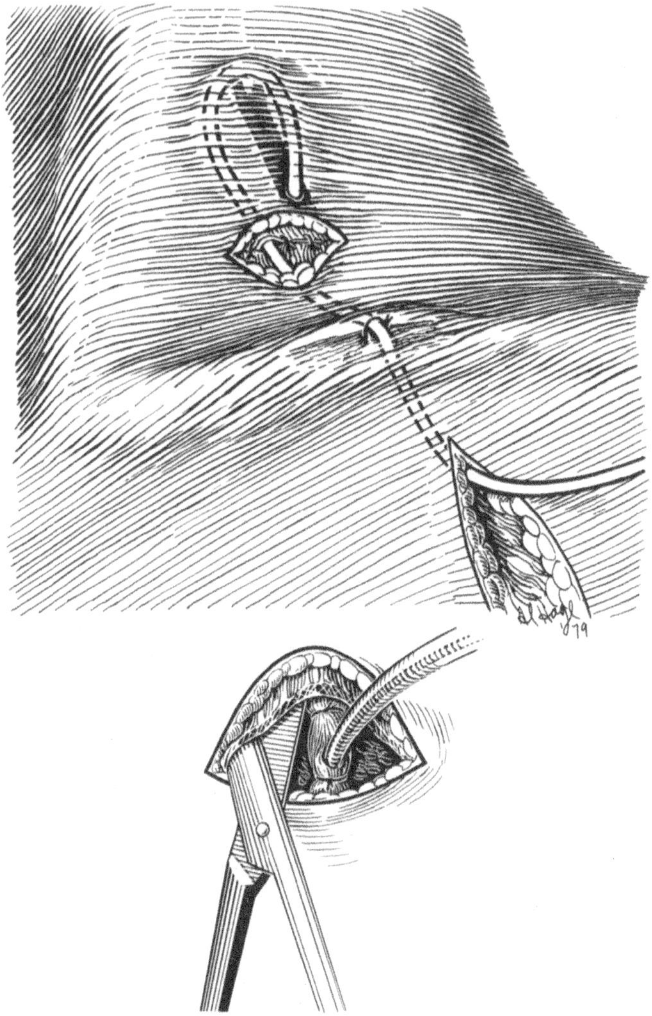

Figure 9: Transparent view of catheter-electrode in place. Retro-platysmal upwards dissection permits an upward looping of the catheter. Under local anesthesia, the catheter is then tunnelled towards the subclavicular incision. A periosteal fixation stitch installed from the upper incision on the clavicula may prevent straightening of the supraclavicular portion of the lead. It is important to close this upper incision in several layers to avoid lead infection.

2.1.2. Intracardiac lead-electrode positioning. Under fluoroscopic guidance, with the help of stylet manoeuvring or body inclination, the electrode is ultimately positioned at the selected endocardial site in the apex of the right ventricle.

Later X-ray views demonstrate intraventricular positioning when the lead extremity bends anteriorly. In a wedged cardiac vein position, the lead's extremity will bend posteriorly (14).

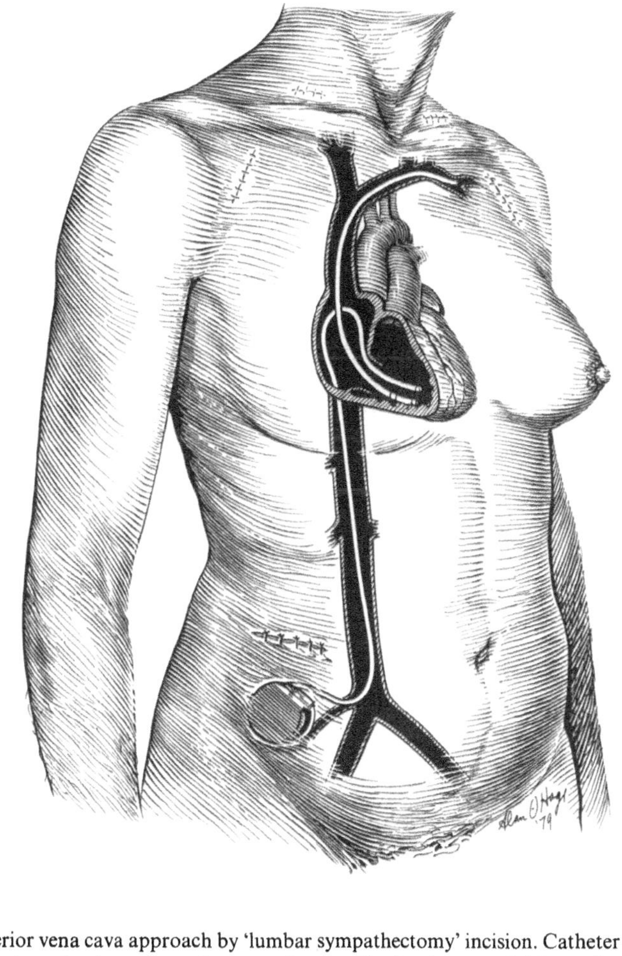

Figure 10. Inferior vena cava approach by 'lumbar sympathectomy' incision. Catheter introduction via a lumbar vein and retroperitoneal pace-maker positioning in case of failure of catheter introduction in the upper caval system.

Under antero-posterior fluoroscopy the catheter will make a small curve through the tricuspid orifice and point leftwards. With a small vertical heart with dextro-rotation the electrode tip will be located close to the configuration of the spine. With a large right ventricle of an horizontal clockwise rotated heart the electrode tip will be further away from the spine and even may reach the apex of the cardiac configuration. Generally the electrode tip will have to be located under the diaphragm configuration.

Valsalva or coughing manoeuvres may improve the stability of the electrode. Various difficulties may arise in electrode positioning as illustrated in Figures 11 to 22. Tricuspid insufficiency, pulmonary hypertension with right ventricular hypertrophy and dilatation are said to be major causes of lead dislodgement.

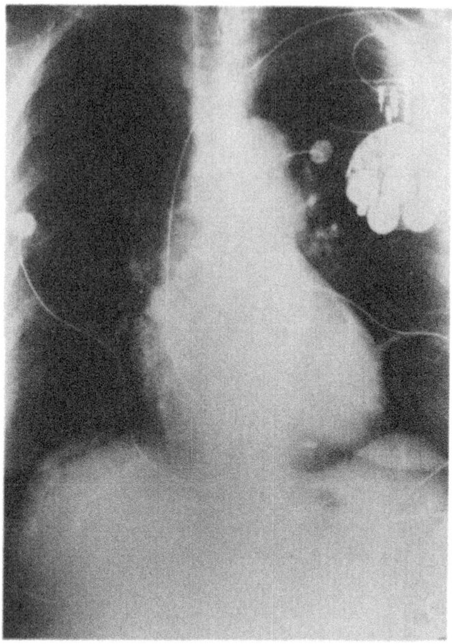

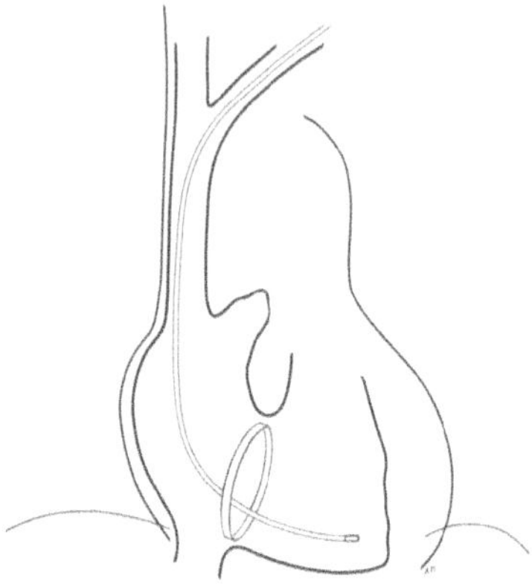

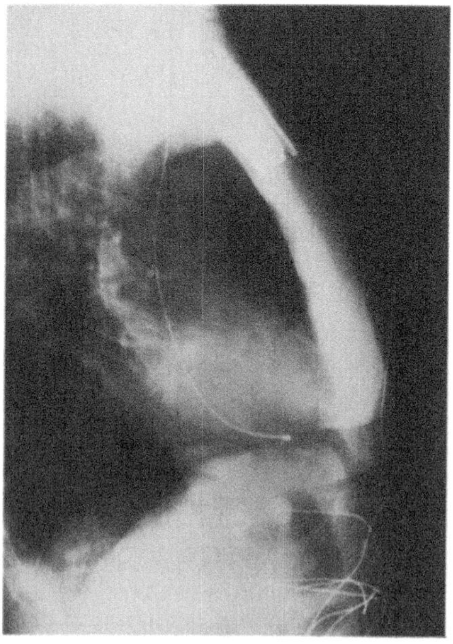

Figure 11. Normal electrode position in the right ventricular in-flow track. Note the smooth curves of the lead in the innominate vein, the superior vena cava and the right ventricle. The electrode tip is lateral to the vertebrae. Lateral incidence confirms adequate positioning.

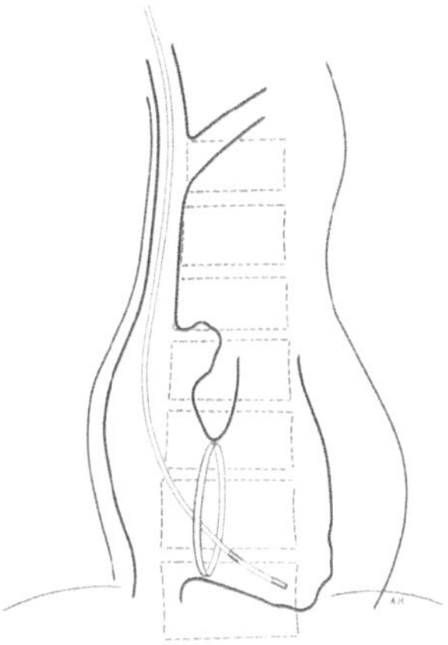

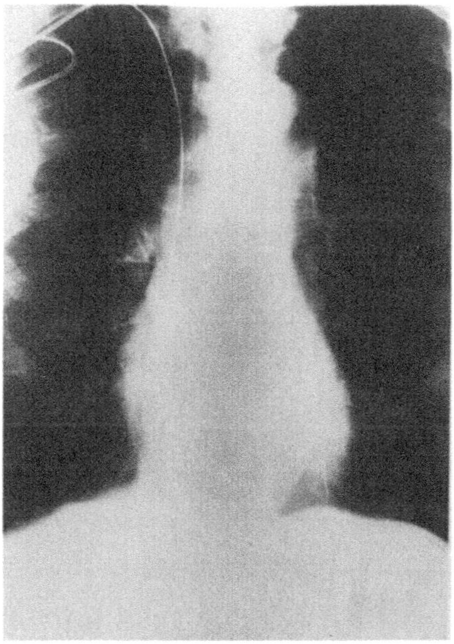

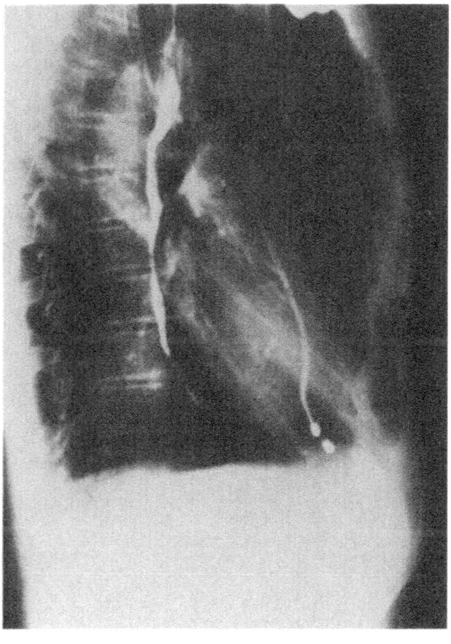

Figure 12. Correct right ventricular endocavitary electrode positioning. The distal electrode tip is superposed on the vertebrae. This more median position is explained by the small vertical shape of the heart. Lateral incidence confirms adequate positioning.

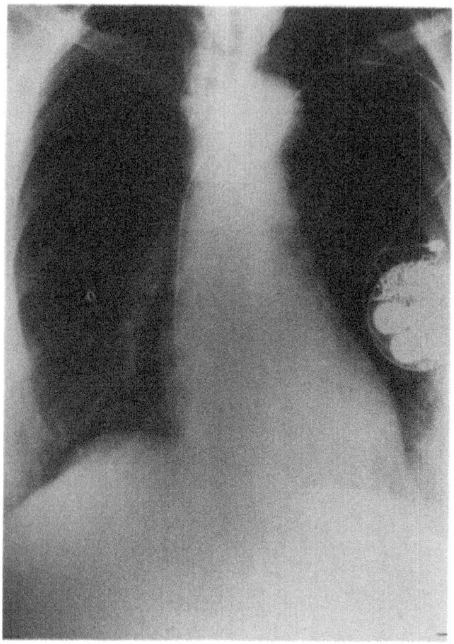

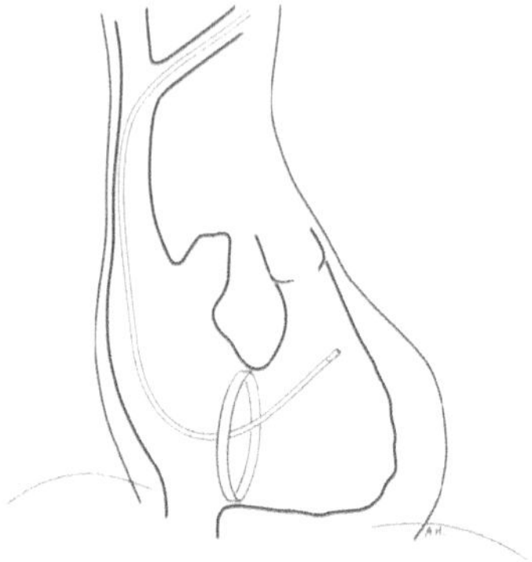

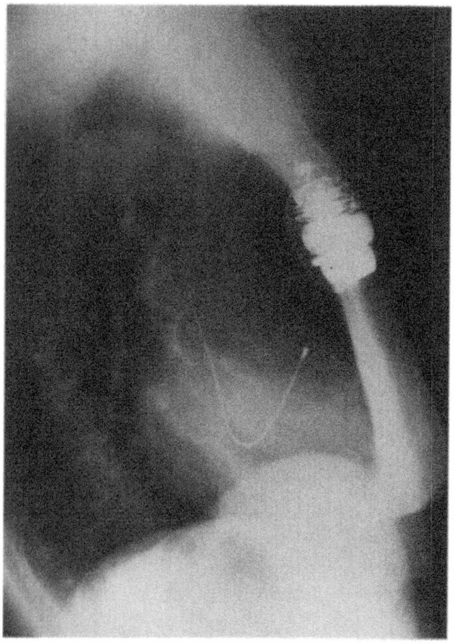

Figure 13. Electrode tip in the right ventricular infundibulum. This frontal view may suggest a coronary sinus positioning. The lateral incidence eliminates the latter possibility by its anterior bending of the lead.

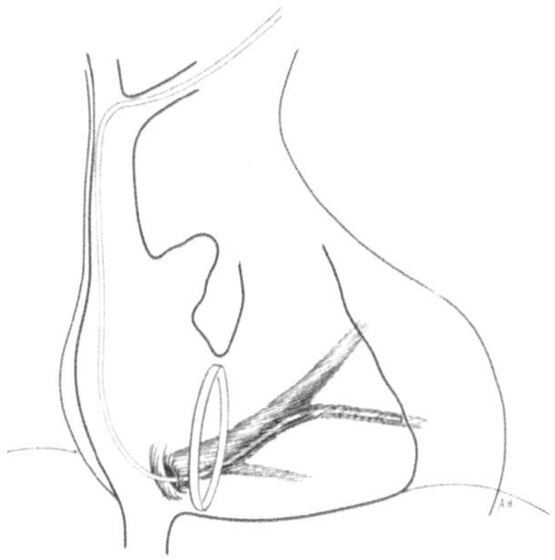

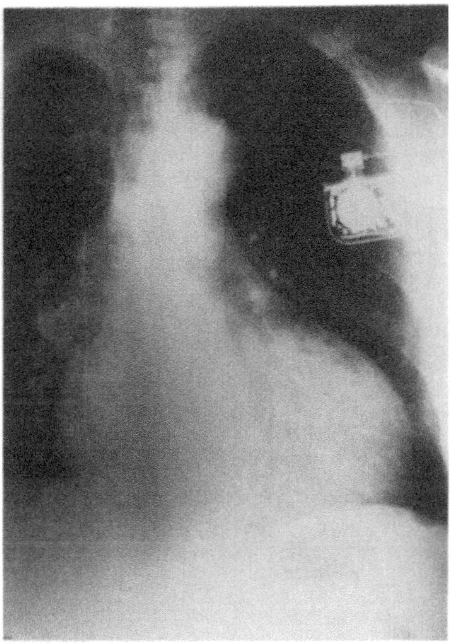

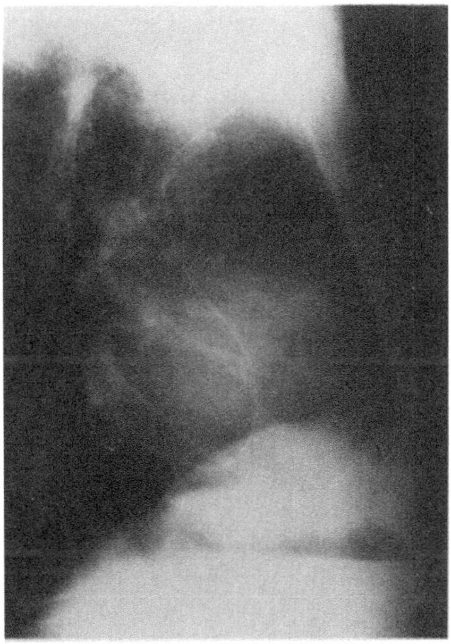

Figure 14. Electrode tip is located in a postero-inferior cardiac vein. In the frontal view, a characteristic square root curve is seen. The lead bends in the right atrium then turns upwards in the coronary sinus and bends again to enter a cardiac vein. The lateral incidence shows the very posterior peripheral location of the distal tip.

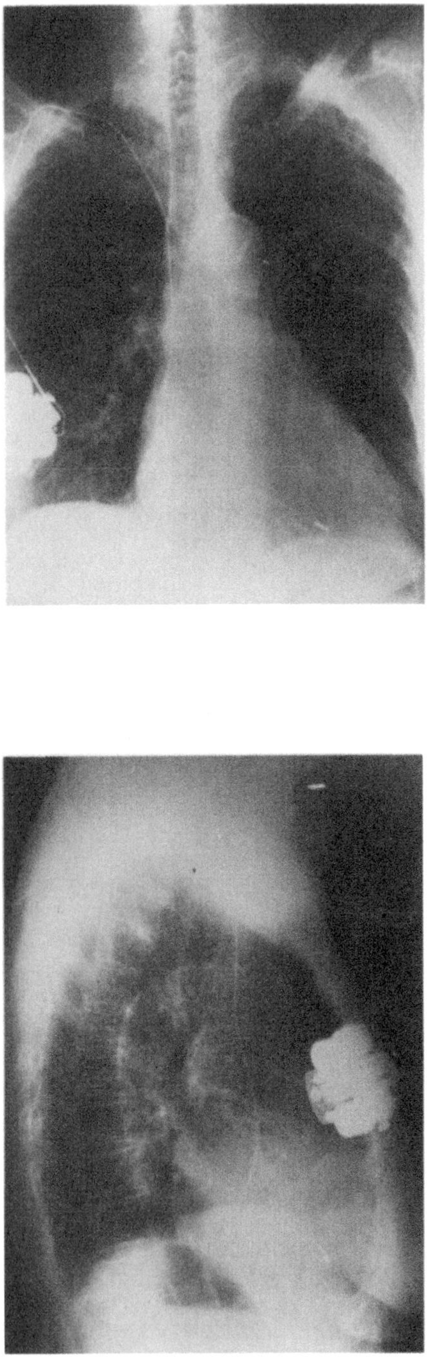

Figure 15. Normal positioning in the right ventricule. The frontal image may suggest an upwards bending towards a cardiac vein. The lateral incidence demonstrates the intraventricular positioning.

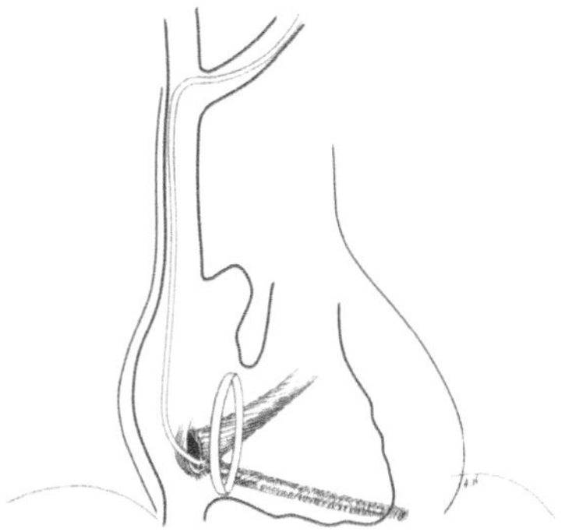

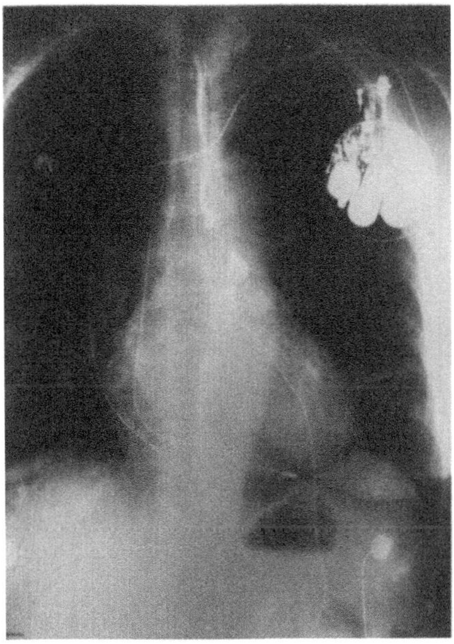

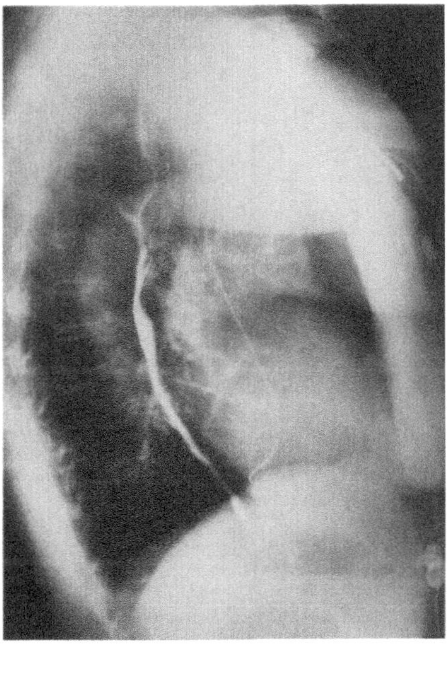

Figure 16. Endocardial lead positioning in the posterior interventricular vein. The frontal view would suggest an adequate interventricular positioning. At the junction of the innominate vein with the superior vena cava, a more accentuated bending is noted. (electrode wedging effect). The lateral incidence demonstrates a posterior peripheral location of the electrode in a ventricular vein draining in the coronary sinus, very close to its origin in the right atrium.

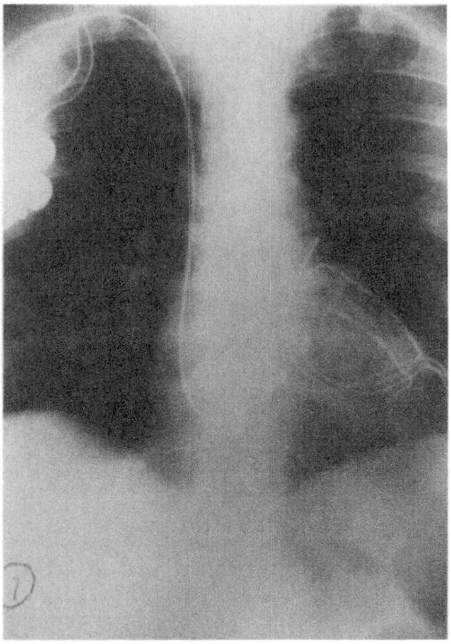

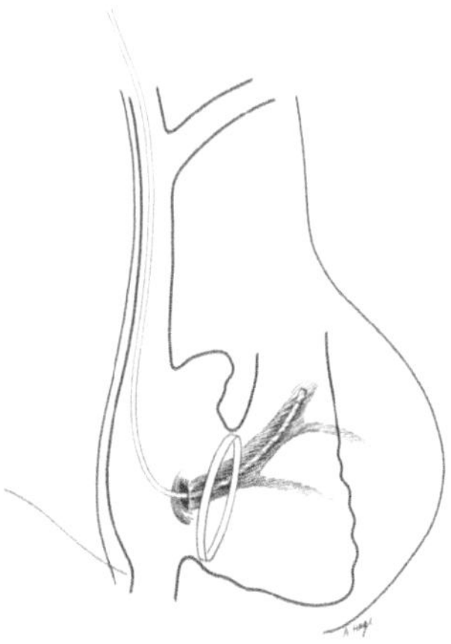

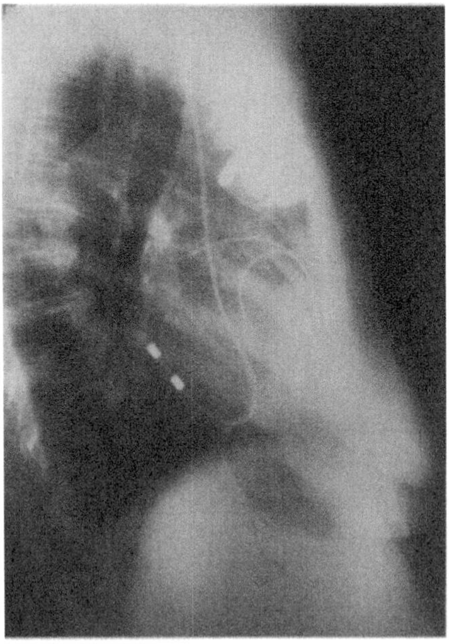

Figure 17. Endocardial lead in the coronary sinus: this position is characteristic in both frontal and lateral views. Differential diagnosis should be made with an endocardial lead in the right ventricular infundibulum (see figure 13).

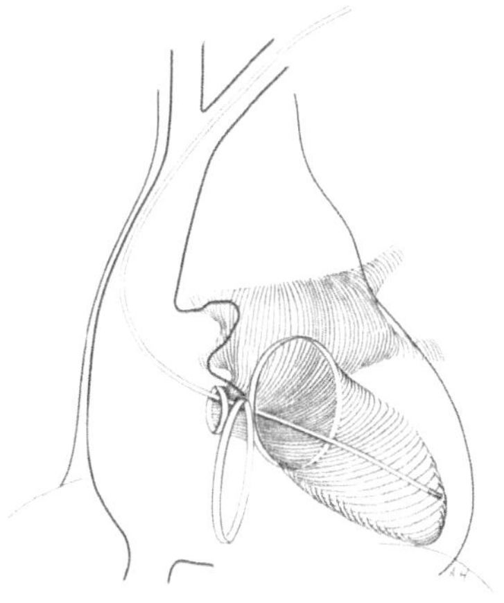

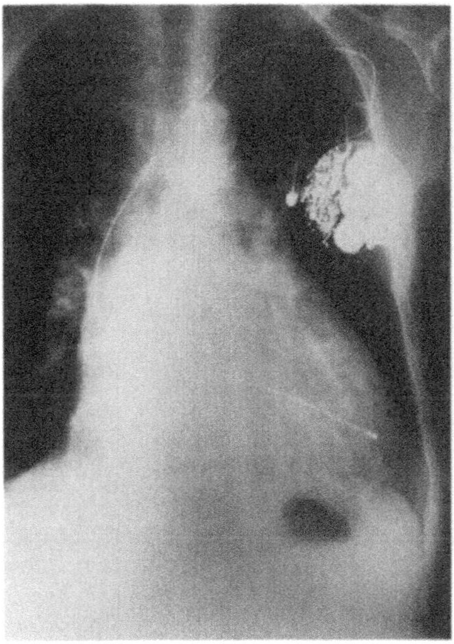

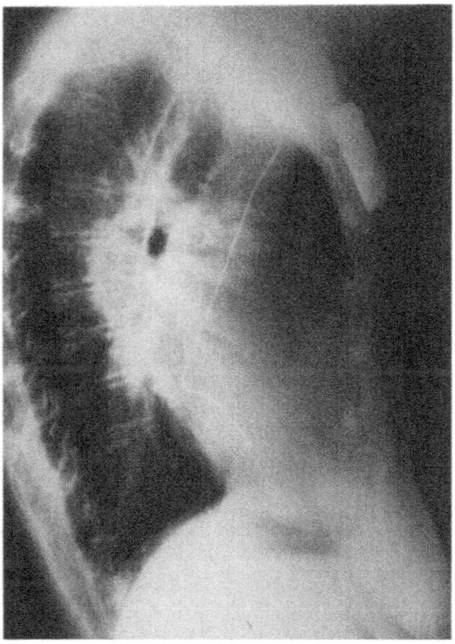

Figure 18. Endocardial electrode positioned in the left ventricle via a foramen ovale. Considering both incidences, this unusual pathway may be suggested by the posterior and very lateral position of the electrode. A cardiac vein positioning might be suggested, but the frontal incidence does not demonstrate a typical square root sign as seen in Figure 14.

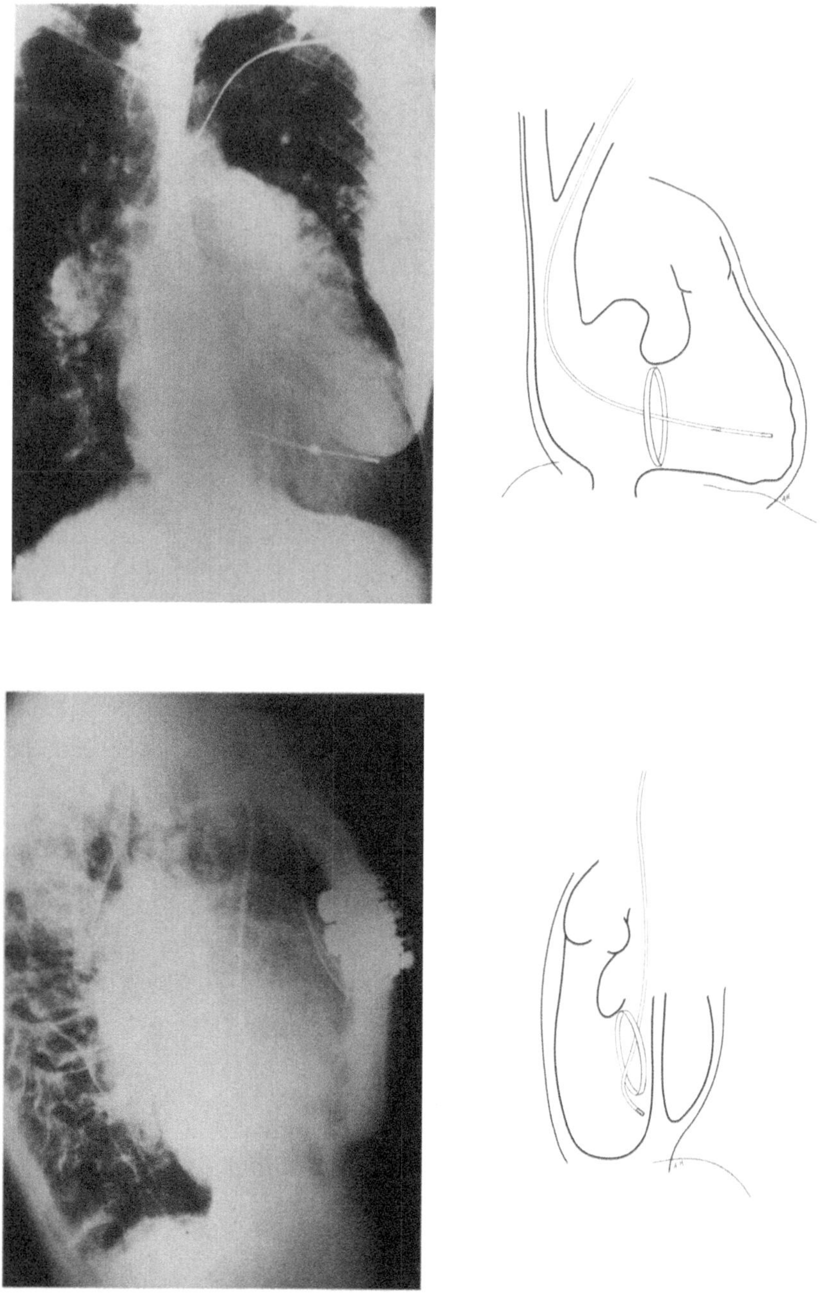

Figure 19. Elderly lady with an ASD and pulmonary hypertension: normal positioning of the electrode in the right ventricle. The distal tip of the electrode is located more posteriorly than usually. Left ventricular positioning through the ASD was suggested. The lateral incidence shows the distal tip of the electrode posteriorly but one has to keep in mind the important dilatation of the right ventricular cavity bringing the septum towards the left and rear.

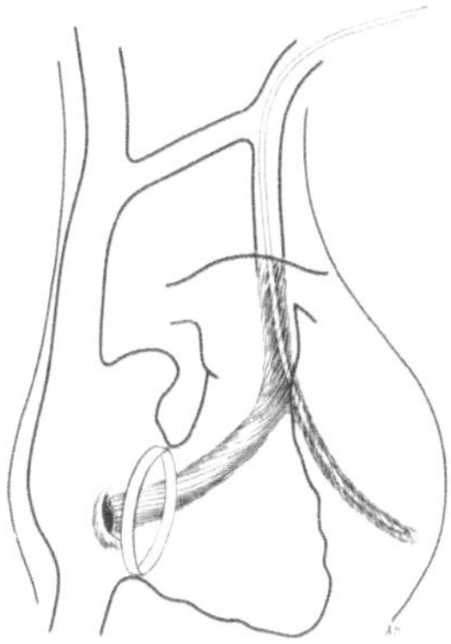

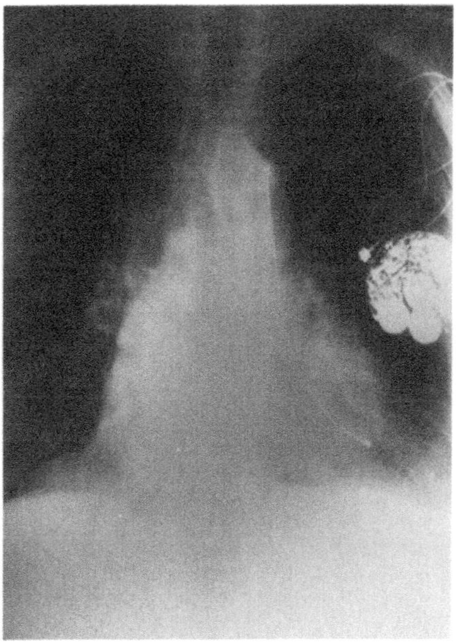

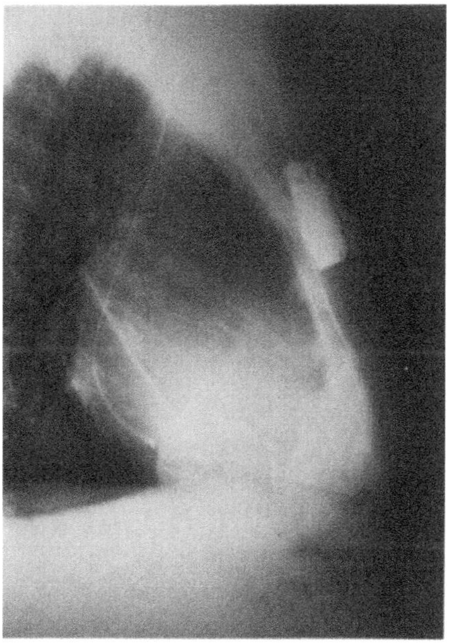

Figure 20. Electrode tip in a left postero-lateral cardiac vein. The lead follows a persistent left superior vena cava, draining in the coronary sinus. The electrode tip follows a natural direction into this vein.

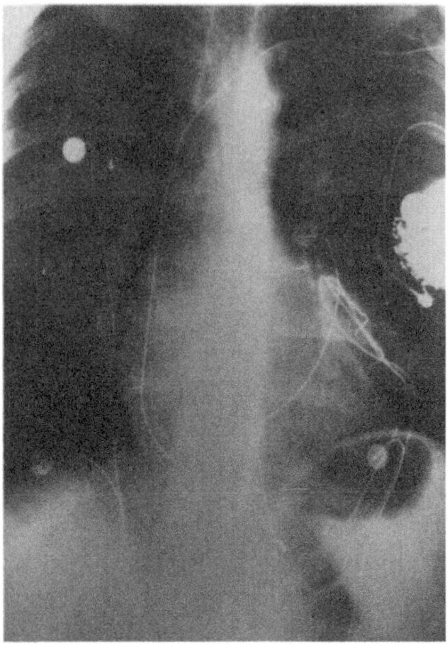

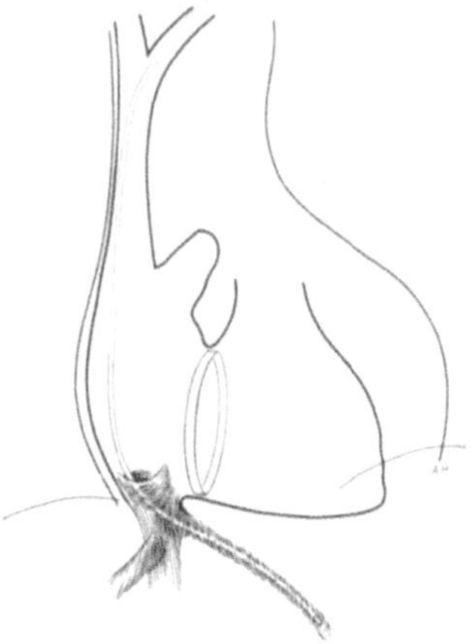

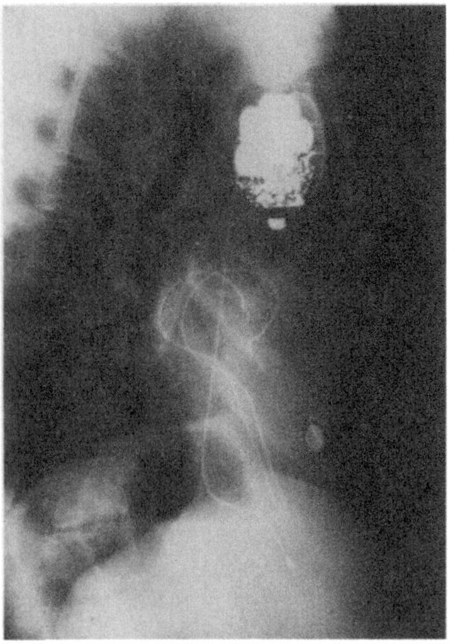

Figure 21. Endocardial electrode located in the left hepatic vein. The extremity of the endocardial lead is slightly vertical and projects in the hepatic area.

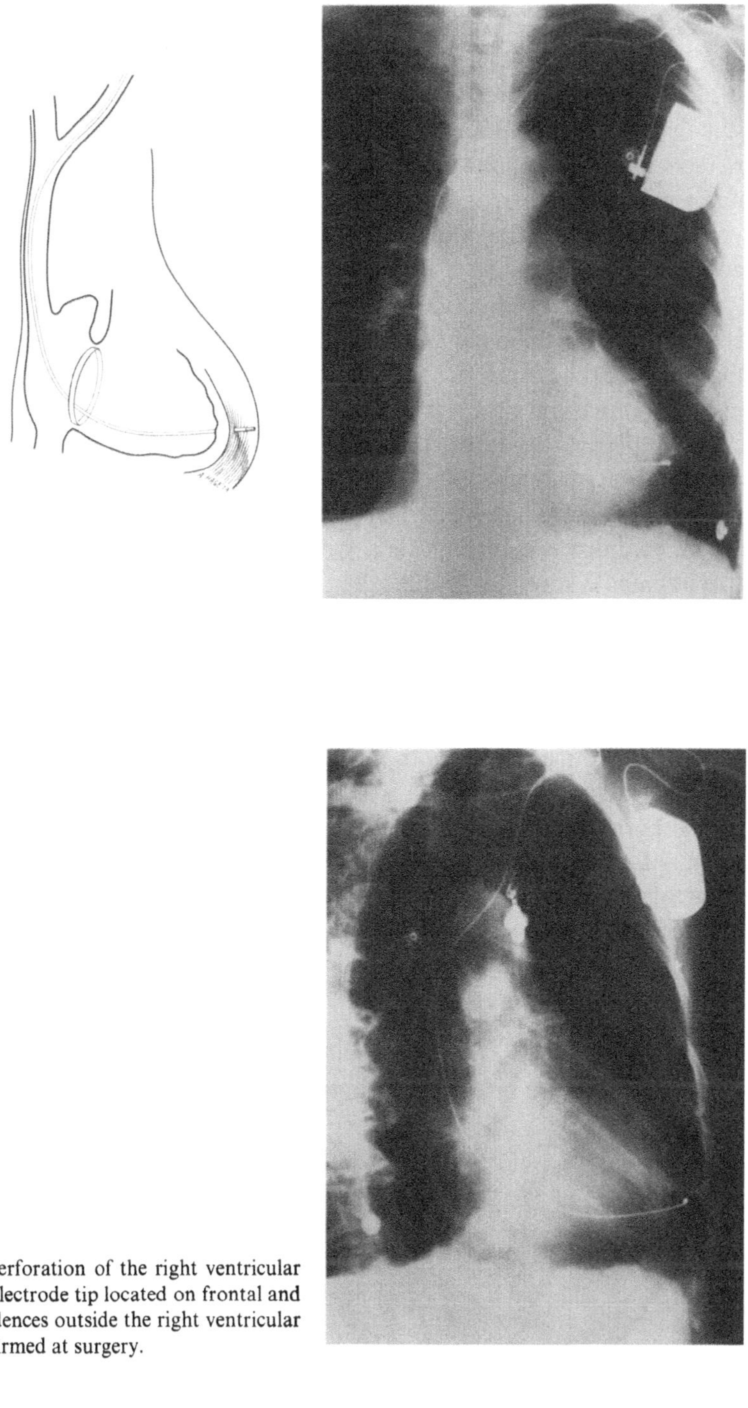

Figure 22. Perforation of the right ventricular wall by the electrode tip located on frontal and oblique incidences outside the right ventricular cavity. Confirmed at surgery.

Ventricular electrode expulsion ends adequate pacing, but lack of pacing may also be observed with an electrode seemingly in the area of the right ventricle.

A minor displacement inside the right ventricle may cause exit blocks presumably by contact with infarcted areas such as the lower septum or the diaphragmatic postero-basal wall. A patch for septum correction is, of course, non-conductive.

Accurate endocardial threshold mapping may lead to optimal positioning away from the commonly accepted apical location.

With electrode positioning close to the tricuspid valve, a slightly downward bending curve of the atrial part of the lead should be allowed, bearing in mind that in the raised-body position the heart descends about 2 cm, potentially dislodging tricuspid electrodes.

Ventricular perforation accompanied by diaphragmatic pacing may not always be demonstrated on X-rays. In rare instances, clinical cardiac tamponade may occur. In other cases, the hemorrhagic distension of the pericardium may induce continuous pain in the left hypochondrium or lumbar area mimicking splenic embolization.

2.2. Endoscopic technique

2.2.1. Suprasternal mediastinoscopic, atrial electrode surface positioning. (Figure 23) Atrial synchronization with a ventricular electrode in place has been performed by Lagergren in 1963 (15). Under general anaesthesia, through a suprasternal horizontal skin incision, a mediastinoscope is advanced to the carina, using the trachea as a guide. The posterior wall of the origin of the right pulmonary artery is encountered distal and ventral to the carina. The atrial electrode is positioned in this extrapericardial preatrial space for P-wave sensing.

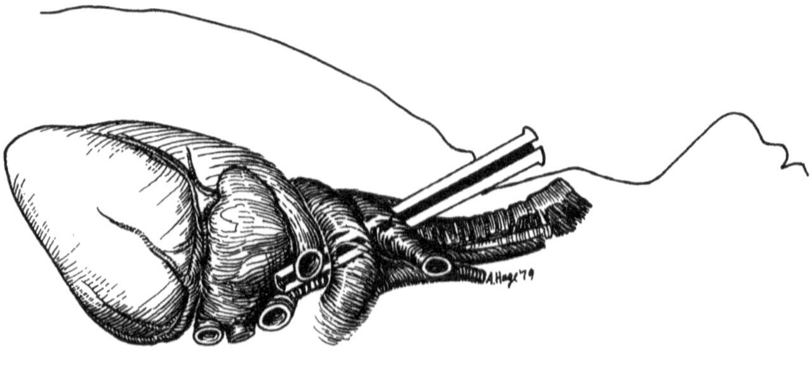

Figure 23. Mediastinotomy for surface positioning of atrial electrode behind the origin of the right pulmonary artery.

2.2.2. Transdiaphragmatic endoscopic, ventricular electrode fixation. A pericardioscope has been described by Crosby during the VIth World Symposium on Cardiac Pacing. The discussion of its merits is to be published in the Proceedings of the Symposium.

2.3. Transthoracic technique

These procedures are usually performed by thoracic surgeons and it is felt of little value to give detailed technical descriptions here. They are summarized below (16, 17, 8) (Figure 24).

2.3.1. Site of direct thoracic approach. The left lateral thoracotomy gives access both to the left ventricle and the left atrium. This route is elected for fixation of an atrial electrode on the left auricular appendage at the time of myocardial implantation.

The anterior thoracotomy through a breast-sulcus skin incision limits the access to the anterolateral lower part of the left ventricle (19) (Figure 25).

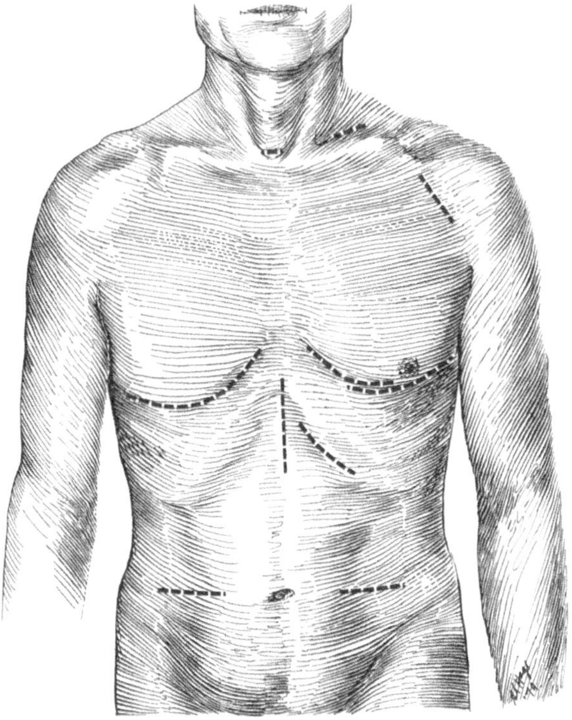

Figure 24. Skin incisions for lead and pacemaker positioning.

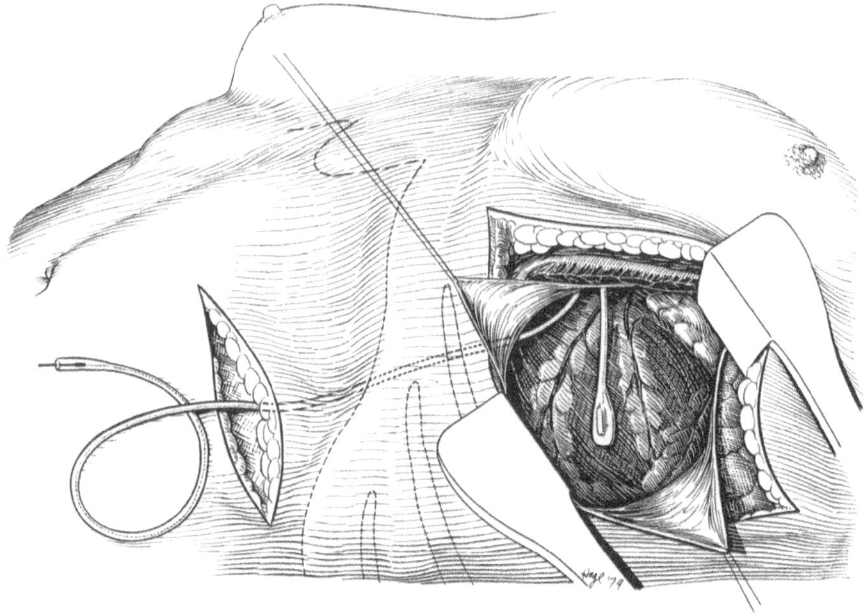

Figure 25. Anterior thoracotomy approach for epicardial electrode fixation on the left ventricle between the left anterior descending coronary artery and its second diagonal branch. One third of the lead remains upwards in the pericardium. The lead is tunnelled through the diaphram to a subcostal pocket for pacemaker connection.

The parasternal mediastinotomy is in fact a laterally restricted anterior thoracotomy (20) with cartilage resection opening the mediastinum and leaving the left pleura intact by gently pushing its anterior edge laterally (Figure 26). The approach to the heart is usually restricted to the right ventricular outflow tract where adequate epicardial electrode fixation may become more problematic due to the thinness of the wall.

Epicardial electrodes should be fixed on a thick, non-fibrotic and fat-free ventricular area. The disadvantages of opening the pleura are less significant than the risks of pacing failure due to improper fixation of the electrode on a thinner area of the right ventricle.

The pericardium or pericardial fat is best reapproximated allowing only a small exit for the lead(s), protecting by this means other epicardial surfaces for future surgery.

Prior to chest closure, the leads are tunnelled towards the pacemaker pocket. Exit from the thorax is transdiaphragmatic for abdominal pacemaker locations. An alternative solution is retromammary pacemaker positioning (Figure 27). Close to the sternum, a small piece of rib cartilage is resected allowing the lead(s) to leave the mediastinum without a 'pinching' effect. This very medial thoracic lead exit probably lessens the lead motion due to respiration.

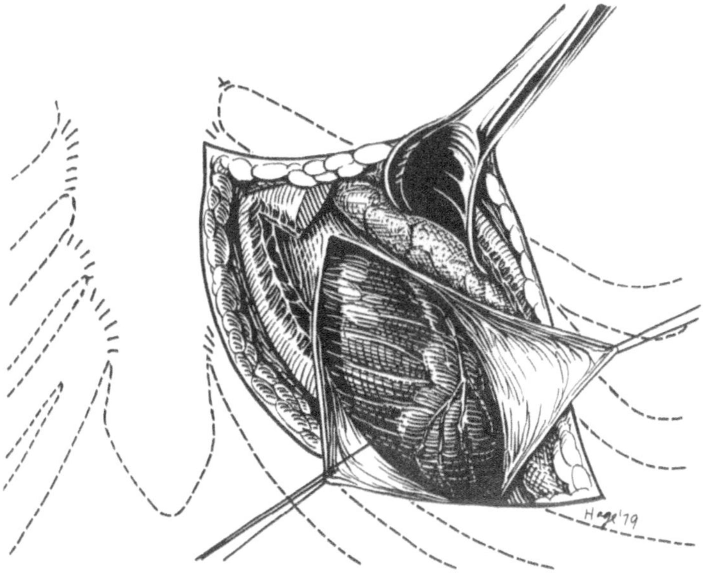

Figure 26. Parasternal mediastinotomy and view limited to the right ventricular outflow tract.

The anterior right thoracotomy, without transsection of the sternum, gives access to the right atrium for more physiologic pacing in cases where functioning ventricular electrodes are already in place (Figure 28).

In addition, if a ventricular electrode is required, a lead may be introduced through the atrial wall or atrial appendage and secured to the atrial wall. An attempt to place epicardial leads with this approach is difficult and hazardous.

The median sternotomy is the appropriate route for most cardiac surgical procedures. Concurrent or iatrogenic A-V disturbances will be corrected by preoperative epicardial electrode fixation.

In all the above mentioned approaches, the adequate epicardial surface may be too small for implantation of a second electrode. In case of unipolar stimulation, is it mandatory to implant a second, spare, epicardial lead?

This commonly accepted policy is debatable. Threshold elevations to exit block levels may occur on dormant electrodes and leads may rupture in the same manner as active leads.

Longitudinal parasternal mediastinal approach. This approach, with removal of three rib cartilages, allows implantation on the right ventricular outflow tract of an implantable receiver coil for a radio frequency pacemaker and has been used in 1964 by Camilli (21).

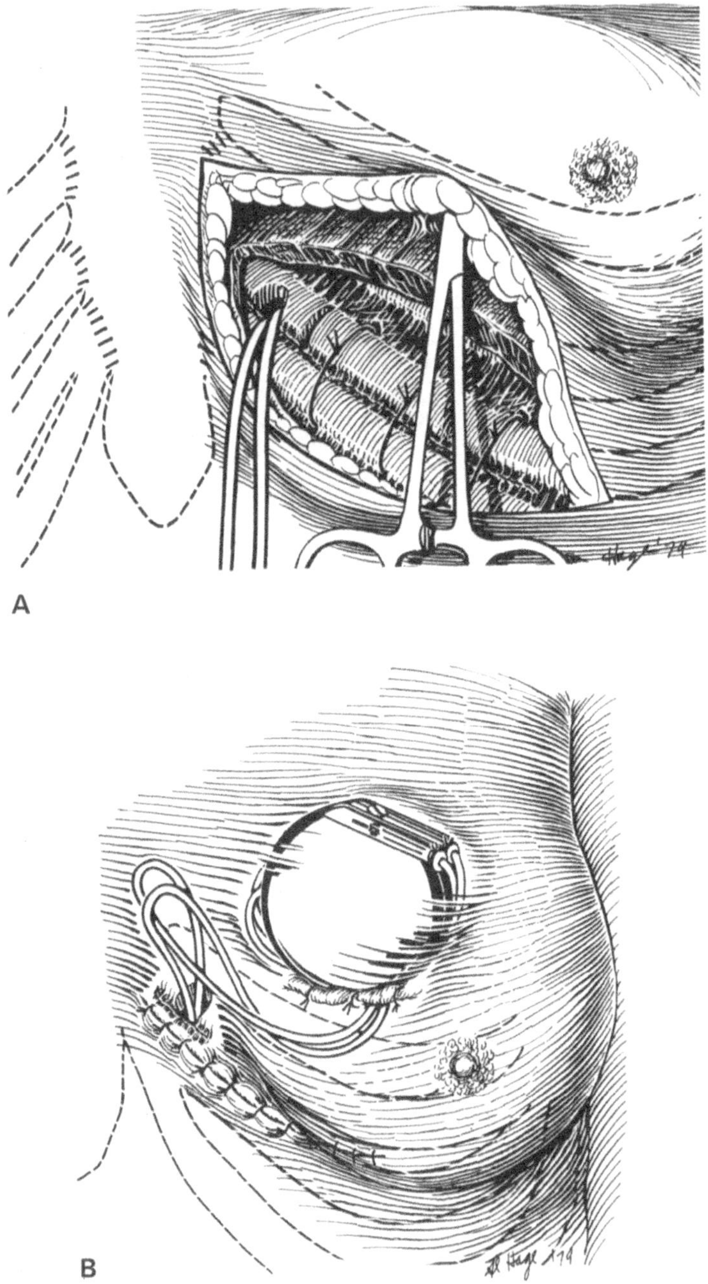

Figure 27. A – Retromammary positioning of the power unit. Medial partial rib cartilage resection allows lead exit.
B – After pectoralis closure the unit is introduced in the retromammary pocket which will be closed 5 cms higher than the skin incision in order to fix the unit firmly in a tight pocket.

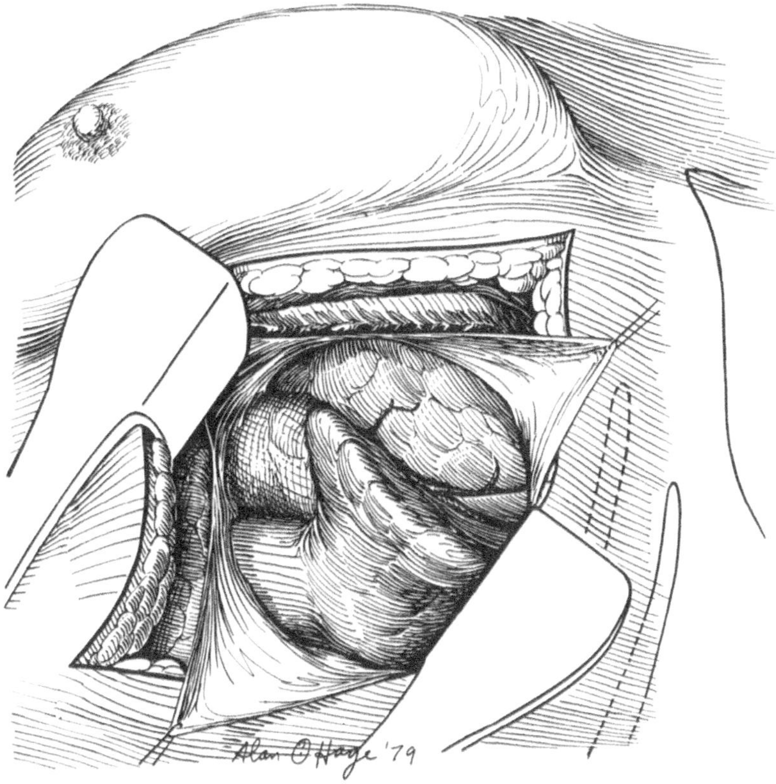

Figure 28. Right anterior thoracotomy allows atrial electrode fixation and endocardial positioning in the right ventricle with fixation at the atrial wall entrance.

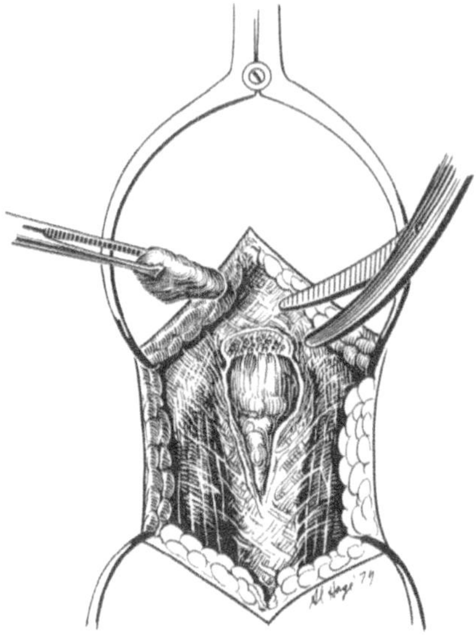

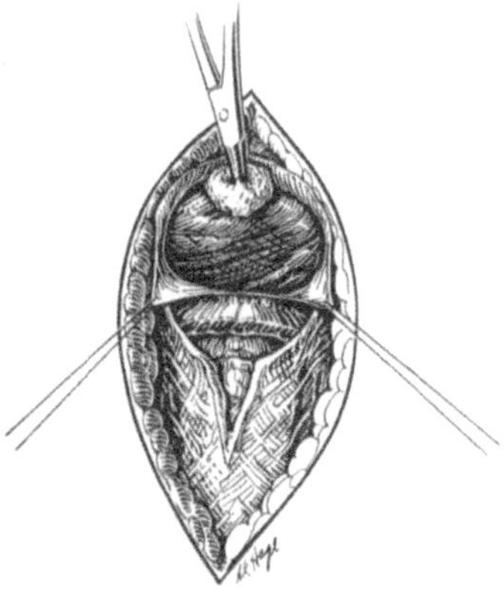

B

A

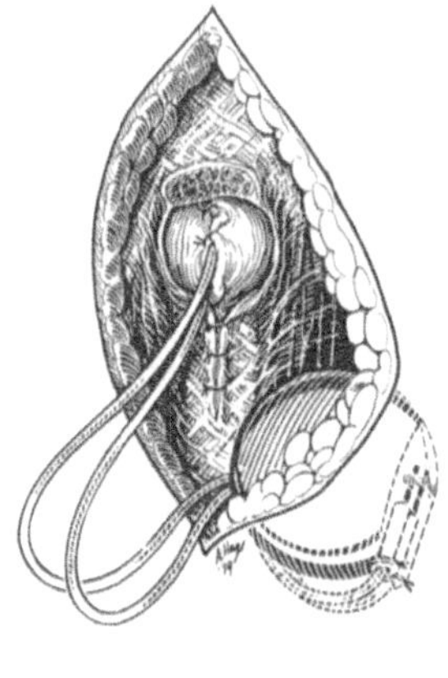

C

Figure 29. A – Epigastric approach. Opening of midline aponeurosis between both recti and resection of xyphoid process.
B – Limited view on exposed diaphragmatic surface of right ventricle.
C – After pericardial closure and pacemaker connection, the unit may be positioned either through the same skin incision or by tunnelling the lead towards a more caudal location.

2.3.2. Site of transabdominal approach. Median epigastric route (figure 29). Access to the diaphragmatic surface of the right ventricle can be gained through this approach (22). The aponeurosis between both recti is opened in its upper part and the xyphoid process is preferably removed. Diaphragmatic muscle fibers are split antero-posteriorly and the pericardium is opened.

Left subcostal route (figure 30). A complete severing of the left rectus muscle from its chondral attachments is first performed. Lateral retraction of the muscle with incision of the posterior sheath is possible. After displacing the peritoneum, the diaphragm and pericardium can be opened (23).

When transvenous and transthoracic pacing are judged inappropriate, the transdiaphragmatic route may be chosen. In case of previous heart surgery, such as aortocoronary bypass, the anterior surface of the heart may be difficult to approach by anterior thoracotomy. Usually, adhesions are less important on the diaphragmatic surface and morbidity from bleeding may thus be lowered considerably by a transdiaphragmatic approach. However, the limited access to the right ventricle is potentially hazardous. A rupture of the right ventricular wall during electrode fixation may need drastic salvaging action. Therefore, this procedure may not be considered a minor surgical act (24, 25, 26). Once the decision is made to approach the heart epicardially, the only adequate epicardial site may be on the left ventricle and hence the abdominal route should be chosen only after rejection of thoracotomy as an alternate route.

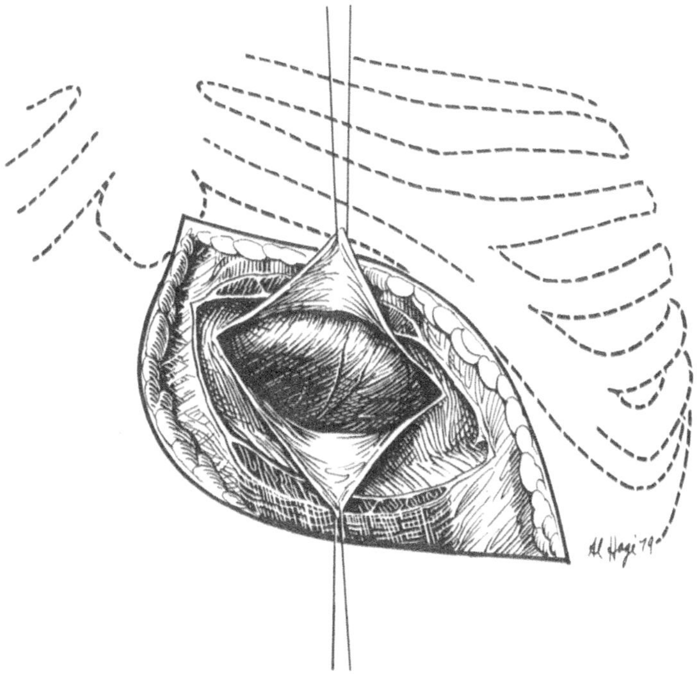

Figure 30. Left subcostal approach with transsection of the left rectus muscle. With lateral retraction of the muscle – which is more difficult to illustrate – one may gain the same access.

2.4. Surgery for the pacemaker unit

Although pacemakers are thinner than in the past, superficial locations cause bulging in the lean patient.

The decision on where to locate a pacemaker should be clearly discussed with the patient after examining the quality of his subcutaneous tissue. Activities such as hunting may contraindicate infraclavicular homolateral location. Automobile seat belts are also to be considered. The patient should be aware that the esthetical benefits of deeper locations most often imply general anaesthesia for battery changes. The younger age group of patients, with the expected increased pacemaker longevity, should be given this choice whereas local anaesthesia might be a prevailing medical choice for the elderly patients. Access to deeper locations such as the retroperitoneal space may necessitate the use of curarizing agents. One has to be aware that unfortunate muscle twitching may occur as the patient awakes.

The various most common pacemaker locations are represented in Figures 31 to 34. The subcutaneous pocket is best dissected before electrode positioning, to allow adequate hemostasis by inside sponge compression. Meticulous hemostasis in anticoagulated patients is of prime importance to avoid wound hematomas with subsequent pacemaker infection.

In a doubtful case, activated collagen may become an important temporary adjunct.

Axillary migration of twitching may occur if the pocket size is much larger than the pacemaker body. On the other hand, the depth of the pocket should exceed by 3 cm the total height of the pacemaker allowing a full closure of the pocket prior to subcutaneous and skin closure. Separating the pacemaker from the subcutaneous suture line may decrease the risks of wound dehiscence. Stitch abcesses may be lessened by using a single subcuticular running stitch. Considering the future surgery of battery replacement (Figure 31), it is important to position the pacemaker in such a way as to protect the connector and lead from accidental future surgical trauma. An effort is made to avoid the presence of the lead in the middle of the incision, the connector being placed caudally and the lead emerging in the very lower part of the skin incision. On reopening the pocket, the scalpel will only be in contact with the metallic part of the pacemaker. The retromammary position is esthetically appealing and may also be used with an anterior thoracotomy. After prepectoralis pocket dissection, the pacemaker is inserted. An important suture line closes the pocket about 5 cm above the skin closure in order to avoid later gliding towards the submammary scar.

Abdominal pacemaker locations are best situated below the belt except for the retromuscular epigastric pacemaker in a lean person. Longer leads may have to be used if the lead enters the venous stream in the upper body, with a pacemaker location on the abdomen (Figure 35).

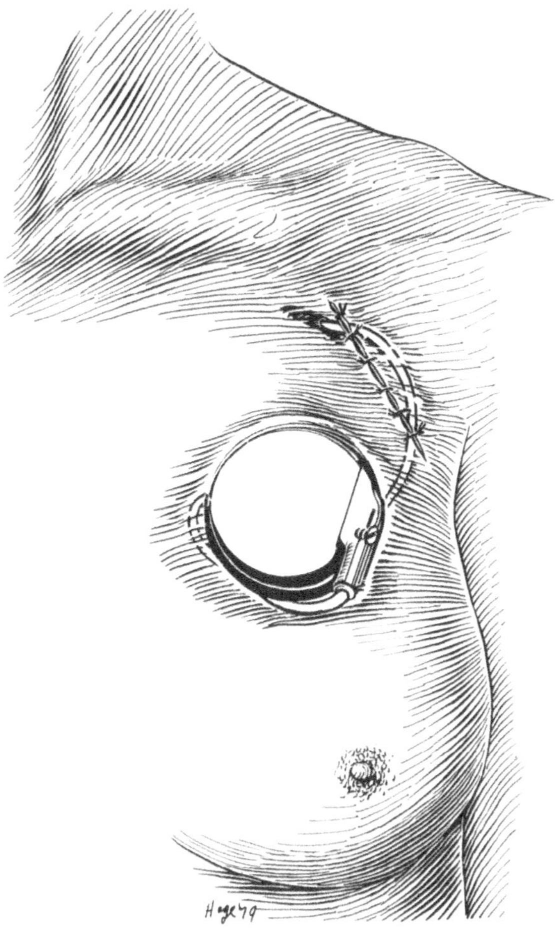

Figure 31. Transparent view of pacemaker positioning in a way as to protect the lead and connection at the time of reopening for battery change.

Through a subcutaneous tunnel, the lead is brought downwards. Some authors routinely measure threshold in this fashion for a given period of time on the permanent lead prior to permanent implantation. Others would limit this technique to exceptional cases such as lack of supporting tissue after radical breast amputation.

In conclusion, techniques for implantation of a pacemaker are various. Problems may arise due to poor general condition, cachexia or to fear of an anatomical deformity by a bulging implanted device. In the elderly-aged group, the morbidity of a thoracotomy and the extended length of hospitalization favour the endocardial transvenous approach. In the presence of right ventricular failure or after unsuccessful endocardial positioning, a thoracic or epi-

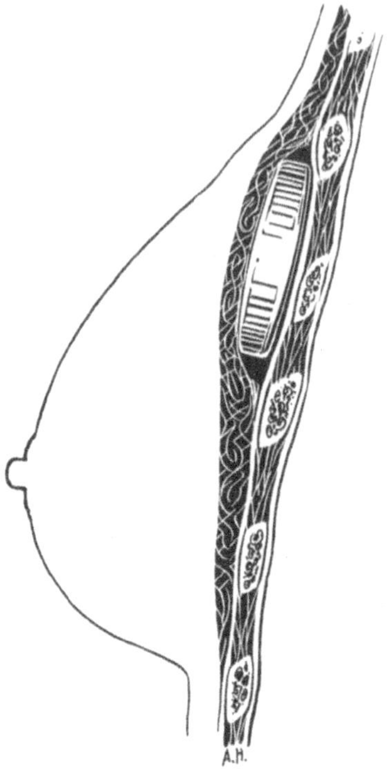

Figure 32. Retropectoralis position of power unit.

gastric approach should be contemplated. In the younger age group, the anterior thoracotomy with left ventricular epicardial fixation may be preferred. Deeply embedded power units are best accepted psychologically even though general anaesthesia is required for battery changes. However, programmability and magnet tests may not be feasible on retroperitoneally located units.

Finally the utmost care should be taken to insure adequate surgical closure since infection around the pacemaker usually requires the complete removal of the system. Usually antibiotics are administered for the first 5 postoperative days. As with temporary pacing anticoagulants are never used unless otherwise indicated.

3. CLOSING REMARKS ON THE RESPONSIBILITIES OF THE IMPLANTING PHYSICIAN

The various approaches to the heart for the purpose of improving or ensuring a continuous and adequate cardiac output by means of electrical stimulation

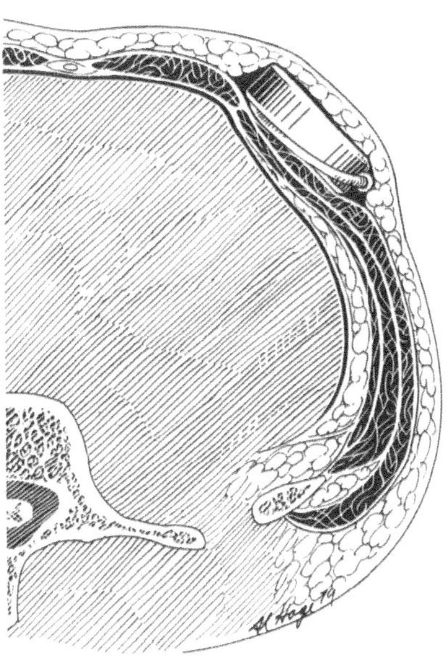

A

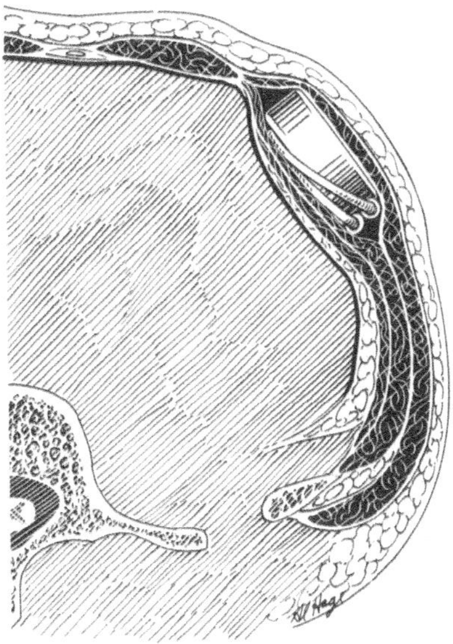

B

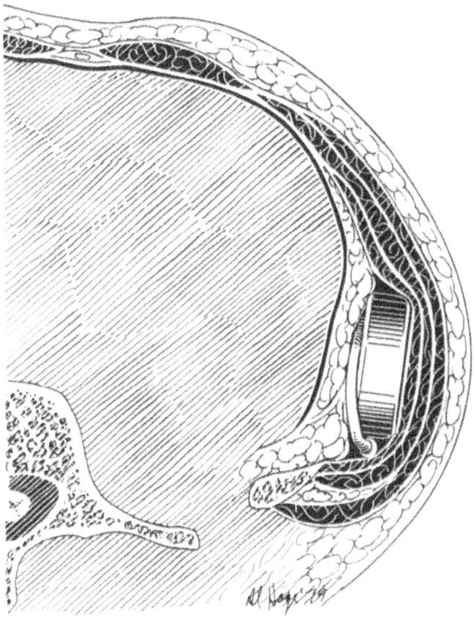

C

Figure 33. Lateral abdominal pacemaker locations: A – Subcutaneous; B – Intermuscular (Bipolar unit); C – Retroperitoneal.

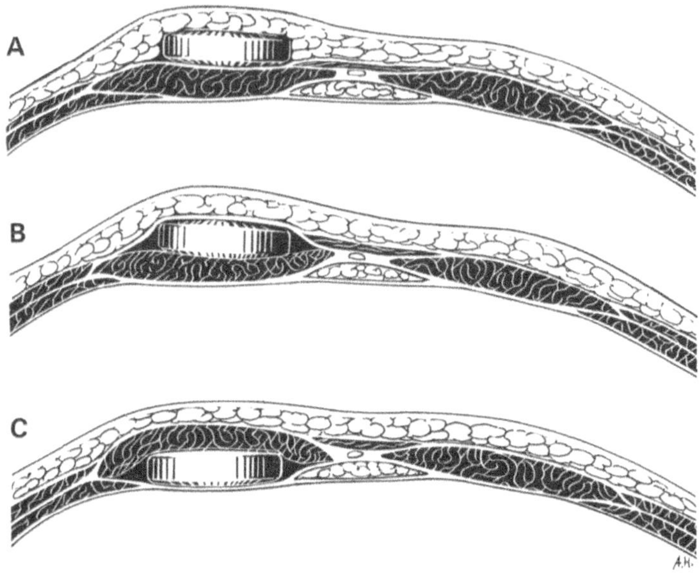

Figure 34. Anterior abdominal pacemaker locations: A – Subcutaneous; B – Behind rectus sheath; C – Behind rectus.

present specific advantages and drawbacks. Moreover, each approach may be preferred for clinical or esthetic or anatomic reasons.

Prevention and treatment of complications are part of the implanting physician's responsibilities (27) although the indications for pacing may have been determined by other physicians. The implanting physician, while faced with a primary implant, should also plan his approach having in mind the projected life span for cardiac stimulation in each patient. Suitable alternate routes for future replacement of electrodes should be considered at this early stage.

The physical environment for cardiac pacemaker implantation also may be influential on postoperative events such as early infection. Limited facilities may eliminate the choice for a more extended surgical approach which might have been a more appropriate choice in specific cases. In other situations, the epicardial approach may be systematically preferred in thoracic surgical units. In both alternatives, the implanting physican should be aware that he may have to justify his particular systematic approach with reference to the overall quality of postoperative evolution of his patients.

Without opening a debate on standards of care for permanent pacemaker implantation, suffice it to say that institutions and physicians involved in cardiac pacing should probably be able to guarantee that all appropriate surgical approaches can be dealt with – if deemed necessary – without potential harmful delay for the patient.

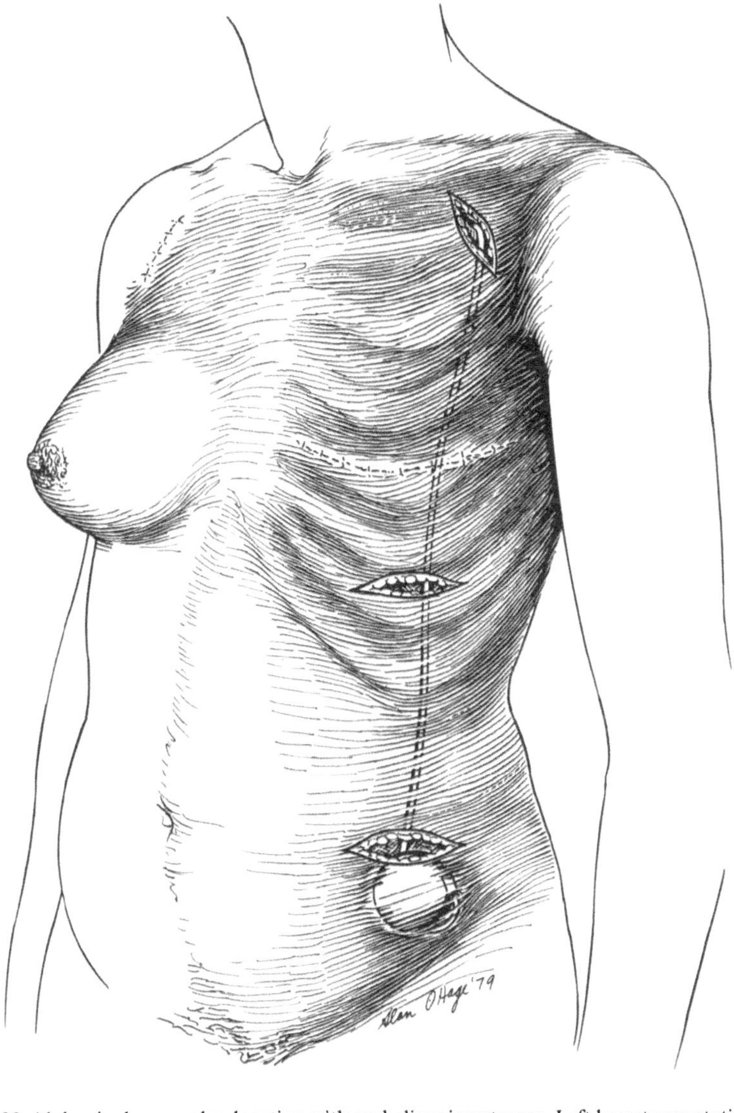

Figure 35. Abdominal pacemaker location with cephalic vein entrance. Left breast amputation and unsuccessful right-sided approach.

The selection of the mode of stimulation is to be determined by the diagnostician whereas the choice of a specific pacemaker device (in consideration of its volume) may be influenced by the implanting physician's appreciation of the patient's tissues.

The physician responsible for the long-term follow-up in his centre, being more aware of the published failure reports, may ultimately be the most influential voice in the committee selecting the pacemaker brands and models in his hospital. However, the implanting physician may never legally be released from the responsibility.

Finally, in an attempt to determine the implanting physician's responsibilities, it should be emphasized that the technical preoperative advice should be given by the hospital bioengineering section.

All of these points should be properly discussed in any hospital considering permanent cardiac pacing therapy, including, of course, the structure of a long-term follow-up system.

In determining standards of care for pacing therapy, the satellite-hospital situation is encountered where by common acceptance, power unit replacements are routinely performed in smaller centres to avoid unnecessary travelling by elderly patients. Unexpected situations may arise in the course of this minor surgical procedure with a final result for the patient that is less desirable than normally expected in the better equipped centres.

These remarks are not meant to cause alarm, but to establish that pacemaker implantation, which is often considered a minor procedure, is nevertheless an act where expertise may avoid major complications. Its iterative nature, whether for correction of tissue complications or device failures, greatly increases the importance of skillful planning and execution.

ACKNOWLEDGEMENTS

I wish to thank Medtronic for underwriting the cost of the drawings done by Al Hage, and my son Bruno for editorial assistance.

REFERENCES

1. Zoll M: Resuscitation of the heart in ventricular standstill by external electrical stimulation. *N Engl J Med* 247: 768, 1952.
2. Chung EK: Indications of temporary pacing. In: *Artificial cardiac pacing – practical approach*, The Williams & Wilkins Company, Baltimore, 1978, pp. 161-172.
3. Pirzada FA, Venkataraman K, Madias JE, Hood WB JR: Prophylactic preoperative pacing. In: *To pace or not to pace*, Thalen HJTh, Harthorne JW (eds.), Martinus Nijhoff Medical Division, The Hague/Boston/London, 1978, pp. 82-90.
4. Moosman DA: The anatomy of infraclavicular subclavian vein catheterization and its complications. *Surg Gyn Obs* 136: 71-74, 1973.
5. Lillehei CW, Levy MJ, Bonnabeau RC, Long DM, Sellers RD: The use of a myocardial electrode and pacemaker in a management of acute postoperative and postinfarction heart block. *Surgery* 56: 463, 1964.
6. Reemtsma K, Delgado JP, and Creech O Jr: Heart block following intra-cardiac surgery: Localization of conduction tissue injury. *J Thorac Cardiovasc Surg* 39: 688-693, 1960.
7. Sowton E, Leatham A, Carson P: The suppression of arrhythmias by artificial pacemaking. *Lancet* 2: 1098, 1964.
8. Furman S: Therapeutic uses of atrial pacing. *Am Heart J*, 86: 835, 1973.

9. Brockman SK: Dynamic function of atrial contraction in regulation of cardiac performance. *Am J Physiol*, 204: 597, 1963.
10. Roth F, Salzmann C, Gurtner HP: Elektrische Stimulation des Herzens über eine Oesophagus-elektrode. *Schweiz Med Wschr* 99: 1661, 1969.
11. Burack B, Furman S: Transoesophageal cardiac pacing. *Amer J Cardiol* 23: 469, 1969.
12. Furman S, Robinson G: The use of an intracardiac pacemaker in the correction of total heart block. *Surg Forum* 9, 1958.
13. Littleford PO, Spector SD: Device for the rapid insertion of a permanent endocardial pacing eleetrode through the subclavian vein: preliminary report. *Ann Thorac Surg* 27: 265, 1979.
14. Moss AJ, Rivers RJ, Cooper M: Long-term pervenous atrial pacing from the proximal portion of the coronary vein. *JAMA*, 209: 543, 1969.
15. Lagergren H, Johansson L, Karlöf I, Thornander H: Atrial-triggered pacemaking without thoracotomy: apparatus and results in twenty cases. *Acta Chir Scand*, 132: 678, 1966.
16. Nathan DA, Center S, Wu CY, Keller W: An implantable synchronous pacemaker for the long-term correction of complete heart block. *Am J Cardiol* 11: 362, 1963.
17. Chardack WM, Gage AA, Greatbatch W: Correction of complete heart block by a self-contained and subcutaneously implanted pacemaker. *J Thorac Cardiovasc Surg* 42: 814, 1961.
18. Tyers GFO, Hughes HC, Torman HA, Waldhausen JA: The advantages of transthoracic placement of permanent cardiac pacemaker electrodes. *J Thor Cardiovasc Surg* 69: 8, 1975.
19. Hunter SW, Bolduc, Long L, Sister Victorine, Quattlebaum FW: A new myocardial pacemaker lead (sutureless). *Chest* 63: 430, 1973.
20. Mobin-Uddin K, Smith PE, Lombardo C, Jude JR: Local anesthesia for insertion of epicardial electrodes. *J Thorac Cardiovasc Surg* 55: 112, 1968.
21. Cammilli L, Pozzi R, Pizzichi G: Radio-Frequency pacemaker with receiver coil implanted on the heart. In: *Cardiac Pacemakers*, Glenn WWL, *Ann N Y Acad Sc* 3: 1007-1029, 1964.
22. Hirsch HH, Scior H, Zipf KE: Über die Pericardiotomia inferior longitudinalis (Sauerbruch) als Zugang zum Herzen für die Schrittmacher-implantation bei Morgagni-Adams-Stokes-Syndrom. *Beitr Klin Chir* 208: 446, 1964.
23. Parsonnet V, Lawrence G, Zucher IR, Assefi I, Millburn NJ: Subcostal transdiaphragmatic insertion of a cardiac pacemaker. *J Thorac Cardiovasc Surg* 49: 739, 1965.
24. Buffle P: Ventricular pacing with epigastric trans-diaphragmatic electrodes: Long-term follow-up and comparison with other implantation methods. *J Thorac Cardiovasc Surg* 72: 226, 1976.
25. Steinke W, Thomas F, Hassan Z, Mendoza R, Gear A: Subepicardial infarction, myocardial impression and ventricular penetration by sutureless electrode and leads. *Chest* 70: 80, 1976.
26. Brenner AS, Wagner GS, Anderson ST, Rosati RA, Morris JJ Jr: Transvenous, transmediastinal, and transthoracic ventricular pacing: A comparison after complete two-year follow-up. *Circulation* 49: 407, 1974.
27. Dreifus LS, Cohen D: Implanted pacemakers: Medico-legal implications. *Am J Cardiol* 36: 266, 1975.

7. ELECTRODES, LEADS AND INTERFACE PROBLEMS

MARIUSZ J. STOPCZYK

A pacemaker lead is defined as: an insulated wire connecting an electrode to a pulse generator. The electrode is an uninsulated termination of the lead which is in direct contact with the heart. The site of contact, with all its electrical and electrochemical characteristic features, and its capability of delivering electric current into the excitable cardiac structures as well as of transmitting action potentials (QRS and/or P waves) in an opposite direction to the amplifier of the pacemaker, is called the pacemaker-heart interface.

TEMPORARY VERSUS PERMANENT ELECTRODES

Temporary transvenous electrodes, usually bipolar ones, are used for diagnostic and therapeutic cardiac pacing, both atrial and ventricular. The electrode is inserted transvenously and connected to a temporary pacemaker. For atrial pacing sometimes the transoesophageal approach is used. Mechanical and electrochemical problems (materials and technology) of temporary electrodes are less critical, since the electrode is usually disposable and is used for a short time period.

The mechanical properties of the permanent lead (wire) are critical for its long-term application. There is a general opinion that the lead is now the most critical factor in the reliability of the whole implanted circuit. The present lifetime of pulse generators is 15-20 years but the electrode-lead technology limits this to 10 years.

For the *permanent transvenous electrode*, the multifilament leads consisting of several metallic ribbons wound around a flexible polyester core seem by now to be the best from the point of view of lead fracture, but their structure is less suitable for endocardial implantation. Helical coil wires with a stainless steel stylet for stiffening during insertion are used most widely for this purpose. This structure is more prone to metal fatigue and wire rupture, but a modern type of this lead with three to four parallel wires seems more reliable and more flexible and entails also the advantage of a lower electric resistance. It is obvious that any sharp kinking of the lead, usually at the site of the pacemaker connector, increases the risk of wire fracture.

The next problem of permanent electrodes, after mechanical resistance of the lead wire, is the choice of an appropriate material for the electrode itself at the tip of the lead. The electrochemical properties of the electrode-heart interface will be discussed below. It is stressed that because of polarization phenomena at the electrode surface only special materials such as platinum-iridium alloys are suitable for this purpose. The permanent *myocardial electrodes*, implanted on or in the myocardium, are usually made of the same wire as the lead but without insulation at the tip. Elgiloy, an alloy composed of six metals, is generally used as a compromise between the electrochemical and special mechanical needs.

The best biocompatible plastic material for *insulation of the lead* is silicon rubber (Silastic), commonly used nowadays since it is long-lasting material which does not harden in course of time.

BIPOLAR VERSUS UNIPOLAR ELECTRODES

The *bipolar elctrode* type, where both electrodes are in direct contact with the heart, is widely used for temporary pacing, but opinion on its applicability for permanent pacing is divided, and presently these electrodes are used almost exclusively in the United States, although their application there is now also decreasing.

The *unipolar system*, where one electrode is in direct contact with the heart and the second (indifferent) electrode is located somewhere else in the body, has several advantages: first of all for the non-heart electrode a large surface anode, which is usually the can of the pacemaker, made of titanium or stainless steel, which in view of the small current density and low resistance prevents electrochemical corrosion. The unipolar electrode is more flexible and resistant to fracture, and it has only one connector to the pacemaker. In case of interference with proper heart activity for a fixed-rate system, the risk of cardiac vulnerability is lower when unipolar pacing is used. This is due to the effect of anodal stimulation in the vulnerable period of the cardiac cycle with bipolar stimulation.

The amplitude of the cardiac potential in a unipolar system is higher and has its peak at a lower frequency, more suitable for the pacemaker circuit and for the band-pass filter construction. Finally, the analysis of the patient with a unipolar unit is simpler, since less sensitive equipment is necessary for photoanalysis or pulse monitoring.

The only disadvantage of unipolar pacing is its higher sensitivity to external interference, including muscle potentials. With the newer pacemakers protected against interference, this problem is of no practical significance. Because of the anti-interference circuit the pacemaker reverts to the fixed-rate mode in case of external interference. In my personal opinion also muscle twitching around the unipolar pacemaker is now less frequently met, due to the introduction of flat metallic can pacemakers without sharp edges and corners.

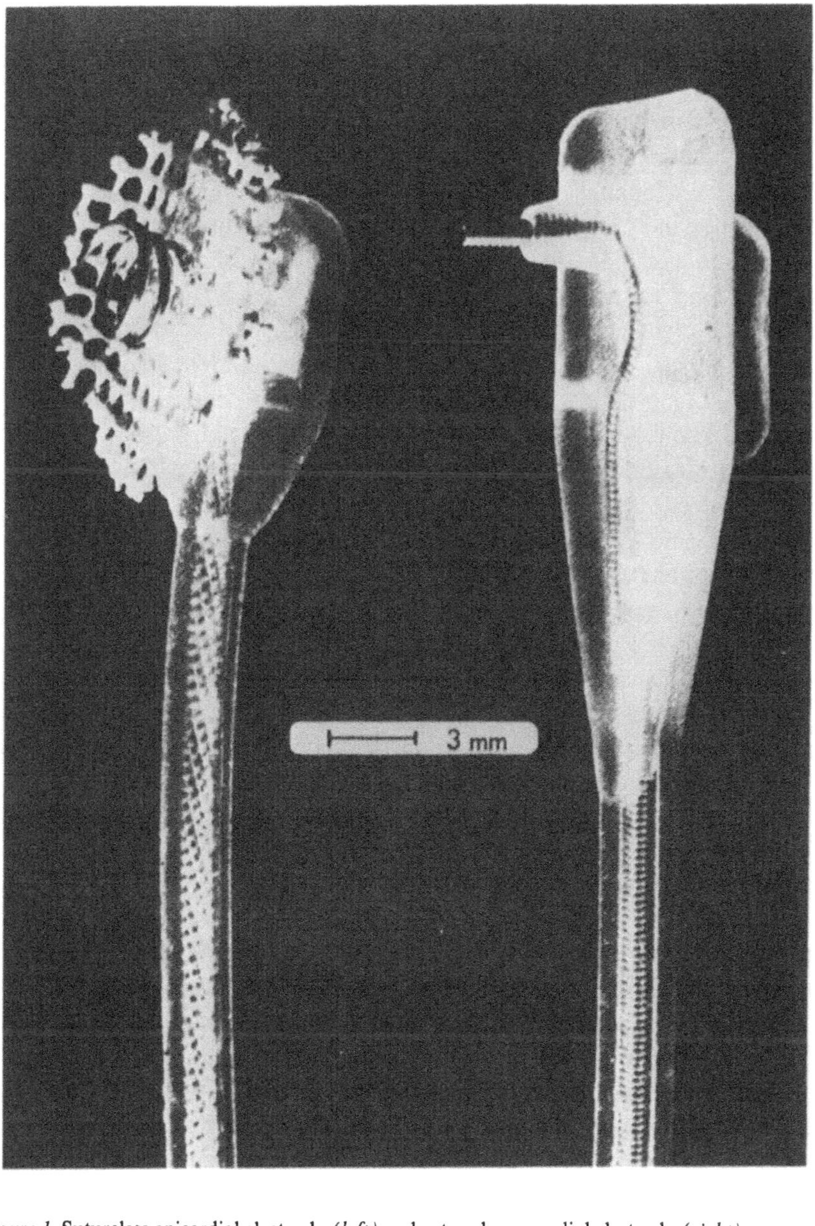

Figure 1. Sutureless epicardial electrode *(left)* and sutured myocardial electrode *(right)*.

ENDOCARDIAL VERSUS MYOCARDIAL ELECTRODES

The advantages of implantation of endocardial electrodes are now evident and commonly recognized. The use of myocardial (intramural) electrodes is acceptable only in case of cardiac operations for other reasons and in small children. This may be true also for some patients with unsuccessful trials of endocardial stimulation, although the number of such cases decreases gradually as a function of experience and progress in the technique of endocardial electrode fixation.

Corkscrew electrodes that can be implanted without a thoracotomy have been introduced and are now mostly used as myocardial leads (Figure 1 left). Endocardial fixation is the next problem; it is very important not only for diminution of electrode dislocation and more successful ventricular electrode implantation, but also in view of more widespread use of new pacemakers, requiring atrial electrodes (atrial-synchronized, sequential, bifocal, atrial-on-demand, and so on) and providing new possibilities for better treatment in more complicated arrhythmias. Several electrode types have been designed and used. Flanged-tip electrodes are widely used as a standard type; special types now include barbed (Vitatron), hooked (Biotronik), ballooned (Elema) and more recently designed electrodes with miniature corkscrew tip: sharp (Biotronik, ELA) or smooth (Vitatron Helifix). The last type seems the most promising one for the near future, especially the version with the possibility of tip rotation without stylet (Medtronic), just by means of an evenly bent lead coil wire. A J-shaped electrode of this type could be very useful for atrial fixation for which the coronary sinus lead and other types (with hooks) are unsatisfactory as yet (Figure 2).

PACEMAKER-TO-ELECTRODE CONNECTION

The pacemaker-to-electrode connection is the second interface in the whole pacing circuit. It is a difficult problem to standardize connection of the electrode to the pacemaker, in view of competition between the manufacturers. On the other hand, no type of connector is yet ideal to be introduced as standard, and further developments are expected. The most common type is a single plug secured with a screw (Medtronic, Cordis). A theoretically ideal connector should engage the lead wire without a plug, since the diameters and types of wires are very similar all over the world. An example of such a connector is the 'Dutch connection' produced by Vitatron.

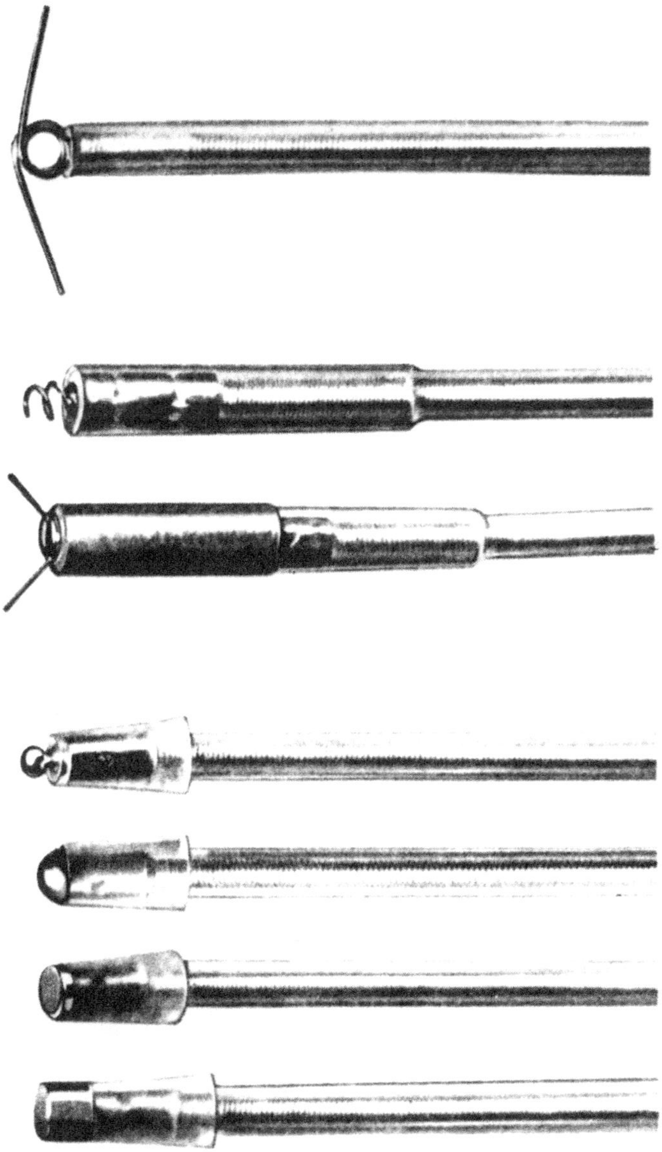

Figure 2. Different types of endocardial unipolar electrode tips. Three in the upper part of the figure: fixation by sticks, screws, and hooks.

ELECTRODE-TO-HEART INTERFACE

Electrochemical problems

Electric charge carriers differ in metals (electrode) and tissues. In metals the carriers are electrons and in tissues this function is performed by electrolyte ions. At the tissue-electrode interface a thin layer of polarized hydrogen ions is formed, the so-called Helmholtz layer, with very high capacitor properties, up to $50 \mu F/cm^2$. Parallel to this capacitor the interface has the character of a resistor (Warburg resistor), whose value depends on the frequency of the passing alternating current. The polarization voltage developing at the site of contact between the electrolyte and metal has no influence as a direct-current voltage cut off by the output capacitor of the pacemaker. This capacitor, charged slowly between pacing pulses and discharged during a pulse, is of a relatively low value

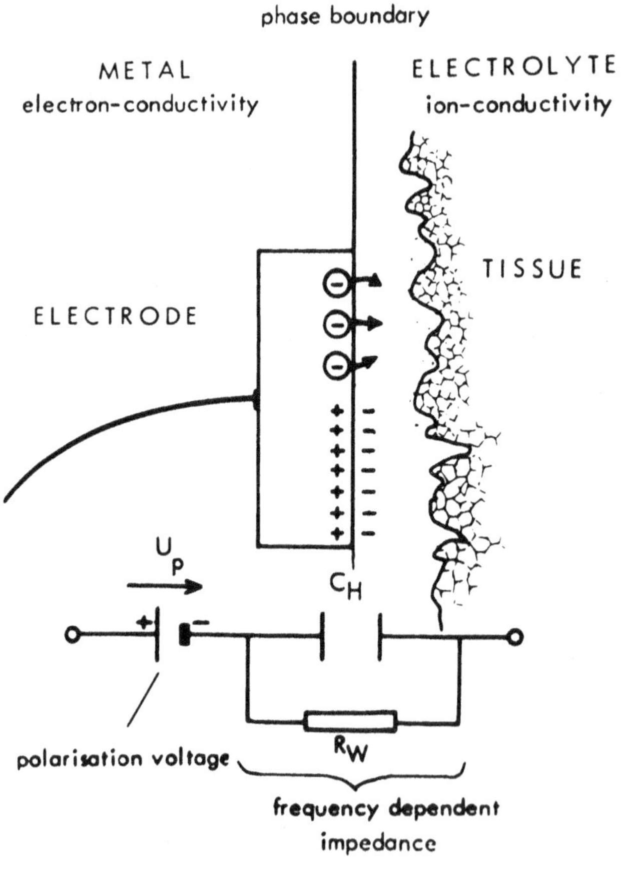

Figure 3. Electrode-tissue interface and its equivalent circuit: C_H: Helmholtz capacitance R_W: Warburg resistor; after Irnich (1).

and assures that the net charge transfer across the electrode during each cycle is equal to zero (Figure 3).

The ECG signals received from the pacing electrode are greatly disturbed by the discharge of the Helmholtz capacitor, if they occur shortly after the pacing pulse. The voltage amplitude of this capacitor discharge can even reach several millivolts, even after 50 msec, and the time constant is very similar to the slope of the QRS signal. The detection of stimulated QRS is thus very difficult and the principle of the threshold tracking pacemaker can hardly be realized. Fortunately, after a time interval corresponding to the usual refractory period of the pacemaker the discharge of the capacitor is over, although in the case of a short pacemaker refractory time, pacemaker recycling may be a problem.

Stimulation threshold

The biological effect of pacing is achieved when a propagated excitation of the cardiac chambers occurs. The minimal electric field strength necessary for producing this effect is called the energy threshold. The energy of the pulse depends on the voltage, current, and pulse width. The energy density at a given point of excitable tissue is inversely related to the square of the distance from the electrode (energy source) and the density of energy at the electrode. This means that the threshold is lower as the area of the electrode surface is smaller (to a certain value of this area, about 0.3 mm^2). Unfortunately, the impedance of the electrode rises as its size diminishes, so a necessary compromise must be reached. In view of Ohm's law this compromise means that the minimal voltage threshold is reached at the point where the benefit derived from the electrode surface reduction is counterbalanced by the impedance rise. As pointed out by Irnich et al. (1), this minimum voltage threshold is related directly to the relationship between the thickness of the nonexcitable tissue surrounding the electrode and its surface area.

Presently electrodes of about 8 mm^2 surface area and 1 kOhm impedance are regarded as optimal. The resistance of the lead may influence the threshold, as is particularly true for voltage pacemakers, and, in view of this, lead impedance must be less than 10 percent of the total electrode-lead impedance.

The current threshold is related only to the electrode area and under normal conditions met with in practice it is independent of electrode and lead impedance. The implantable pacemakers are mainly of the voltage- or current-limited type. It is obvious that during implantation not only the current threshold but also the voltage threshold must be measured.

The threshold value is particularly important at the time of electrode implantation, since it provides, together with radiological control and ECG voltage measurement (from the electrode), the most important information about electrode fixation. The absolute threshold value for any particular electrode is important, as well as the difference between the first capture beat and the full effectiveness of pacing. This must be of the same order when good fixation is achieved.

During the first two weeks after implantation the threshold is rising because of fibrotic tissue growth around the electrode. There is no direct relationship between the initial and the later threshold value. This is the reason why the value of the acute threshold is of little importance for the later treatment of the patient, and why presently this value has been excluded from the data in the patient card. After a small decrease of the threshold in the third week it remains stable with a well-known twenty-percent range of changes caused by physical activity and so on (Figure 4).

A rise of the threshold above the available energy of the pacemaker pulse is called exit block. This phenomenon appears as loss of capture and is at first incomplete, with effective pulses situated in the hyperexcitability period just after the T wave of the spontaneous beat, before complete block develops. If

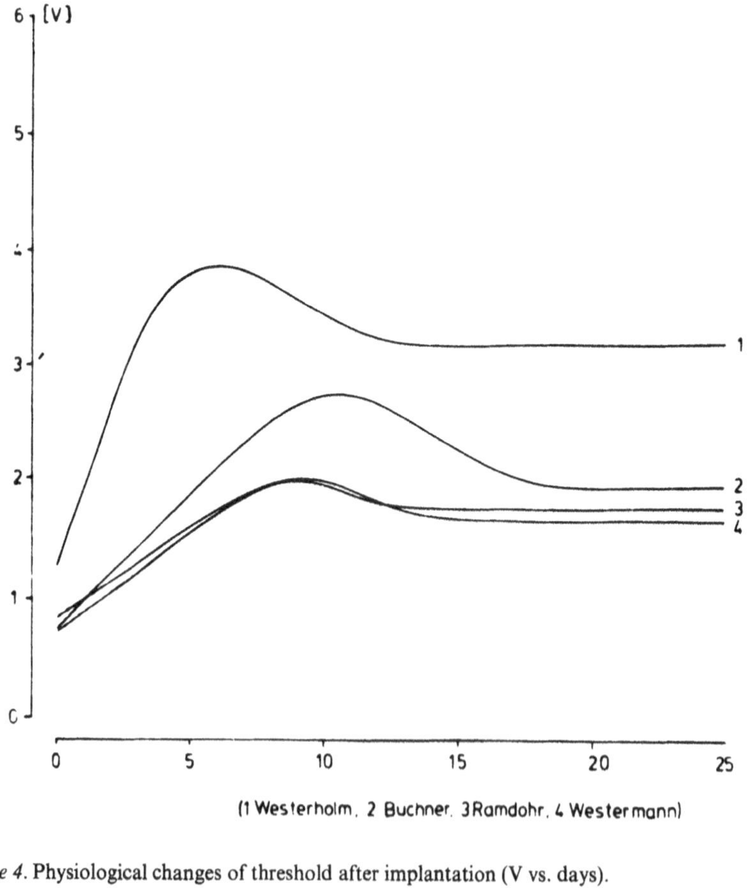

Figure 4. Physiological changes of threshold after implantation (V vs. days).

pharmacological treatment with steroids and potassium is insufficient a new electrode must be inserted. Fortunately, exit block is presently very infrequent in cases treated with endocardial electrodes.

A sudden rise of threshold can be observed if acute coronary ischaemia develops at the site of electrode insertion. We have observed such a case in which the pacemaker had to be removed and replaced with a higher-energy unit. After one year, during which scar formation in the myocardium has been completed, it could be replaced with a low-output pacemaker. We were also able to confirm in animal experiments the appearance of a transient but very high threshold rise during brief reversible coronary ischaemia (2). This mechanism can certainly explain some cases of sudden death of pacemaker patients with coronary artery disease.

ENDOCARDIAL ELECTROGRAMS

The last feature of electrodes is their use as catheter leads, transmitting spontaneous cardiac activity to the amplifier of the pacemaker. The lead/electrode and amplifier/input impendance ratio is essential information for this purpose. To spare the voltage amplitude of the ECG a high input impedance and low lead impedance with a coefficient as high as 10:1 is needed, and this need is met in modern pacemakers. The electrode/lead resistance and capacitance act as a band-pass filter influencing the actual frequency range of the intracardial ECG signals. This is taken into consideration in the construction of the pacemaker circuit. During implantation the electrograms taken by the inserted electrode must have an amplitude of about 5-10 mv, at least, and slew rate (*dv*/*dt*) of about 1-3 v/s but not below 0.5 v/s. A unipolar electrogram has a greater amplitude but a slightly lower slew rate than a bipolar electrogram. The shape of the QRS complex is usually qrS, qRS or qR..

In case of electromagnetic interference (EMI) the electrode acts as an antenna, and the metal shielding of the pacemaker circuit may be insufficient to protect against EMI inhibition. To prevent this inhibition a special HF filter is now provided in several pacemakers at the input of the electrode. Atrial potentials are usually of smaller amplitude, even with stable electrode position. The input of an atrial pacemaker (atrial-triggered, atrial-inhibited, bifocal) is usually more sensitive (up to 0.5 mv).

REFERENCES

1. Irnich W, Mindt W, Schaldach M, Hurzler Ph, De Caprio V, Furman S: Stimulation electrodes. In: *Advances in pacemaker technology*, (Schaldach M, Furman S, (eds), Berlin, Springer, 1975, ch. 4.
2. Pieniak M, Zochowski J, Stopczyk M: Rising threshold of electrical stimulation in ischemic areas of the heart. Proc. 4th Int. Symp. on Cardiac pacing (Thalen, H.J.Th. ed.) Van Gorcum, Assen, 1973.

8. PACEMAKER TECHNOLOGY

DAVID L. BOWERS

1. INTRODUCTION

Since the implantation of the first pacemaker in 1959 the pacemaker circuitry has increased in complexity and the trend will continue. There are many reasons why the pulse generator circuits became more complex: among others, there was a need to adapt the generator to heart demands (demand pacemaker), provide for functional adjustment (programmable pacemakers with rate adjustment) and achieve greater circuit efficiency which extends generator life.

The various techniques used for construction of the pacemaker circuit and the package systems applied to adapt the circuit for implantation in the human body will be discussed.

2. CIRCUIT STRUCTURE AND CONSTRUCTION

2.1. Discrete circuits

Early pacemaker electronics were simple in design and easy to construct. Electronic assemblies were constructed using individual or discrete components such as resistors, capacitors, diodes, transistors, reed switches and inductor coils. The type of circuit structure used to mount and electrically interconnect the discrete circuit components was one of two structures; a printed circuit board (PCB) with an electrical conductor pattern etched on the board surface with components mounted on the PCB surface, or strung between two PCB's. The latter circuit construction method is referred to as 'cordwood construction' and provides the best component to volume density ratio of the two construction methods. Because the circuit assembly and components were encapsulated in epoxy, certain design constraints were required to prevent cracking or mechanical stress to components during the epoxy curing phase. Fragile components like glass diodes

This chapter is compiled from a contribution of the author in 'Pacemaker Technology' (edited by Hilbert J.Th. Thalen and Jozef Cywinski) and is to be published by Martinus Nijhoff Medical Division, The Hague, 1980.

and reed switches were carefully mounted to the PCB relieving mechanical stress on the component leads, and in some cases extra protection was required to relieve stress by applying silicone rubber around the component.

Various circuit construction techniques were developed to reduce the affects of electrolyte migration and free-ion contamination from coming in contact and affecting circuit components and the electrical interconnect pattern. One unique technique was to completely eliminate the printed circuit board and support the components with an electrical conductor interconnect pattern. The purpose for this type of free-space construction is to use the conductor elements to support the components and therefore eliminate any interaction due to electrical impedance shunts between the components and the conductor paths (Figure 1).

2.2. *Hybrid circuits*

The evolution in circuit construction followed closely the evolution in pulse generator packaging. A wider variety of circuit construction techniques became available when the electronics was placed in a hermetic or controlled environment and not subjected to the non-hermetic environment associated with epoxy pulse generators. One advance construction technique suitable for pacemaker application is the 'hybrid' circuit. A hybrid circuit can be defined as a circuit structure which combines various technologies to form a complete electronic circuit. For example, in hybrid construction thick-film technology is used to make circuit resistors combined with semiconductor technology to form active devices like transistors. This combination of technologies to form a hybrid circuit is an effective technique to construct high density and sophisticated pacemaker circuits.

Figure 2 shows various hybrid circuits comprising the electronic section for a fixed rate or asynchronous pacemaker. The circuit illustrates the relative size of various electrical components and the type of layout pattern used to electrically interconnect the components. A thick-film process is used to construct this circuit and is the preferred process for producing today's pacemaker electronics.

Here is a simplified description on how a thick-film hybrid circuit is produced. The circuit components (resistors, capacitors, inductors, transistors and diodes) are either attached or printed on a thin wafer-like structure called a substrate. The substrate is a diaelectric or nonconductive sheet material, usually made of alumina, used to support circuit components in similar fashion as a printed circuitboard (PCB) supports discrete components but on a much smaller scale (approximate 1/5 PCB area).

The first process is to print a conductor pattern on the substrate surface using gold or a conductive ink. The printing technique for the conductor pattern and the following steps for thick-film resistors are similar to the old art of silk screening where the pattern is printed through an exposed portion of a fine wire

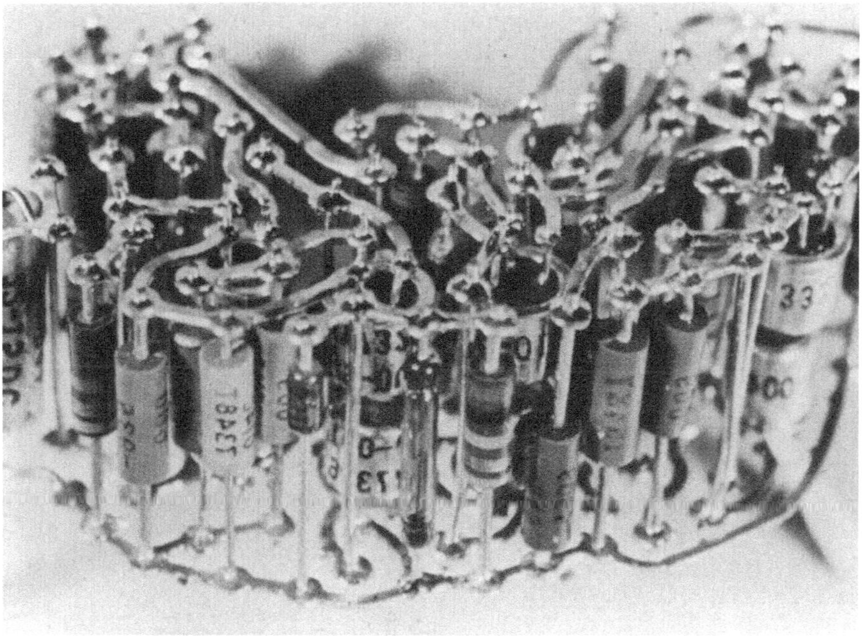

Figure 1. Early pacemaker circuit assembled with standard components. (Courtesy Medtronic)

mesh screen. After each printing step or cycle the substrate and pattern are cured in an oven at elevated temperature.

The next processing step is to print the circuit resistive elements. To print all the various resistor values comprising a hybrid circuit may require one or more printing cycles where each cycle uses a different resistive ink (ohms per square) to make a wide selection of resistor values. The value of a thick-film resistor for a particular resistive ink is determined by its dimensional physical shape. When all the resistors are printed and cured, the next step is to electronically measure and trim the resistors to a given value.

After the trimming process is completed the remaining circuit components are mounted to the substrate. The terminals of the chip capacitors are either soldered or attached using a conductive epoxy to the gold conductor pattern. The semiconductor chips (transistor, diodes and integrated circuits) are epoxied to the substrate and then small conductor wires, about one-half the diameter of a human hair, are connected (bonded) between the appropriate terminal pads on the semiconductor chip and the substrate conductor pattern. In some cases the semiconductor devices are directly attached to the substrate conductor pattern, without wires, referred to as beam-lead bonding.

At this stage the circuit can be functionally tested and dynamically trimmed to

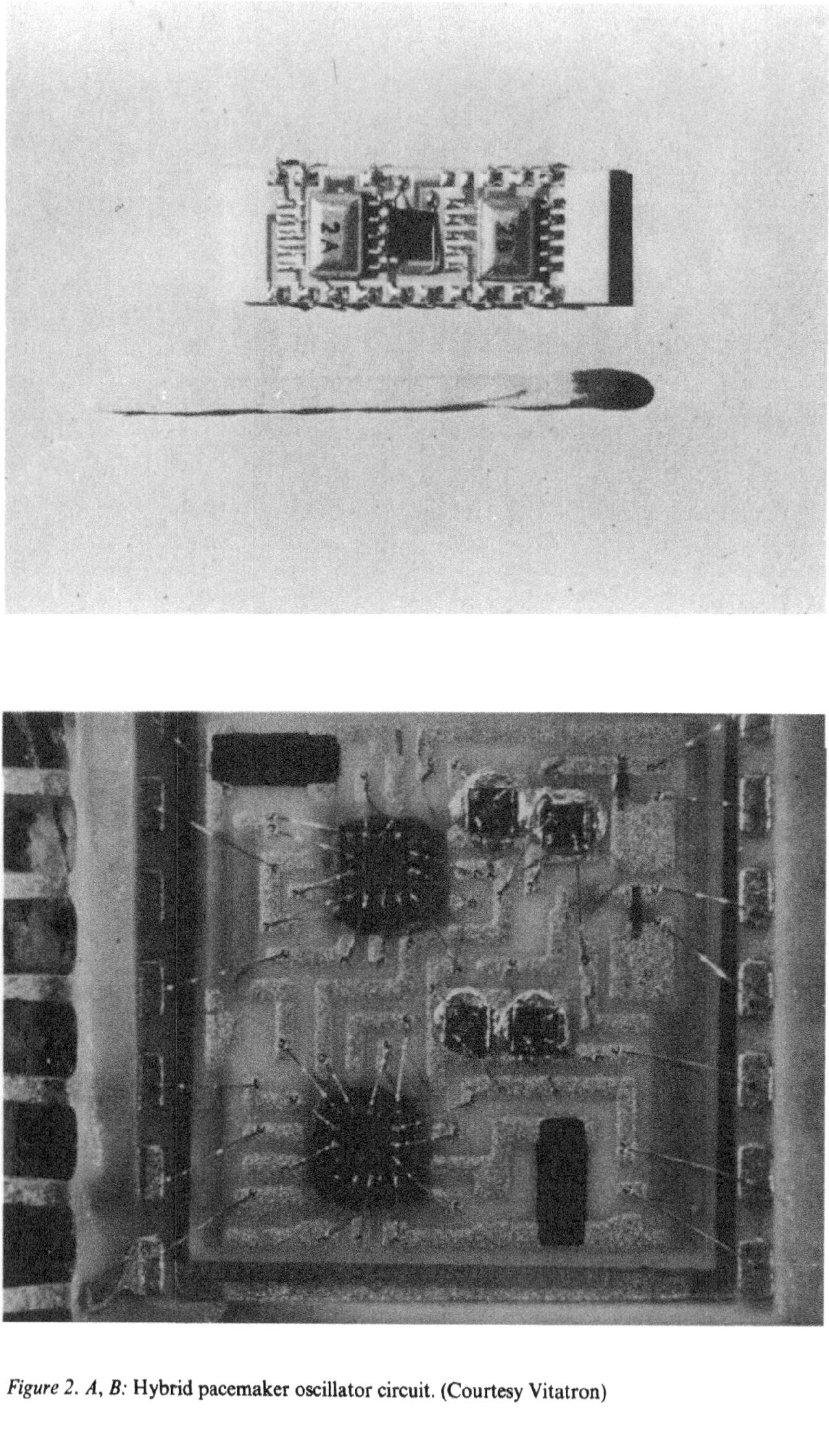

Figure 2. A, B: Hybrid pacemaker oscillator circuit. (Courtesy Vitatron)

meet selected design specification. Throughout the manufacturing process the hybrid circuit is subjected to many rigorous tests and inspections to insure circuit quality and reliability. The final process step is to mount the substrate in a package and make the package hermetic.

Another process used to construct pacemaker hybrid circuits is the thin-film or monolithic process where the entire pacer electronics are contained on or within (diffused into the material) a thin wafer sheet similar to a thick-film substrate. In the thin-film process the resistors and conductors as well as capacitors are vapor deposited on the thin diaelectric wafer instead of printing the resistors and conductors on the substrate as done in thick-film processing. Simply stated, the difference between thick-film and thin-film hybrid circuits is the methods used to construct the components; in thick-film the components are printed on the substrate while in a thin-film process the components are vapor deposited onto the base material. If the base substrate material is a silicon wafer, transistors, diodes and other semi conductor devices can be diffused into the silicon material producing all the active components while vapor deposition on the material surface can produce the passive components and the electrical interconnection pattern. In some cases the resistors are also diffused in the silicon base material. Therefore, the thin-film plus the diffusion processes have the potential of placing the entire circuit, including active (semiconductors) and passive (resistors and capacitors) components on one silicon chip. This single monolithic chip circuit enables reduction of the size of the pacemaker electronics over the hybrid circuit, and therefore reduction of the entire pacemaker package size

2.3. *Epoxy-encapsulated pulse generator*

The pulse generators built in the 1960's and the first part of the 1970's were powered by mercury-oxide zinc (HgO Zn) batteries. The HgO Zn battery is not a hermetic or totally sealed package but contains a pressure vent allowing hydrogen (H_2) gas and occasionally liquid electrolyte (Na OH) to escape when the internal pressure exceeds the sealing pressure of the vent. Therefore, a package material had to be selected which would easily pass hydrogen gas but contain the escaped electrolyte fluid. The package material selected to pass hydrogen gas and contain the electrolyte was a polymer epoxy resin. The epoxy resin was relatively inert and body compatible and provided a good and rugged mechanical structure which firmly retained the electronic and battery assembly. Package size and shape are also important especially for a foreign object such as a pacemaker implanted in the body. The pulse generator should conform to body tissue and contain no sharp edges or protrusions which would cause skin erosion or tissue trauma. With the use of epoxy material it was easy to mold the pulse generator package into any shape having rounded corners and a smooth conforming surface. Unfortunately pulse generator package shape is not solely dependent on physiological considerations but determined by the size and shape of technical components such as the power source and electronics.

2.4. Hermetically-sealed pulse generator

In a total hermetic pacemaker, the electronics and power source are sealed into a controlled environment and designed to retain this environment for the design life of the pulse generator. An advantage for a controlled environment is that it makes possible the use of advanced electronic circuits such as thick or thin film hybrids and special semiconductor devices which were impossible to use in an epoxy encapsulated device. The term 'hermetic' implies that the control environment within a sealed package is gas-tight as well as fluid-light and will not be influenced by the gas or fluid environment outside the package. To achieve this isolation between the inside and outside environments requires the use of a metallic package or can. Hermetic feedthrough devices are one of the critical components used for the purpose of making electrical connection through the metallic can between the inside electronics and the outside world.

The electronics and power source are mechanically supported in the metallic can and are electrically connected together. If the metallic can is used as the indifferent electrode, it is electrically connected to the electronics. The can material selected for pacemaker application should have the following properties:

1. Compatible with body tissues
2. Non-corrosive and non-toxic
3. Easy to form into a pacemaker package
4. Easy to seal, retaining the controlled or hermetic environment

Some of the selected materials used for can construction are titanium, stainless steel and special alloys such as Haynes 25R. Besides the selection of the can material, it is also important to properly prepare the metallic surface, especially if it is to be in contact with body tissue. The reason for surface preparation is to remove any foreign or residual material which may have contaminated the basic material during the forming and manufacturing process. In some pacemaker applications where the metallic can is not used as one of the electrode surfaces, it is covered with thin electrical insulated coating such as silicone rubber or a thin coating of epoxy resin.

The controlled or inert environment in the hermetic package should not be altered during the operating life of the pulse generator, at least not for its intended design life. If the environment is altered, it should not change pacemaker performance either in function or longevity. To achieve a stable environment in the can requires careful processing of the can assembly during manufacturing. It is important to eliminate moisture from inside the can which may be retained on the can inner surface, the electronics and power source assemblies. A procedure used to remove moisture and other gas contaminates from the can is to bake-out the unsealed can assembly in vacuum at elevated temperature. After the vacuum bake-out procedure, the can assembly is then back filled with a dry inert gas or mixture such as nitrogen, argon or helium. Keeping the can assembly in the dry inert environment, the next procedure is to properly seal the can making it hermetic.

The sealing procedure is a critical process. Various welding methods are used to close the package without altering the enclosed environment or affecting the non-corrosive property of the can material. The welding methods range from the sophisticated electron-beam and laser welders to simple resistive and electrode welding equipment. The type of welding method selected will depend on the can material, size and shape of the can, and production quantities. Regardless of the type of welding method selected, the welded can must retain hermeticity under chemical attack and high mechanical stress.

One of the important steps in the manufacturing process is to test and verify that the sealed can is truly hermetic. The test methods normally used are designed to check for both large and small cracks or holes in the can assembly. A gross-leak test procedure using the Freon bubble method is designed to check for large holes with gas leakage rates between 10^{-2} to 10^{-5} cubic centimeters per second. The fine-leak test procedure uses a helium gas mixture in the controlled environment, testing for a low-leakage rate from 10^{-4} to 10^{-10} standard cubic centimeters of helium per second per atmosphere. A technical guideline for the maximum leak-rate for a generator hermetic can which will have minimum influence on the controlled environment, is a leak-rate less than 1×10^{-8} std cm^3 of He per sec per atm. Yes, it is a very low leak-rate but necessary if the pulse generator is to retain its controlled environment over a 10 to 15 year operating life.

In addition to all the test precautions in verifying package or can hermeticity, it is equally important to make sure the components used inside the can do not alter the controlled environment. Therefore, the power source selected for use in a hermetic package is either a self-contained hermetic battery system or one designed not to evolve gas or leak electrolyte. The cleaning and handling procedures for the electronics used in a total hermetic package are similar for the electronics encapsulated in epoxy resin. One major advantage in placing the electronics in a dry and moisture free environment is to eliminate the effects of residual surface ion contamination from altering circuit performance.

The total hermetic pulse generator having the electronics and power source sealed in a stable and controlled environment will give the pacemaker circuitry and battery the best conditions to achieve realistic longevity, an important feature if we are to design 10 to 20 year pacemaker systems without having to wait 10 or 20 years to verify system performance.

These modern techniques have enabled the construction of long lasting pacemakers that fulfill one of the goals set in early days of pacing: 'the life-time pacemaker'. They also enable the development of sophisticated automatic or external adjustable pacemakers that will not only improve the quantity but also the quality of the patient's life.

9. ENERGY SOURCES

WILSON GREATBATCH

The groundwork for pacemaking was laid in 1932 when Hyman reported a hand-cranked generator set which successfully stimulated a heart (1). Zoll, in 1952, poineered the first clinical pacemaker with an external device which stimulated the heart with 150-volt pulses delivered transcutaneously through the closed chest wall (2). Zoll's device was very painful and resulted in severe skin damage under the cutaneous electrodes. Few patients could endure treatment more than a few days. Nevertheless, Zoll's remarkable device saved countless lives and remained in extensive clinical use for many years.

From 1957 to 1960, five timely developments foretold the shape of a subsequent decade of pacemaking. First, Weirich et al. placed stimulating electrodes directly on the exposed epicardium (3). Then Bakken designed a hand-held transistorized stimulator to drive the epicardial electrodes at an energy level many orders of magnitude below that of Zoll's device and far below any level of pain sensation (4). Next, Furman and Robinson reported clinical stimulation of a human heart with a temporary endocardial catheter, driven by a hand-held stimulator of Bakken's design (5). Furman's concept anticipated the transvenous approach to pacemaking, which is widely accepted today. Then Abram in England made an important contribution with a completely implanted passive stimulator, with epicardial electrodes and a coil loop driven by induction from outside the body (6). Lastly, the first cardiac pacemaker was implanted in an experimental animal by our group on 7 May 1958 (7).

We believe that the first successful long-term clinical implant took place in Buffalo on 6 June 1960 and was reported by our group later that year (8). This device operated without incident for 18 months, after which it was surgically replaced.

A prior clinical implant was reported by Senning in Sweden (9), but this unit worked only a few hours (10) and Senning later recommended abandonment of the procedure (11).

Our VOO asynchronous device consisted of a simple two-transistor, transformer feedback blocking oscillator, powered by a battery of ten Mallory RM1 zinc-mercury cells. This cell was a modification of the original Rubin zinc-mercury battery developed for Second World War military use.

Weirich's original electrodes were simply pieces of surgical stainless steel wire,

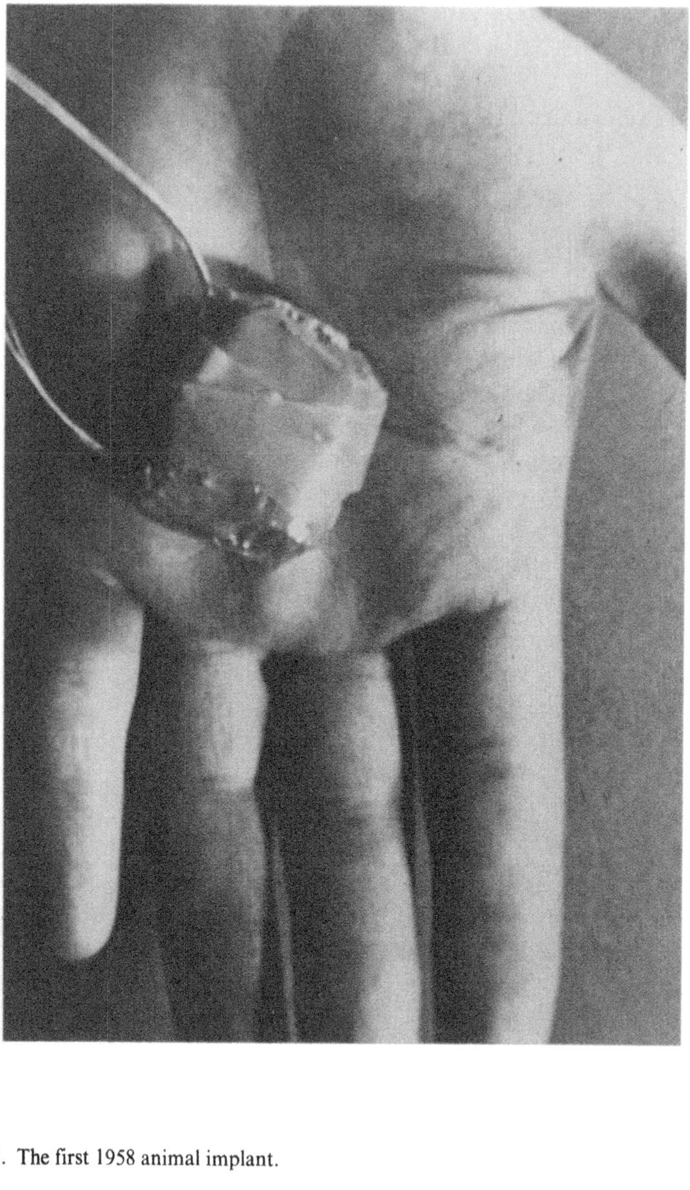

Figure 1. The first 1958 animal implant.

sewn into the myocardium. Hunter et al. later combined these into a silicone patch containing two stainless-steel bipolar pins (12). We used these in our initial clinical implants. Anodal corrosion proved to be a formidable problem on the positive pin and on the positive wire. Chardack then introduced his spring-coil platinum-iridium myocardial electrode (13) and later adapted this design to a permanent transvenous catheter (14). Chardack's catheter eliminated the need for a thoracotomy with its attendant prognosis of ten percent early mortality.

Within five years the implantable cardiac pacemaker had become universally accepted as the treatment of choice for complete heart block, and in May 1965, Dr. William Chardack was able to host a worldwide symposium in Buffalo on cardiac pacemaking. Lagegren for one, was able to present a total of 305 cases reported from five European centres (10).

At about this same time, our group introduced the implantable VVI (R-wave-inhibited) pacemaker into clinical practice (15).

THE RUBIN-MALLORY ZINC-MERCURY BATTERY

Nearly all early pacemakers depended on the Rubin-Mallory zinc-mercury battery. The original cell used an aqueous potassium hydroxide electrolyte. The medical cell used a less active sodium hydroxide system. A small amount of manganese dioxide was added to inhibit internal self-discharge in storage prior to use. Later, silver was added to the mix, to amalgamate with the liquid mercury that evolved as the cell was discharged. A very rigid quality control program was used on the medical cell production line. Although it was eventually superseded in the seventies by other more reliable systems, we must not forget that it was this cell that made pacemaking possible. It quickly became the industry standard and remained so for some fifteen years.

X-RAY ANALYSIS OF BATTERIES

In earlier years there was no way to evaluate the condition of zinc-mercury batteries non-destructively. It was the practice of the military to take a sample from their warehouse stocks, destructively analyze the sample, and then decide on the disposition of the stock from this sample. In 1963, during a visit to the Mallory factory in North Tarrytown, New York, I saw an X-ray of a flashlight battery that had been sent from England. All the internal parts were clearly discernible. I asked if X-ray might not tell something about the condition of zinc-mercury cells and was told that it could not, that cell exhaustion did not change the X-ray picture.

I found this hard to believe and upon returning home, I discharged a number

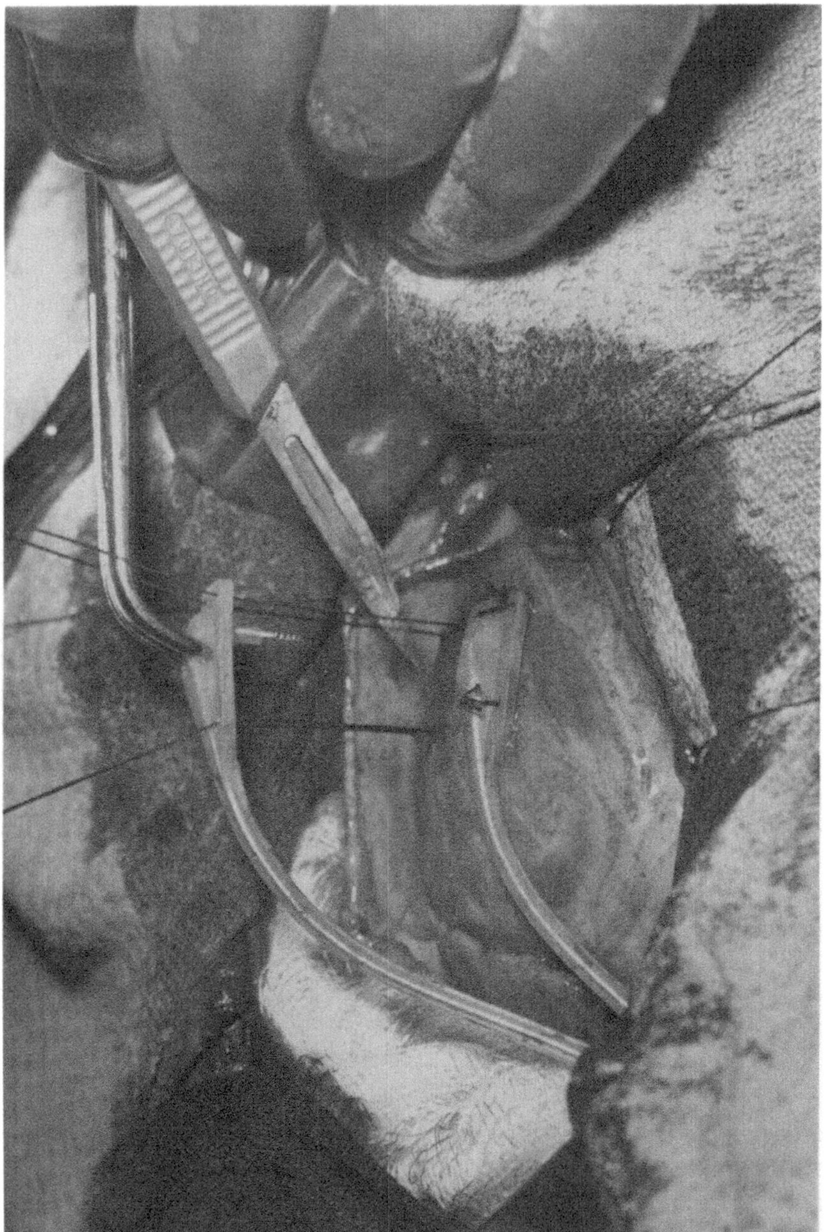

Figure 2. Early Chardack spring-coil electrodes (Ref. 13, 14).

of RM1 cells to 10, 30, 50, and 100 percent exhaustion. I had them X-rayed at a local foundry that used an X-ray machine to look for hairline cracks in castings. I found that a new cell showed a crisp, clear delineation of the anode and cathode structures. At 10 percent discharge, the edges became noticeably fuzzy. At 30 percent discharge, the exhaustion residues had obliterated the first of two annular rings between anode and cathode. These rings were undoubtedly due to some structural discontinuity in the metal case. At 50 percent discharge, both rings were obliterated. At 100 percent charge, most of the area between the anode and cathode was quite opaque and drops of liquid mercury could be seen in the hollow zinc anode.

We published these findings (16) and this method of cell analysis then became a standard procedure for most of the pacemaker manufacturers.

Naturally, we tried the same methods on our lithium batteries, but we were disappointed by our findings. We did find that any problem with structural faults in the lithium cells and, in particular, any leakage of iodine between insulator structures could be detected. Thus, we have continued to X-ray each battery at least once during manufacture and continue to depend on X-ray for data prior to destructive failure analysis. It would appear, however, that the microcalorimeter is a more useful tool with lithium batteries.

From manufacturer's data we had calculated a probably battery life of five years but by 1970 Furman reported an average pulse generator lifetime of only two years with most clinical explants being necessitated by premature failure of the battery (17). Several mechanisms contribute to this problem. The electrolyte is sodium hydroxide, which is very corrosive. It attacks the separator and the zinc anode. The separator itself is one or more layers of webril, an organic material which is not invulnerable. Zinc oxide tends to migrate through the cell, forming conductive paths which drain it. Liquid mercury forms dendrites which also create shorting paths. Side reactions inevitably generate hydrogen gas which normally rises to pressures of 300 p.s.i. innocuously vents through the neoprene seals, then through the epoxy pacemaker structure, and into the body. Such cells cannot be hermetically sealed and pacemakers containing them can be hermetically sealed only by going to engineering extremes that we ourselves find unacceptable.

Thus, it became clear that the zinc-mercury battery was the limiting factor in pacemaker reliability and little improvement could be expected until we had better batteries. This search for a better battery took three directions: nuclear batteries, rechargeable batteries, and new high-performance chemical cells.

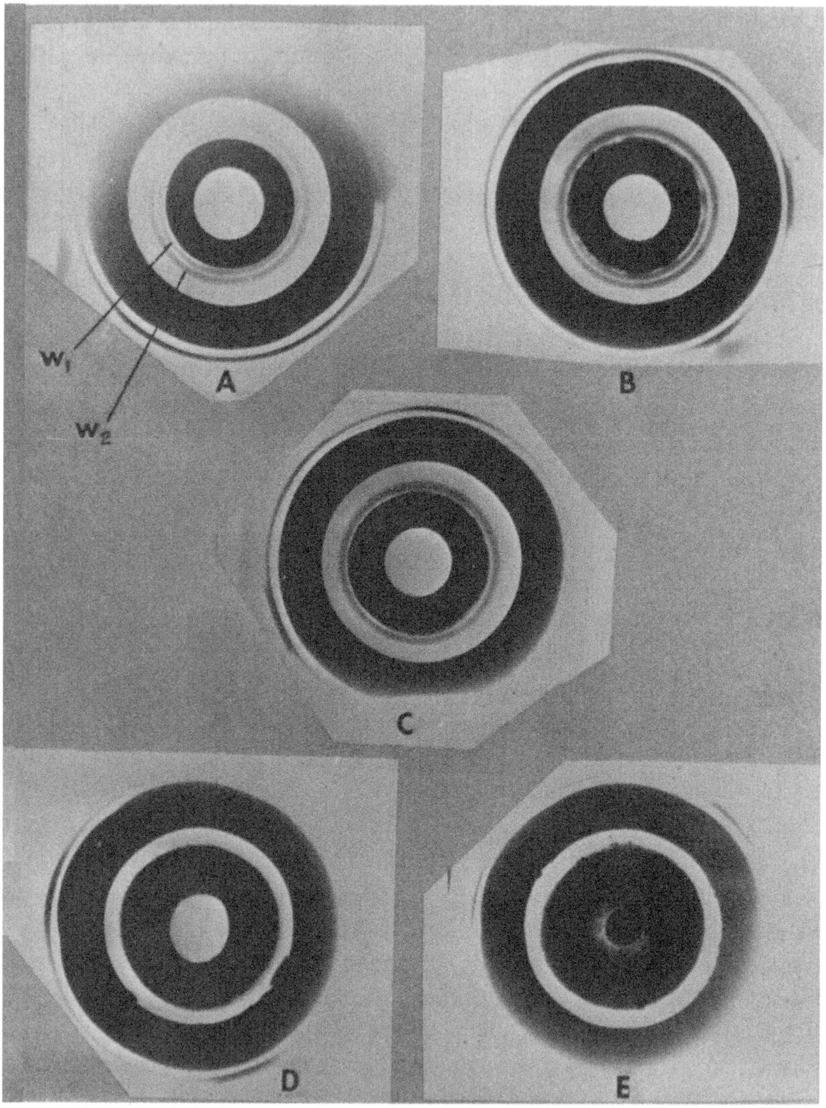

Figure 3. X-ray views of new and fully discharged mercury cells (Ref. 15).

ANODE	$Zn + 2\,(OH)^- \rightarrow Zn\,(OH)_2 + 2e^-$
CATHODE	$HgO + H_2O + 2e^- \rightarrow Hg + 2\,(OH)^-$
COMBINED	$Zn + HgO + H_2O \rightarrow Hg + Zn\,(OH)_2$

Figure 4. Zinc-mercury cell reactions.

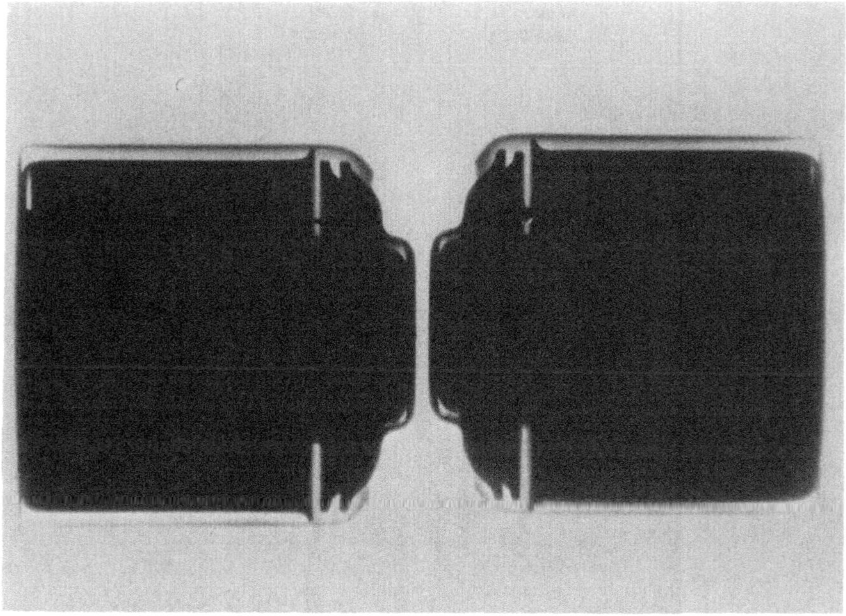

Figure 5. Mercury dendrites in falied RM1 zinc-mercury cells (x-ray photo).

NUCLEAR BATTERIES

The source of all terrestrial energy is the sun and it is only natural that man would try to emulate the atomic processes by which the sun warms us. Nuclear energy can be obtained in three ways, by fission as in the A-bomb, by fusion as in the H-bomb, and by nuclear decay. The energy inherent in an element is a function of its position in the atomic table. Very light elements like hydrogen have enormous energy. Mid-table elements have much lower energy. Very heavy elements like plutonium and uranium have again high energy, but much lower that that of hydrogen.

The splitting of a plutonium atom into elements of smaller atomic number releases a great deal of energy. The A-bomb and our nuclear power generating plants operate on this basis. The joining of two hydrogen atoms into a helium atom releases much more energy, but to date no means has been found to contain this reaction into a continuous process. In fact, it requires the energy of an A-bomb to force the two hydrogen atoms into close enough proximity to trigger the fusion reaction into a H-bomb explosion. Of the three mechanisms, the only one suitable for pacemakers is the decay reaction. Three isotopes have been

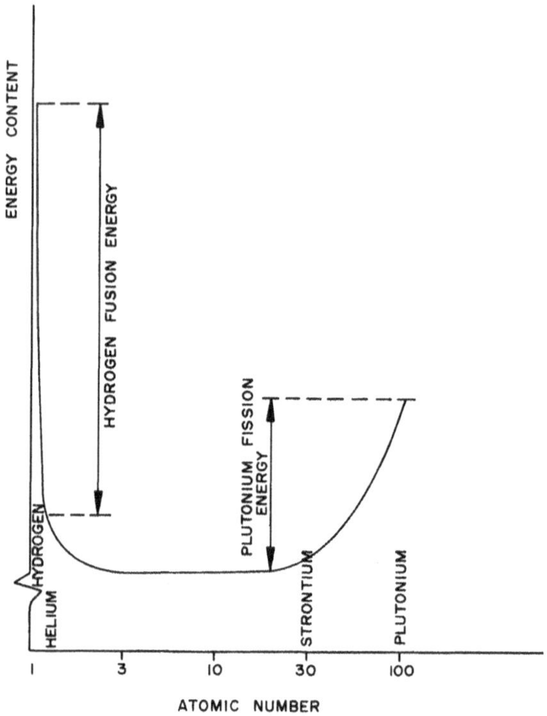

Figure 6. Energy vs. Atomic number of nucleides.

considered and/or used for powering pacemakers. These are the decay of plutonium 238, promethium 147 and tritium (H^3).

Promethium 147 is a beta (electron) emitter with a half-life of 2.7 years. High-velocity electrons are emitted which impact on a photosensitive surface where current is generated. Since current must flow from within the primary containment, a hermetic feed-through connector must be provided. This inevitably weakens the primary containment structure and represents a major disadvantage of the system. The other major disadvantage is the short half-life of the isotope. To achieve a ten-year power supply, much more promethium must be provided than would be needed to supply sufficient current for the pacemaker initially. Since all radioactive isotopic pacemakers have some nuclear leakage, this extra fuel means unwanted radiation. These factors led to rather early abandonment of the promethium system, although a number of such pacemakers were clinically used in Europe (18). The promethium pacemaker is not competitive with the plutonium types, but rather with long-life chemical systems, which have now eclipsed it.

Plutonium 238 is an alpha (helium ion) emitter. Its high-velocity ions impact on the container wall and generate heat. The heat is converted into electric energy by means of thermopiles, either of dissimilar metals or of dissimilar doping of a

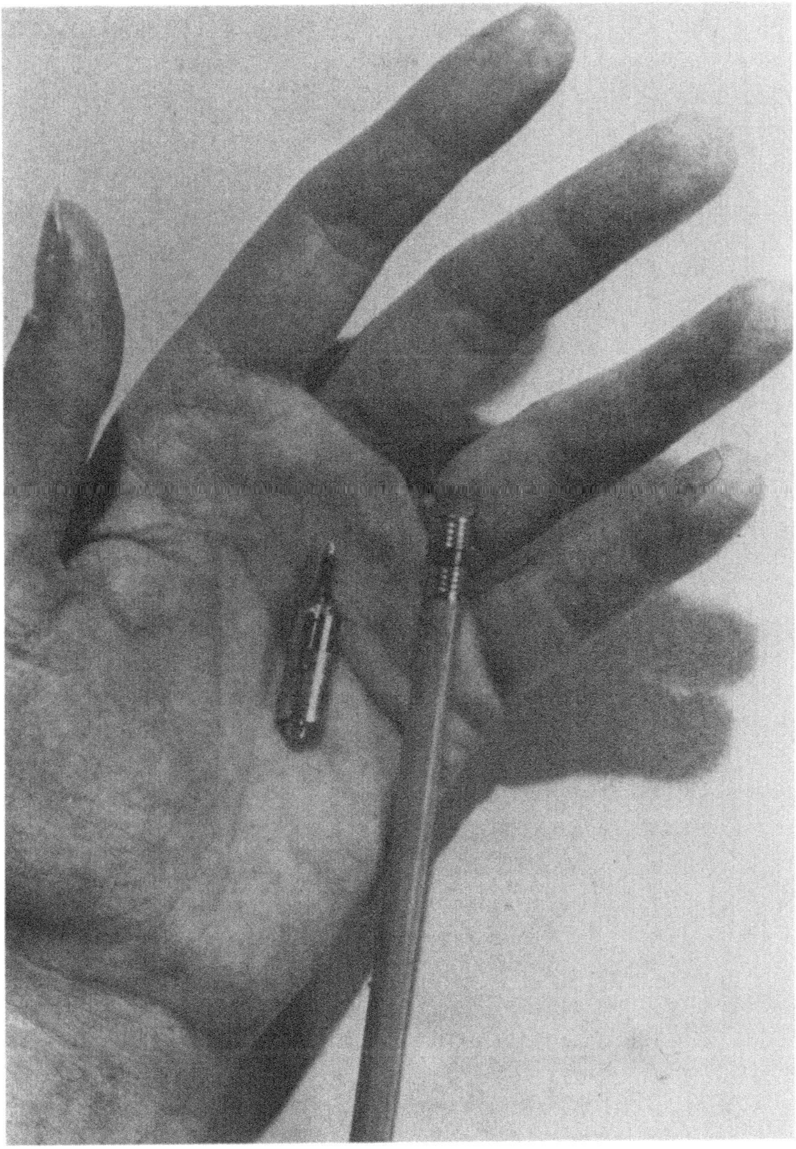

Figure 7. Endocardial catheter Pm^{147} nuclear pacemaker (Ref. 18).

semiconductor such as bismuth telluride. Nuclear pacemakers today exclusively use plutonium 238 (19, 20, 21), usually as an oxide. The fact that the energy output of the isotope is heat eliminates the need of an electrical feed-through insulator through the primary fuel containment. This eases the containment design problem. The primary technical disadvantage of plutonium 238 is its excessively long half-life of 87 years, which means that a lost pacemaker could be a serious hazard a millennium later. Thus severe regulatory government control is exerted to insure that no device is ever lost.

Lastly, tritium (H^3) has been considered by us and others (22). Its half-life of 13 years is ideal but the low specific energy (only 17 KeV), which makes it so safe,

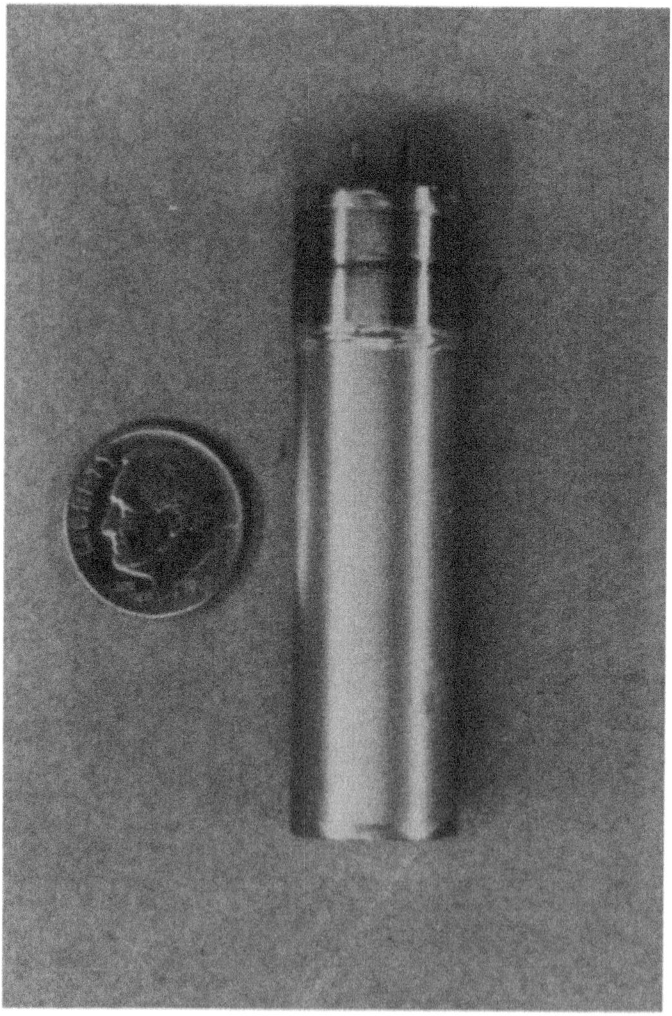

Figure 8. Pu^{238} 'Atomcell'. Courtesy Hittman Corp.

at the same time introduces thermical energy conversion problems which have never been solved.

We believe that nuclear pacemakers are safe, efficacious and cost-effective, but the regulatory compliance aspects have been so severe that few physicians will bear them. Thus, the nuclear pacemaker has never achieved more than a fraction of one percent of the world pacemaker market.

RECHARGEABLE BATTERIES

Sennings's first implant in 1958 used a rechargeable nickel-cadmium battery (a). This system proved unsatisfactory and it was soon abandoned. Since that time, each year has produced at least one or two papers purporting to solve the problems inherent in this philosophically attractive approach. Two questions must be answered. Is the lifetime of the battery as good, with recharging, as the lifetime of a comparable primary battery, without recharging? Second, is it medically acceptable to both physician and patient to give the patient controls of the recharging function? The answer to *both* questions must be yes if the rechargeable system is to be usable. It was not until the early seventies that a serious challange appeared from the proponents of rechargeable systems. Fischell et al., at John Hopkins University, reported the adaptation of an aerospace nickel-cadmium rechargeable battery to clinical pacemaker use (23). Furman (personal communication, 1977) disapproved the treatment concept, but others disagreed with him. The present author has not yet seen sufficient clinical data to answer the question of the battery's technical adequacy, but the clinical aspect has probably been answered in the negative since this system too has never achieved more than a fraction of one percent of the pacemaker market.

LITHIUM BATTERIES

The third area of battery development was in new high-performance lithium cells. These are all alkali-halogen systems. Lithium is the most active of the alkali metals: it is rather easily handled and all the new pacemaker battery systems use it. The new systems differ from each other principally in their halogen cathodes and the way in which the halogen is used.

The first to appear (24), and by far the most used today is the lithium iodine system which was introduced into pacemaker work by our group (25) in 1971. The cell reactions are:

$$Li \rightarrow Li^+ + e^-$$
$$I^2 + 2e^- \rightarrow 2I^-$$

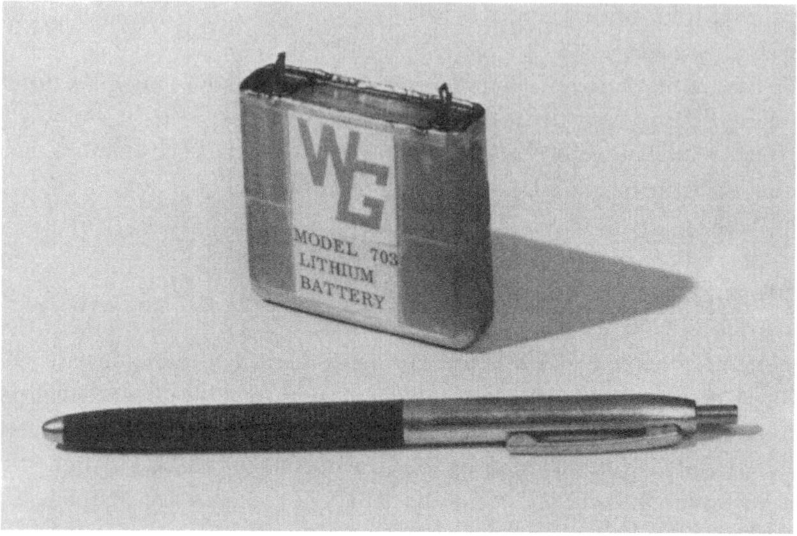

Figure 9. Lithium-iodine battery.

The combined reaction is:

$$2Li + I_2 \rightarrow 2LiI$$

The cathode material is a complex of iodine and poly-2-vinylpyridine (P2VP). Neither is a conductor of electricity so neither alone can make a cell cathode. However, when mixed together and held at 300 °C for three days, they become a black, tarlike, viscous paste which is electronically conductive. About one mol/mol is required to form the complex. This is not retrievable in the cell reaction, so extra iodine is added, generally up to about 10:1 to 20:1 by weight. As iodine is used, the impedance of the depleted cathode first falls somewhat and then rises. At beginning of life (BOL) the lithium iodide electrolyte impendance increases linearly with the first phase of discharge and is much greater in magnitude than the cathode impedance. In the second phase of discharge, the cathode becomes starved of iodine and develops a higher impedance than the lithium iodide electrolyte. This produces the familiar shoulder of the discharge curve after which the loaded voltage falls more rapidly with discharge. However, if the load is removed for a reasonable period (three days) during phase I or phase II of discharge, the open-circuit voltage (OCV) of the cell will return to within millivolts of its original 2.80-volt level. During the third phase the concentration of available iodine in the cathode has dropped so low that the Nernst equation is no longer satisfied for the 2.80-volt level. OCV then begins to drop. This third phase occurs well beyond the normal-design EOL of the cell. Probably one of the best indications of an exhausted cell is low OCV, assuming that there are no intrinsic loads from internal shorts and so on.

The three principal problems that led to the demise of the zinc-mercury battery are nonexistent in the lithium iodine cell. First, there is no gas generation. The zinc-mercury cell operated at some 300 p.s.i. of hydrogen pressure which periodically vented off through a neoprene seal. This leads to the second problem of hermeticity. The lithium iodine cell is hermetically sealed in a metal can with a glass-metal feedthrough. Thus, no body moisture can enter and no battery effluents can get out. By our own definition, a true hermetic seal will not pass more than 30×10^{-9} cm^3 of helium per second after an overnight bomb of helium at 60 p.s.i. No organic material will meet this test. Thus a true hermetic

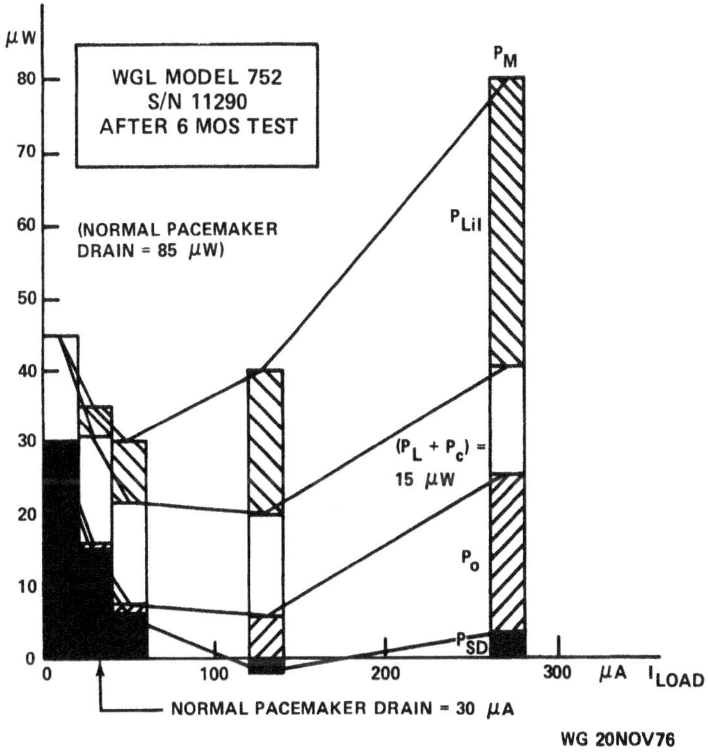

Figure 10. Three phases of LiI battery discharge. Phase 1 – Lithium-Iodide electrolyte growth; Phase 2 – Iodine depletion of cathode; Phase 3 – Insufficient iodine remains to satisfy Nernst equation requirements for 2.8V OCV.

$$E = E^\circ - \frac{RT}{nF} \ln \frac{(aLi+)(aI-)}{(aLi)(aI_2)^{\frac{1}{2}}}$$

Where: aX is the activity of the species

Since only (aI_2) changes and other (aX) are near unity, we may approximate:

$$E = E^\circ - \frac{RT}{nF} \ln \frac{1}{(aI_2)^{\frac{1}{2}}}$$

$$E = E^\circ - \frac{RT}{ZnF} \ln (aI_2)$$

Therefore:

$$aI_2 = \exp \frac{E - E^\circ}{0.013357} = \exp 75\,(E\text{-}E_0)$$

Since the JANAF value for $\triangle G = -64.450$ Kcal/mole, we can tabulate:

aI_2	E_{ocv}
100%	2795 mv
47%	2785 mv
11%	2765 mv
2.4%	2745 mv

Figure 11. Nernst equation.

seal can be achieved only with glass, metal or ceramic. The third problem deals with separator degradation. The lithium iodine battery eliminates with separator degration. The lithium iodine battery eliminates this problem since it has no fabricated separator. When lithium comes into contact with iodine complex, during manufacture, a mono-molecular layer of lithium iodide forms. This spontaneously formed separator grows in thickness as the battery is used. Should it be pierced or shattered for any reason, new lithium iodide will form to replace it. Thus, the separator is self-healing. These three factors permit a pacemaker cell which has a proven reliability much better than the older zinc-mercury battery.

Subsequent to the introduction of the lithium iodine cell, no less than six other lithium batteries with other halogen systems were introduced into clinical practice. Their pertinent characteristics are listed in the Table 1. Each of these systems has demonstrated so marked an improvement over the older zinc-mercury battery that any differences between them in reliability are probably masked by the emergence of the electrode as the principal failure mechanism. The pacemaker battery is no longer a significant clinical problem. Most surgical interventions today are electrode-related.

FUTURE PACEMAKER BATTERIES

There exists a rapid speed of development in pacemaker technology which will reflect changing requirements in power sources with higher pulse-current capability. Many of the new designs are digital devices which are locked to a quartz crystal and cannot run away (26). Programmability has enabled not only complete non-invasive control of many therapeutic functions, but also control of many diagnostic functions, such as battery condition and electrode impedance, telemetering them out to an auxiliary receiver. We foresee the possibility of using sensors such as the platinum endocardial electrode tip as a pO_2 sensor. Certainly, the endocardial electrogram can be telemetered out. Core temperature and intracardiac pressure perhaps could also be read out. The imminent availability of one-chip low-current microprocessors expands, nearly without limit, the computing possibilities in the pacemaker itself. The number of things a pacemaker will be able to do will be limited only by the sensors available and by the physician's evaluation of the cost-effectiveness of the measurement or the control.

To meet these new requirements, pacemaker power sources will require higher voltages and higher pulse-current capability. Our group has already described a lithium bromine type battery with 3.5 volts and a pulse-current capability of two amperes for 20 msec (27). The energy density of such systems will approach 400 Wh/kg.

MICROCALORIMETRY OF BATTERIES

Microcalorimeters have been used in biochemistry and in nuclear chemistry to identify and quantify chemical and nuclear reactions by the amount of heat developed or absorbed (28, 29). However, microcalorimeters had not been used for battery analysis prior to 1976. Recently, Thoren et al. (30) and Prosen et al. (31) reported preliminary results of tests on small batteries with small-aperture microcalorimeters originally designed for biochemical work.

We have now built several large-aperture microcalorimeters suitable for testing pacemakers and pacemaker batteries (32). The first, completed in May of 1976, has been in continual 24-hours use since that time. Our design closely follows that of Prosen, but with modifications to adapt it to our use. Three concentric heat sinks are thermally insulated from each other.

Table 1. Lithium battery systems.

	Hg/Zn	LITHIUM IODIDE					
		WILSON GREATBATCH					
	Mallory RMI	702E (+CRC)	752	755	761/23	761/15	762
Anode	Zn	Li	Li	Li	Li	Li	Li
Electrolyte	NaOH+Ag	LiI	LiI	LiI	LiI	LiI	LiI
Cathode	HgO	I_2+P_2VP	I_2+P_2VP	I_2+P_2VP	I_2+P_2VP	I_2+P_2VP	I_2+P
Voltage-open circuit/cell	1.35	2.8	2.8	2.8	2.8	2.8	2.8
Battery weight (grams)	13.8	80	27	33	27	17	30
Battery volume (cm^3)	3.0	31	9.5	9.5	7.6	4.6	8.6
Energy density gravimetric W-H/kilo	100	110	140	230	230	190	208
Volumetric W-H/cm^3	.45	.28	.39	.79	.82	.71	.73
Self discharge	Yes 23 μa	10% in 10 years	10% in 10 years	10% in 10 years	less than 10% in 10 years	less than 10% in 10 years	less t 10% i 10 ye
Capacity (B.O.L. A-H)	1.0	3.5	1.5	3.0	2.5	1.3	2.5
Energy (W-H)	1.35	8.75	3.75	7.5	6.25	3.25	6.25
Hermetic seal	No	Yes	Yes	Yes	Yes	Yes	Yes

OTHER LITHIUM							
CATALYST RESEARCH			SAFT	GTE/ARCO	MALLORY	DUPONT	WILSON GREATBATCH
802/23	802/35	810A/23	210 Silver Chromate	Thionyl Chloride	LSA-900-6	Cordis	Bromine 766
Li	Li	Li	Li	Li	Li	Li	Li
LiI	LiI	LiI	$LiClO_4$ + Propylene Carbonate	$LiAlCl_4$ + $SOCl_2$	LiI + Al_2O_3	$LiClO_4$	LiBr
I_2+P_2VP	I_2+P_2VP	I_2+P_2VP	Ag_2CrO_4	$SOCl_2.C$	PbI_2 PbS+Pb	CuS	$Br_2.P_2VP$
2.8	2.8	2.8	3.45	3.66	1.9 (5.7)**	2.11 (6.3)**	3.45
30	54	25.6	9.0	16	40	17 (51)**	27
11.2	19	8.6	3.1	6.6	10	6.0	9.5
200	190	220	210	410	120	.217	440
.53	.53	.64	.61	.97	.46	.61	1.25
10% in 10 years	10% in 10 years	less than 5% in 10 years	None measured	1% in one year	None measured	None measured	10% in 10 years
2.3	4.3	2.1	0.61	1.9	0.91	1.8	3.5
6.0	10.0	5.51	1.9	6.6	4.5	3.7 (11.1)**	12
Yes	Yes	Yes	No	Yes	Yes	No	Yes

** Voltage of battery (more than 1 cell).

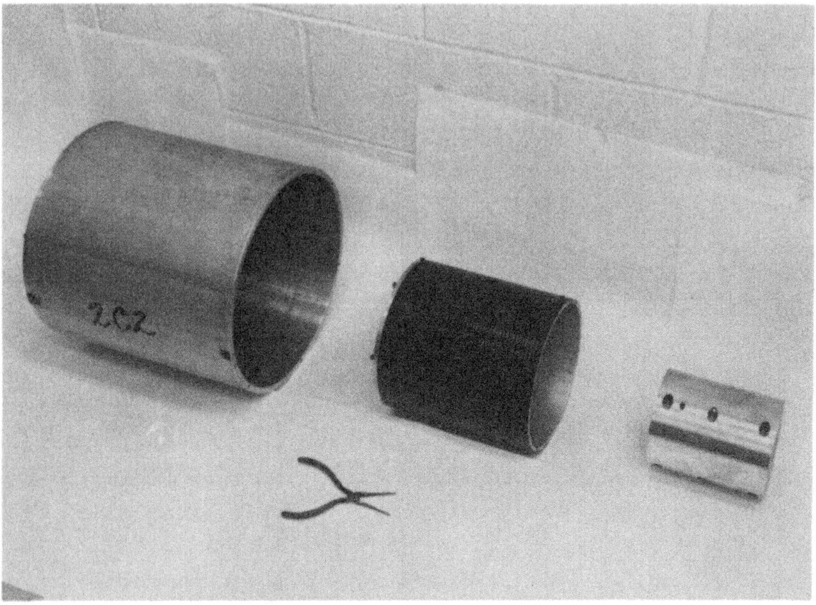

Figure 12. Exploded view of microcalorimeter.

In the centre of the third heat sink is a tight-fitting capsule made of high-purity copper. Bismuth telluride thermopiles surround the capsule and separate it from the third heat sink. The battery to be tested is placed into this capsule, where it fits snugly. Any heat flow from the battery passes through the series-connected thermopiles which develop about 0.2 μv for each microwatt of heat flow. An internal operational amplifier raises this signal to the millivolt level. The amplified signal is brought outside to a strip-chart recorder. Room temperature is held to 23 °C $\pm$ 0.5 °C.

The microcalorimeter is calibrated by passing a known current through a precision resistor placed in the capsule. Calibration is stable to $\pm$ 10 percent. We can reliably measure heat as little as one microwatt (a germinating grain of rice generates 15 microwatts!).

Direct assessment of internal self-discharge is hampered by the presence of other exothermic reactions in the battery. New cells exhibit much higher heat evolution than do mature ones. Much of this has been traced to innocuous side reactions such as the curing of plastic materials and adhesives used in battery construction. For example, three drops of epoxy adhesive, cured for three days at room temperature and then placed in the microcalorimeter show a heat evolution of 25 μW at 37°C.

Microcalorimetric measurements of heat evolution are significantly lower in older batteries than in newer cells. For example, four 1.5 Ah Model 752 batteries manufactured in early 1977 showed an average heat evolution of 27 μW, whereas five similar cells manufactured in mid-1975 showed an evolution of 2 μW a year later. Both the completion of the curing reactions mentioned above, and the increasing thickness of the lithium iodide electrolyte layer, account for this reduction of internal heat of the batteries. A similar trend was seen in the 3.0 Ah Model 755 cells.

More recently Hansen and Hart have described an improved microcalorimeter design with two major advances (33). It is a differential type, measuring the difference between an unknown and a control. This minimizes the effect of ambient thermal variations. Secondly, they use a liquid bath which is much more stable than our dry system. Although we still make extensive use of our prototypes in our own testing program, we have not made any more of them and we now routinely use Hart's superior device[1] for much of our own work.

POWER SOURCES FOR OTHER PROSTHETICS

With pacemaker usage at a world level of US $ 500 millions per year for apparatus alone, we sometimes tend to forget about all the other physiological stimulators that have developed along with pacemakers. Here, we will skip over such areas as pain control, bladder stimulation, and direct stimulation of the brain, to dwell on the exciting new field of bone growth stimulation (BGS).

Yasuda (34) in Japan and Bassett et al. (35) in New York in the fifties showed that negative current could accelerate the healing of a bone fracture, while positive current desorbed bone. Becker and Spadaro (36) in Syracuse, New York, found that this effect was not specific to any metal, but that when they used positively driven anodes of silver, the metal corroded slightly and created a germicidal silver-ion environment. With positively driven silver electrodes he was able to cure some tissue and bone infection. The germicidal effect was observed with a broad spectrum of bacteria and also with some floating tumour cells.

From my personally biased point of view, I see the sixties as the decade of pacing and the seventies as the decade of lithium batteries. I see the eighties as the decade of electrical control of growth (both positive and negative) of tissue (both hard tissue, such as bone, and soft tissue) and control of infection. I see the development of a new integrated science that will include the generation of electrical stimulations, their introduction into the body through the metal-tissue electrode interface, and the study of the fundamental physiological mechanisms mediating the control. One might call such a science biophysical electrochemistry since each of these disciplines is involved in the integrated whole. Our

[1] Tronac Inc., Salt Lake City, Utah.

present interest is three-faceted, in the design of totally implantable BGS devices, power sources to drive them, and the study of the electrochemistry of the metal-tissue interface.

The outputs of these devices are DC. The magnitude of current required is still highly controversial. Brighton et al. (37) in Philadelphia use 80 microamperes. Becker and Spadaro (36) prefer nearer one microampere. Yasuda in Japan has reported osteogenesis with Teflon electrets (38). These are electrostatic equivalents of permanent magnets which operate at current levels of 2×10^{-22}amp. When the literature reports optimum current levels which differ by so many orders of magnitude, we wonder if the mediating mechanisms might not be actually quite different, depending on the current level used. The higher sub-necrotic levels, under 100 microamperes, may well be an irritant mechanism. It has been suggested that oxidized chemical intermediaries may provide chemical signals to the growth cells. Electret energy levels are down in the range where the body itself operates and some suggest that direct instructions are being sent to the cell's DNA doublehelix genetic apparatus to adopt a different growth pattern. Obviously much work remains to be done.

Power sources for such devices may be smaller versions of our present pacemaker power sources. More likely, they will be new approaches such as electrets or biogalvanic couples. Certainly we will need new concepts of electrochemistry which may have to combine power generation concepts with the electrochemistry of the electrode interface, not only in saline and in tissue, but in the physiologically active and osteogenic vascular bed.

CONCLUSION

The performance of implantable pacemakers was limited largely by the performance of their batteries up until a few years ago. We have traced the early history of pacemakers and their powers sources from the first implants in 1958 to the present. We have hazarded some predictions of what the future might hold, not only in pacemakers, but in some other prosthetic devices. While the present pacemaker power sources seem to be nearly ideal and much more trouble-free than electrodes, we still predict further improvements in size reduction and in reliability, probably whether the industry wants them or not! Microprocessors foretell great advances in the programmability, interrogability and telemetry of pacemakers. We see pacemakers becoming diagnostic devices as well as therapeutic devices.

REFERENCES

1. Hyman, A: Resuscitation of the stopped heart by intracardiac therapy, ... *J Am Med* Ass 99:1888, 1932.
2. Zoll P: Resuscitation of the heart in ventricular standstill. *New Eng J Med* 247:768, 1952.
3. Weirich W, Gott V, Lillehei C: Treatment of complete heart block, ... *Surg Forum* 8:360, 1957.
4. Lillehei C, Gott V, Hodges P, Long D, Bakken E: Transistorized pacemaker for treatment of complete heart block. *J Am Med Ass* 172:2006, 1960
5. Furman S, Robinson G: The use of an intracardiac pacemaker in the correction of complete block. *Surg Forum* 9:245, 1958.
6. Abram L: A surgical approach to the management of heart block, ... *Lancet* 1372, 1960.
7. Greatbatch W, Chardack W: A transistorized implantable pacemaker, ... In: *Transactions of the NEREM conference* 1:8, Boston, 1959.
8. Chardack W, Gage A, Greatbatch W: A transistorized, self-contained, implantable pacemaker, ... *Surgery* 48:643, 1960.
9. Elmqvist R. and Senning A: *Proceedings of the second international conference of the IFME*, Paris, 1959.
10. Lagergren: How it happened: my recollection of early pacing. *PACE* 1:140, 1978
11. Senning A: Discussion of a paper by Stephensen. *J Thor Surg* 38:639, 1959.
12. Hunter J, Roth N, Berneardes D, Noble J: A bipolar myocardial electrode for complete heart block. *Lancet* 79:506, 1959.
13. Chardack W: A myocardial electrode for long-term pacemaking. *Ann NY Acad Sci* 111:893, 1964.
14. Chardack W, Gage A, Federico A, Schimert G, Greatbatch W: Five years clinical experience with an implantable pacemaker. *Surgery* 58 (5):915, 1965.
15. Greatbatch W: Cardiac implantable demand pacemaker. United States patent 3, 478, 746, 1969 (filed 1965).
16. Greatbatch W: X-ray technique for evaluation of exhaustion and detection of mechanical defects in implantable mercury batteries. *Med Electron and Biol Engin* 3:305, 1965.
17. Furman S, Escher D: Transtelephone pacemaker monitoring, five years later. *Ann Thor Surg* 20:326, 1975.
18. Knapp D: Thermionic and betavoltaic nuclear power sources. *Trans Am Nucl Soc* 13 (2), 1970.
19. Laurens P, Piwnica A, Reidemeister C: Applications cliniques d'un stimulateur cardiaque radio isotope. In: *Proceedings of the second international symposium, on power from radioisotopes* En/IB 47, Madrid, 1972.
20. Greatbatch W, Bustard T: A PuO_2 nuclear source for implantable cardiac pacemakers. *IEEE Trans BME* 5:332, 1973.
21. Poole MJ, Myatt J, Brown M: Miniature nuclear batteries, a review of work in the U.K. *Trans Am Nucl Soc* 13 (2), 1970.
22. Greatbatch W: Device for conversion of nuclear energy to electrical energy. United states patent 3836798, 1974 (filed 1970).
23. Fischell R, Lewis K, Schulman J, Love J: A long-lived reliable rechargeable pacemaker. International Symposium on Advances in Pacemaker Technology, Erlangen, 1974.
24. Moser J: Solid state lithium-iodine primary battery. United states patent 3660163, 1972 (filed 1970).
25. Greatbatch W, Lee J, Mathias W, Eldridge M, Moser J, Schneider A: The solid-state lithium battery, ... *IEEE Trans BME* 18 (5):317, 1971.
26. Greatbatch W: Digital demand pacer. United States patent 3870050, 1975 (filed 1973).
27 Liang C: A new high energy density lithium battery system. Twelfth International Conference on Medical and Biological Engineering, Jerusalem, 1979.
28. Monk P Wadso I: *Acta Chim Scand* 22:1842, 1968.
29. Pennington S, Brown H, Berger R, Evans W: *Analytical Biochemistry* 32, 1969.

30. Thoren A, Lodin A: Test results for long-life batteries for cardiac pacemakers. In: *Cardiac pacing: proceedings of the fifth international symposium*, Watanabe Y (ed), Amsterdam, Excerpta Medica, 1977, p 466.
31. Prosen E, Goldberg R, Staples B, Boyd B, Armstrong G: Microcalorimetry applied to biochemical processes. In: *Thermal analysis*, Kambe H, Gern PD (eds), New York, John Wiley and Sons, 1974, p 253.
32. Holmes W, McLean R, Greatbatch W, Holmes C: The use of microcalorimetry in characterization of lithium pacemaker batteries. Twenty-eighth Power Sources Symposium, Atlantic City, New Yersey, 1977.
33. Hansen L, Hart R: The characterization of internal power losses in pacemaker batteries by microcalorimetry. *J Electrochem* 125 (6):842, 1978.
37. Yasuda I: On the piezo-electric effect of bone. *J Physiol Soc* (Japan) 10:1158, 1957.
35. Basset A, Pawluk R, Becker R: Effects of electric currents in bone in vivo. *Nature* 204:652, 1964.
36. Becker R, Spadaro J: Treatment of orthopaedic infections with electrically generated silver ions. *J Bone and Joint Surg* 60A (7):871, (1978).
37. Brighton C, Friedenberg Z, Mitchell E, et al: Treatment of non-union with constant direct current. *Clin Orthop* 124:106, 1977.
38. Yasusa I: Electrical callus and callus formation by electret. *Clin Orthop* 124:53, 1977.

10. DETECTION OF PACEMAKER MALFUNCTION

Harry G. Mond, Lyndel Sutton and J. Greame Sloman

The success of an implanted cardiac pacemaker is dependent upon the establishment of a harmonious relationship between the artificial pacemaker and the human receiver. Failure of a pacemaker system may arise from an electronic or mechanical defect of the pacemaker, a physiological problem, or from a poor relationship between the normal function of pacemaker and host. Such malfunctions may necessitate the repair, replacement, or repositioning of a pacemaker component or removal of a source of external interference. True pacemaker malfunctions must be clearly distinguished from pseudo-malfunctions, where there is no pacemaker system defect. These situations may, variously, require the repair of faulty testing equipment, reassessment of falsely interpreted test data, or treatment of the patient for an unrelated disorder. For simplicity, this paper will be confined to malfunctions associated with the synchronous ventricular inhibited pacing system. It can be seen from the complexity of the situation that proper investigation and interpretation of data is critical to the comprehension and correction of a pacemaker problem.

RATIONALE OF TESTING

Until recently, the safety of a pacemaker implant was dependent on the rapid detection of malfunctions as they arose. The electrocardiograph (ECG) helped confirm an intact pacing system and the oscilloscope was used to visualize the pulse artifact and establish end-of-life characteristics. By these means, prediction of impending pacing failure could theoretically be determined in most patients, but in practice these methods were unreliable. Hence many pacing centres explanted pulse generators on an elective basis, rather than waiting until end-of-life characteristics emerged.

Modern electronic pacemaker circuitry has coupled reduced pulse generator voltage output with a concomitant reduction in pulse repetition rate and often with an increase in pulse width. These changes maintain a safe level of delivered energy whilst enabling power source failure to be anticipated. This predictability and safety has revolutionized testing techniques and today there is little place for routine elective replacement of pulse generators. Consequently, the basis of all testing is accurate determination of an intact pacing system by the routine use of the ECG, together with regular accurate determination of the pulse repetition rate and pulse width. However, testing begins in the operating room when the pacemaker is implanted.

TESTING PROCEDURES AT PACEMAKER SYSTEM IMPLANTATION

Testing at the time of implant serves to verify the correct placement of pacing leads and a normally functioning pulse generator. This has, in recent years, been responsible for a marked reduction in the incidence of pacemaker systems malfunctioning soon after implantation.

With endocardial leads, once the electrode has been positioned at the apex of the right ventricle, testing should be performed with a pacing system analyser. There is now no place for haphazard testing of the pacing threshold with a temporary external pulse generator. The threshold voltage, resultant current, and impedance can be determined at a variety of pulse widths. However, it is essential to use a pulse width equal to that of the pulse generator about to be implanted. A

ROYAL MELBOURNE HOSPITAL

PACEMAKER IMPLANT NO: ....

NEW IMPLANT .... REPLACEMENT ....

PACEMAKER GENERATOR TYPE:.. ....

ASYNCHRONOUS RATE: .... BPM MAGNET .... BPM

LEAD TYPE:

PACING THRESHOLD (0.5M/SEC) ....VOLTS

LEAD RESISTANCE ....OHM.

R WAVE AMPLITUDE ....MV

LEAD SITE ....

GENERATOR SITE ....

CONNECTOR (IF USED) ....

DEATAILS (INCLUDING COMPLICATIONS) BELOW

Figure 1. Pacemaker implant stamp used on the operation sheet to detail the results of testing at pacemaker implantation.

threshold voltage less than 1 volt (v) or a current less than 2 milliamperes (ma) is necessary for most lead types. The average impedance is 400-600 ohms. Once a satisfactory threshold has been obtained, R-wave sensing through the lead is performed. This can be done by the pacing system analyser or it can be measured from an intracardiac electrogram recording. A minimum of 4 millivolts (mv) is required.

Although it is rare to find a malfunctioning pulse generator at implant, electronic component malfunction may occur during shipment. Thus, it is also necessary to test the pulse generator. The results must be compared with those specified at room temperature by the manufacturer.

The results of lead and pulse generator testing should be recorded and kept in the patient's file with the pacemaker clinic records. The form for full testing may be complex – we have devised a simple stamp which is used with the patient's operation sheet (Figure 1).

ROUTINE TESTING OF AN IMPLANTED PACEMAKER SYSTEM

Regular monitoring of the pacemaker system is necessary to detect any malfunction developing after implant. Commonly, such failures are due to the inevitable end-of-life battery depletion. However, defects in manufacture, poor surgical technique, or changes in the patient's physiology, may unpredictably cause a malfunction. Essential pacemaker testing involves the establishment of baseline levels and then routine follow-up with ECG and electronic pulse generator testing. Oscilloscope display of the pulse artefact and fluoroscopic and radiographic chest examinations may also be carried out shortly after implant to provide baseline data for future investigations.

Pacemaker electrocardiography

The ventricular pacemaker QRS depolarization consists of a stimulus artefact and the subsequent ventricular response (Figure 2). The stimulus artefact represents the voltage delivered by the pulse generator, and is seen on the ECG as a perpendicular voltage deflection of the baseline. The size of this artefact differs according to the ECG leads: potentially larger with unipolar compared with bipolar pacing systems. The stimulus artefact may on occasion be seen on the ECG without a ventricular response. If the artefact is large, deflection of the ECG baseline simulating a QRS complex occurs, and therefore it is important to confirm true ventricular depolarization by noting a subsequent T wave. The deflection of the ECG baseline will also deform or modify the subsequent ECG. Thus in determining the QRS frontal plane axis, the first 40-80 msec should not be analysed. This can be illustrated by reversing the electrical polarity

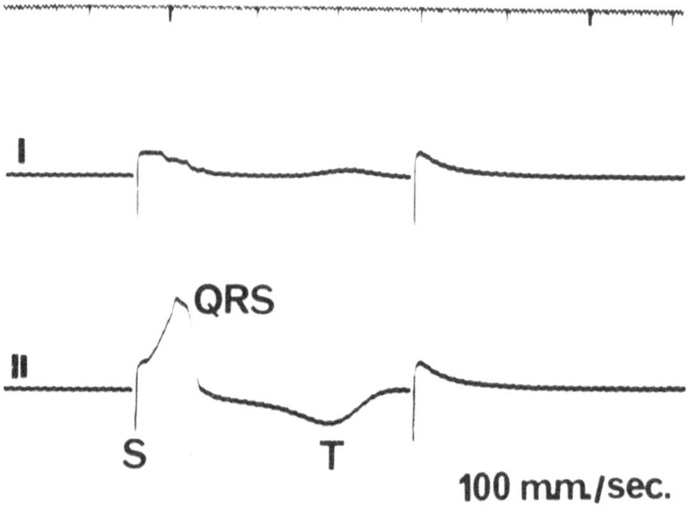

Figure 2. The pacemaker ECG consists of spike or pulse artefact (S), depolarization (QRS) and repolarization (T wave). In lead I the pulse artefact is followed by a smaller QRS and T wave. The second complex is composed of a pulse artefact and no QRS or T wave, i.e., a failed paced beat. The pulse artefact deforms the baseline and this could be misinterpreted as a QRS. However, there is no T wave. This example illustrates the value of taking more than one lead in interpreting the ECG in patients with pacemakers. It also highlights the deformity of the baseline caused by the pulse artefact.

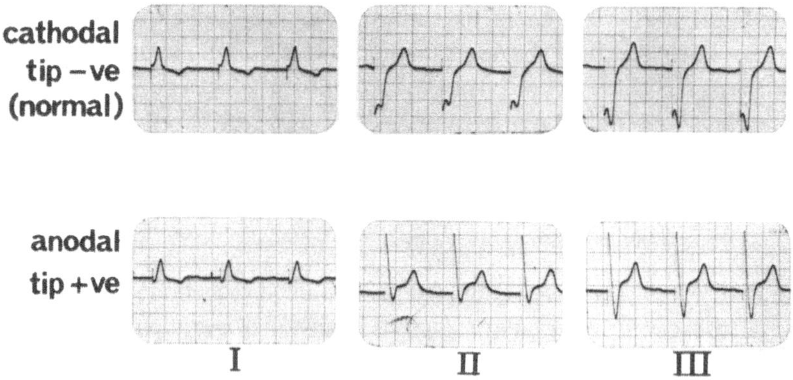

Figure 3. ECG leads I, II and III with a unipolar electrode system and an external pulse generator. The top tracing illustrates the axis of the pulse artefact to the extreme left, when the stimulating electrode is cathodal. The subsequent QRS axis is also to the extreme left. By reversing the poles of the pulse generator, the stimulating electrode is anodal and the axis of the pulse artefact is also reversed. However, the electrode is still at the apex of the right ventricle, and thus, the wave of depolarization or QRS should not change. With anodal stimulation there appears to be marked changes in the QRS axis. This is attributed to the marked pulse artefact deformity of the QRS. For this reason the first 60-80 msec of the QRS should not be included in determination of axis; only the terminal part of the QRS should be used in axis determination. If this is done, the axis is still to the extreme left.

of the pacemaker system and thus reversing the deflection of the pulse artefact (Figure 3).

Vector analysis of the pacemaker QRS reveals typical characteristics when pacing is established from various parts of the heart. Knowledge of various configurations is very valuable in clinical pacing. Unipolar endocardial pacing from the apex of the right ventricle results in the anterior chest leads showing a left bundle branch block configuration and the frontal plain vector is to the extreme left (Figure 4). If the endocardial electrode becomes displaced towards

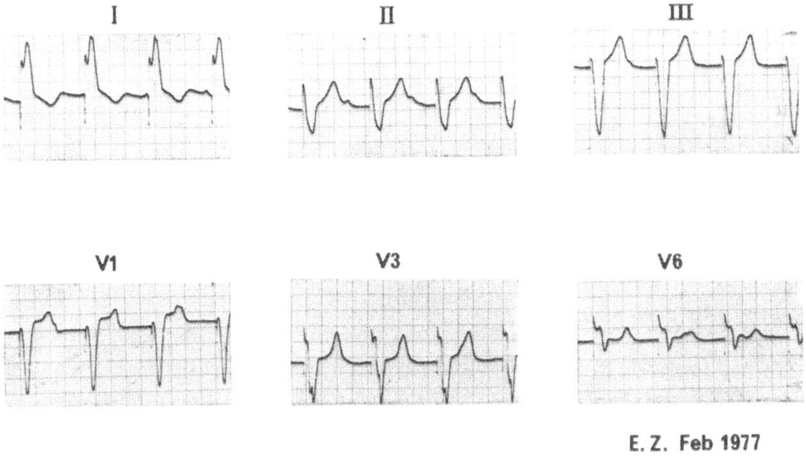

Figure 4. ECG of a unipolar endocardial pacing system with the electrode at the apex of the right ventricule. There is a left bundle branch block configuration and a QRS axis to the extreme left.

the right ventricular outflow tract, then an axis shift occurs. The axis now becomes normal or even extreme right (Figure 5).

On rare occasions, with right ventricular apical endocardial pacing, the appearance of a right bundle branch block (RBBB) configuration is seen on the ECG. The pattern so obtained has been explained by a number of mechanisms. Other causes of RBBB configuration include perforation of the anterior right ventricular wall with the electrode in the pericardial cavity, inadvertent placement of the transvenous lead in the coronary sinus and, very rarely, perforation of the intraventricular septum.

Epicardial left ventricular pacing has an RBBB configuration. Because these leads are implanted at varying positions on the anterior left ventricular surface, the axis will be variable.

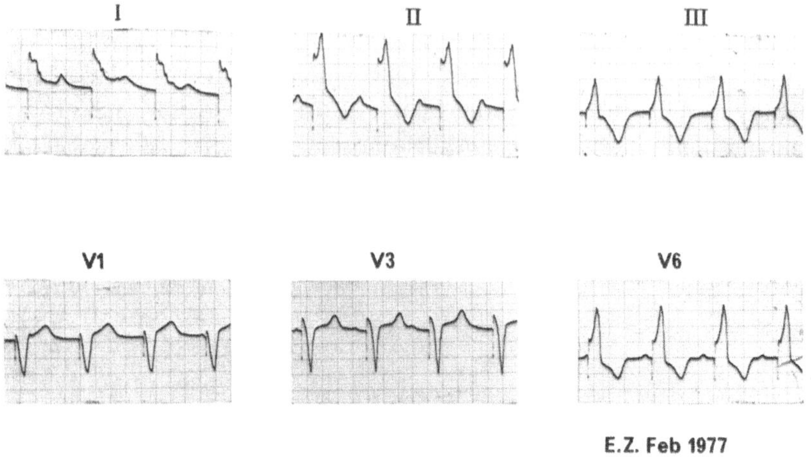

Figure 5. ECG of a unipolar endocardial pacemaker system with the electrode in the right ventricular outflow tract. There is a left bundle branch block configuration and the axis is now between 0 and 90°.

Electronic pulse generator testing

The pulse repetition rate and pulse width can now be very easily measured using a variety of inexpensive commercially available testing devices. If the patient is pacing, testing is performed with the pulse generator in the synchronous mode; testing is repeated in the asynchronous mode using a magnet applied over the pulse generator. The results are then compared with previous recordings, and may be used to detect impending power source depletion.

During the late 1970s the lithium anode became the major power source used for cardiac pacemakers. The most commonly used cathode is iodine, and lithium iodide forms between the two poles as the power source becomes depleted. The internal battery impedance rises and the voltage output falls. This fall occurs gradually from the time of implant and is coupled electronically to a corresponding fall in pacing rate. With most pulse generators a fall of 6-8 beats/min represents impending power source depletion. As the predicted life of these pulse generators is from 5-12 years there should be a theoretical fall of 0.5-1 beat/min/year.

To date, such theoretical falls have been shown with the large 702 lithium iodide power source. However, pulse generators incorporating the smaller lithium iodide batteries have not shown such consistent results. A major problem has been miniaturization of electronic components. Timing circuits have often shown maturation changes with a rate drift in the first six to twelve months of pulse generator use. Thus there has been difficulty in establishing adequate baseline levels for these implanted pulse generators.

Other less commonly used power sources show characteristic changes on power source depletion. The voltage output of the lithium silver chromate power source is stable until it falls acutely towards the end of life to a second voltage output plateau. Pulse rate changes remain stable until this second plateau is reached. Usually the pulse generator has two batteries in series and manufacturers have differing pulse rate changes to demonstrate impending depletion of the first and second battery.

The pulse artefact width is also valuable in the routine testing of pulse generators. Consistent changes, however, are not always incorporated into pulse generators by manufacturers. Usually the pulse width is made to increase as the voltage output falls. This safety mechanism allows for constant energy to be delivered to the heart, and is particularly important in patients with high pacing thresholds.

INVESTIGATION OF A SUSPECTED PACEMAKER MALFUNCTION

In the management of patients with suspected pacemaker malfunction, the initial investigations are those performed at routine testing, accompanied by a clinical examination. In most cases, sufficient information has been obtained from these simple investigations to diagnose the general cause of malfunction. On occasion, further investigations may be necessary. For instance, a fractured lead with intermittent contact may be detected by combining provocative movements with various monitoring techniques, or by long-term ECG monitoring. Lead perforation may be identified using fluoroscopy and intracardiac electrography. Finally, surgical exploration and testing of an explanted pulse generator may be necessary to diagnose a suspected pacemaker malfunction. Some of the methods used in the investigation of a suspected pacemaker malfunction are outlined below.

Clinical findings, including history and examination

An unwell patient is examined clinically. Those patients who are normal in their routine testing, but are continually symptomatic, can usually have their symptoms traced to a non-pacemaker cause. Typical examples are cardiac or renal failure, vertebro-basilar insufficiency, or postural hypotension. However, should the patient history indicate the return of symptoms experienced before the pacemaker implant, for example Stokes-Adams attacks, then the possibility of an intermittent failed pacemaker system should be entertained.

Provocative movements

Specific movements likely to reproduce symptoms should be performed with ECG monitoring. These include rapid arm movements for skeletal muscle inhibition (Figure 6), or unusual postures to demonstrate a fractured lead. An intermittent proximal lead fracture or poor connection between set-screw and lead pin can also be demonstrated by abruptly moving the pulse generator or any palpable lead beneath the skin. Concomitant ECG monitoring and fluoroscopy are essential. On occasion, oscilloscopic analysis may be helpful.

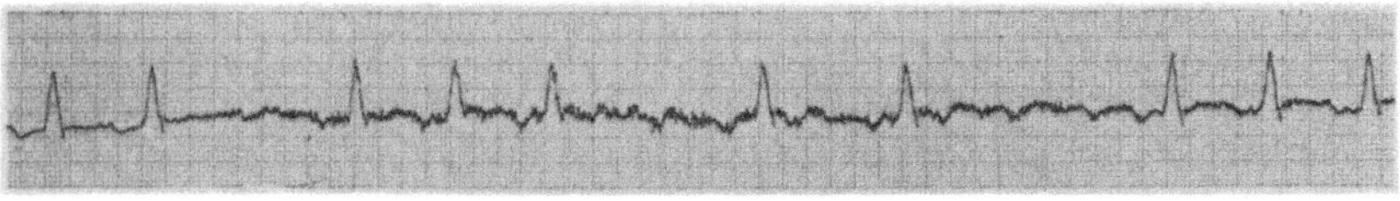

Figure 6. ECG showing skeletal muscle myopotential inhibition of ventricular inhibited pacemaker. A unipolar pulse generator was implanted subcutaneously above the pectoralis major muscle. Rapid arm movements by the patient resulted in near syncopal turns. This ECG illustrates the coarse artefact produced by the arm movements and the subsequent pulse generator inhibition.

ECG monitoring

In cases of suspected intermittent pacemaker system faults, prolonged ECG monitoring may be very valuable. Such systems include 24-hour ambulatory monitoring, ECG telemetry, direct bedside monitoring, and telephone transmission of the ECG.

Chest wall stimulation

Electrical stimuli, too weak to affect the heart, will inhibit an implanted synchronous ventricular inhibited pulse generator, thus testing its demand function. These electrical signals can be applied to the chest wall by an external pulse generator.

Surgical exploration with radiological screening

On occasion, surgical intervention is necessary as a means of investigation of suspected pacemaker malfunction. Many cases of pacemaker malfunction determined by other means will also require surgical intervention in order to rectify the malfunction. Whether a cause has been established or not, the procedures performed during surgical intervention remain essentially the same. Pulse generator and lead system are mobilized and inspected; both are tested using the pacing system analyser. The lead system is inspected carefully using fluoroscopy, and where necessary, tension is applied to the lead to demonstrate fractured ends. Any site where non-absorbable suture material is tied around the lead should be very carefully inspected. Blood inside the lead insulator suggests a break and a possible site for current leakage.

Intracardiac electrography is essential in all cases of suspected ventricular perforation. Where necessary, pulse generator testing should be performed in the electronics laboratory to confirm the findings found at surgical intervention and also to demonstrate possible intermittent electronic faults (see below).

Intracardiac electrography

The unipolar intracardiac electrogram is a simple means of recording electrical potentials from the heart. Using a battery operated ECG machine, the V lead is attached to the exposed terminal pin of the implanted lead and a recording is taken. With a bipolar lead system, a bipolar recording can be obtained using lead 1 of the ECG; the terminal pin from the distal electrode is attached to the right-arm lead and the terminal pin from the proximal electrode to the left-arm lead. When the electrode makes contact with the right ventricular endocardium 'a current of injury' pattern characterized by ST elevation and T-wave inversion occurs. In contrast, coronary sinus recordings have no such pattern. This current of injury disappears with time leaving T-wave inversion. In about 60 percent of cases, the unipolar ventricular electrogram is biphasic with the R-wave amplitude at least 10 percent of the S-wave. In 30 percent of cases, the R-wave is less than 10% of the S-wave. In the remaining 10 percent there is a dominant R wave without a discrete S wave.

As well as being useful for lead placement at implant, such electrograms are valuable for correct diagnosis of right ventricular perforation. Recordings are performed as the electrode is withdrawn from the epicardial surface (Figure 7).

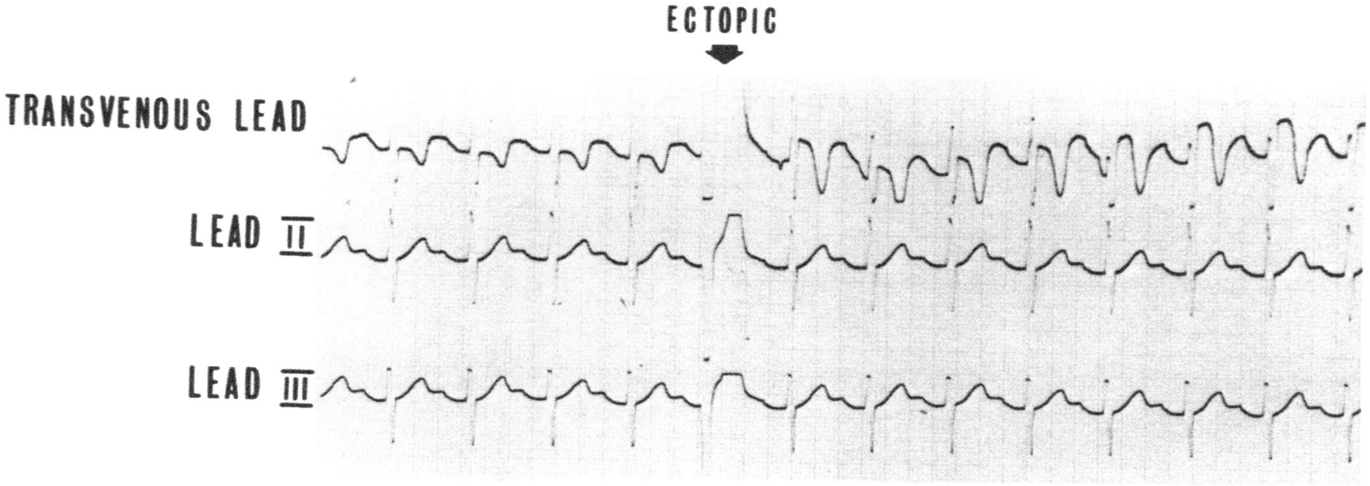

Figure 7. ECG (three simultaneous channels) during withdrawal of a pacemaker lead. The top strip is a unipolar electrogram from the distal electrode and shows a biphasic QRS. On gradual withdrawal of the lead, the pattern changes from an epicardial to an endocardial 'current of injury' pattern. The second and third strip and standard leads II and III. A ventricular premature ('ectopic') beat occurs as the tip of the electrode passes through the myocardium.

Testing of an explanted pulse generator

The explanted pulse generator prior to testing should be thoroughly washed in detergent and water and then soaked in 10-percent formaldehyde. This procedure prevents transmission of any infective agents such as hepatitis B Virus. Pulse generator testing must be performed at body temperature using a water bath or an incubator. The characteristics examined should be compared with the initial test performed and those specified by the manufacturers. These test are divided into three major categories.

Pulse generator output. Pulse generator output is tested is 37° under a 510-ohm load. Testing is performed with and without the magnet:

1. Output pulse voltage shape and pulse width (msec) are examined with an oscilloscope; the leading and trailing edge voltages and pulse width are recorded.
2. Pulse repetition rate (msec) is recorded by an accurate rate counter.

Demand function. Demand function is tested using a simulated QRS complex having the characteristics of approximately 25 Hz and using 4 mv amplitude where necessary. Both positive (R) and negative (S) waves should be used for the test.

1. R-wave sensitivity (mv): this is the minimum simulated QRS necessary to inhibit the pulse generator.
2. Refractory period (msec): this is the period of non-recognition of the simulated QRS after a pacemaker impulse.
3. Interference frequency: this is the frequency of a sine wave which converts a ventricular inhibited pulse generator to the asynchronous mode.

Missing pulse detection. If a pulse generator passes the above tests but there is doubt about performance over a long period, the unit should be tested specifically to identify intermittent failure of operation. The pulse generator must be tested continuously in an incubator at body temperature often for at least 24 hours.

A typical testing system comprises a programmable pulse counter, an event counter, and associated control logic. The programmable counter displays the pulse repetition rate of the pulse generator under test. A duration of approximately 10 msec greater than this pulse interval is programmed into the counter. An output is given if the pulse repetition rate of the pulse generator under test becomes equal to or greater than the programmed interval. The event counter acting through a separate programmable pulse generator counts and displays the number of missed pulses.

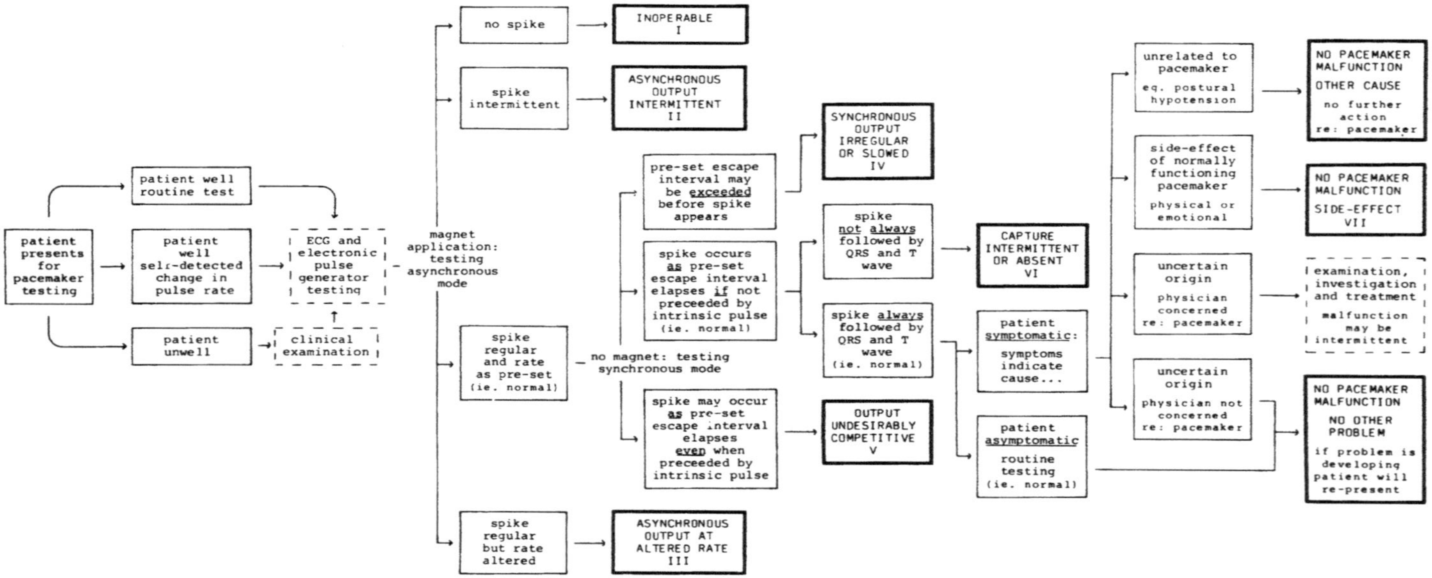

Figure 8. Flow diagram illustrating the procedure for investigating pacemaker patients. *Explanation of terms used:* electronic pulse generator testing – determining the accurate repetition rate and width of the pacemaker pulse artefact; spike – pacemaker pulse artefact; preset escape interval – predetermined pulse repetition rate; intrinsic pulse – spontaneous patient ventricular depolarization.

CAUSES OF PACEMAKER MALFUNCTION

In most cases, sufficient information is obtained from routine testing and a clinical examination to diagnose the general cause of a malfunction. A flow diagram (Figure 8) has been developed to illustrate this initial diagnostic process. Three outcomes are possible: the problem may be pacemaker-related, pacemaker unrelated, or of uncertain origin with further investigation indicated. Should further investigation, using ECG monitoring, discover an intermittent fault, a general diagnosis can then be made by proceeding once more through the flow diagram. If a problem is recognized as being 'pacemaker-related', the table indicated in the particular flow diagram outlet can be consulted for a listing of possible causes.

The tables are divided into true malfunctions and pseudo-malfunctions. In this context, pseudo-malfunction represents all forms of malfunction where there is no specific problem with the pacemaker system, but the investigator interprets the results obtained from testing as a malfunction. In general, pseudo-malfunctions are ECG misinterpretations, but in these tables there is a broader use of the term to include the electronic testing equipment, faulty recordings, and poor understanding of the pacemaker system.

The tables refer to the most common form of pacemaker system, the synchronous ventricular inhibited. On occasion, reference is made to the asynchronous or synchronous ventricular triggered forms of pacing, especially in ECG misinterpretations.

Inoperable pacemaker system

When there is no detectable pulse generator output even after a magnet has been applied the pacemaker system is described as 'inoperable'. There are three major true malfunctions (Table 1): power source failure (either expected or accelerated), random component failure in the output circuit, or a break at some point in the pacemaker-patient electrical circuit. Clarification of the actual malfunction is difficult by routine noninvasive testing as the pulse artefact is absent. Chest radiography and fluoroscopy is usually diagnostic for electrode-lead system fractures with complete discontinuity. The other causes require testing of the exposed pacemaker system at surgery.

In all cases, treatment requires surgical intervention. A pulse generator fault must always be treated with a new pulse generator. Premature power source depletion due to an electrode-lead system fault will also require repair or replacement of the lead. On occasion, non-contact of the set-screw of the pulse generator with the lead pin may lead to failure of pacing and here, the electrode-lead system and the pulse generator both function normally. On tightening the set-screw, the malfunction is corrected. Failure at surgery to make contact between body tissues and the indifferent electrode plate of a unipolar pulse generator will lead to an inoperable system. This is of extreme importance in patients without an intrinsic rate and thus critically dependent on the pacing system.

Pseudo-malfunctions are extremely important because surgical intervention is

Table 1. Pacemaker malfunctions: inoperable – no outpur even after magnet applied.

Malfunction	Frequency	Treatment
True Malfunction:		
1. Power source failure		
– expected end of life	○○○○	nP
– accelerated discharge causes premature depletion		
• asynchronous discharge with competition	○○○○	nP ± nL
• low impedance leads – high electrode surface area	○○○○	nP ± nL
• loss of insulation		
– pulse generator		
• non-hermetically sealed	○○○○	nP
• faulty hermetic sealing	○○○	nP
– lead	○○○	nP ± rL or nL
– adapter sleeve	○○	nP ± nA
– connector	○○	nP
– set-screw (absent cap)	○○	nP
• manufacturing fault, e.g. internal battery short circuit	○○○	nP
2. Output circuit – random component failure	○○○	nP
3. Pacemaker-patient electrical circuit incomplete		
– indifferent electrode plate of unipolar pulse generator not in contact with body tissue	○○○	care at surgery
– electrode-lead system fracture with complete discontinuity	○○○	rL or nL
– non-contact of set-screw with lead pin	○○	tighten screw
Pseudo-malfunction:		
4. Misinterpretation – ECG		
– pulse artefact overlooked	○○	
5. Testing equipment problem		
– equipment faulty	○○○	
– equipment battery failure	○○○	
– equipment misuse		
• magnet not operating reed switch (pulse generator remains inhibited)	○○○	
• poor contact between equipment and patient	○○○	

Frequency: ○○○○=common; ○○○=uncommon; ○○=rare; ○=very rare. *Treatment*: n: replace with new component; r: repair; p: reposition; g: reprogramme; o: observe. *Equipment:* P: pulse generator; P (vt): ventricular triggered pulse generator; P (vi): ventricular inhibited pulse generator; P (asy): asynchronous pulse generator; P (hvo): high voltage output pulse generator; P (prog)) programmable pulse generator; L: electrode-lead system; A: adapter.

not indicated. Pacemaker clinics should not be dependent on only one electronic pulse generator testing device.

Asynchronous output intermittent

When the pulse generator output in the asynchronous mode is intermittent, the stimulus artefact intermittently is not recorded on the ECG or detected with the electronic testing equipment (Table 2). True malfunctions may involve a random component failure in the timing or output circuit, or an intermittent non-contact at some point in the pacemaker-patient electrical circuit. In this group, diagnosis or detection of the fault may be very difficult and prolonged ECG monitoring may be essential. Treatment and pseudo-malfunctions follow the principles as in Table 1.

Table 2. Pacemaker malfunctions: asynchronous output intermittent.

Malfunction	Frequency	Treatment
True Malfunction:		
1. Timing or output circuit – random component failure	○○	nP
2. Pacemaker-patient electrical circuit intermittently incomplete		
– indifferent electrode plate of unipolar pulse generator in poor contact with body tissue	○○○	care at surgery
– electrode-lead system fracture – intermittent contact	○○○	rL or nL
– set-screw not tightly in contact with lead pin	○○	tighten screw
Pseudo-malfunction:		
As in Table 1 – problem intermittent		

Frequency: ○○○○ =common; ○○○ =uncommon; ○○=rare; ○=very rare. *Treatment*: n: replace with new component; r: repair; p: reposition; g: reprogramme; o: observe. *Equipment:* P: pulse generator; P (vt): ventricular triggered pulse generator; P (vi): ventricular inhibited pulse generator; P (asy): asynchronous pulse generator; P (hvo): high voltage output pulse generator; P (prog)) programmable pulse generator; L: electrode-lead system; A: adapter.

Asynchronous output at altered rate

Pulse generator output in the asynchronous magnet mode can develop an altered rate on ECG and electronic pulse generator testing (Table 3). True malfunctions in this group are peculiar to the pulse generator. Causes include changes in the power source or timing circuit. Minor changes are common and may represent

Table 3. Pacemaker malfunctions: asynchronous output at altered rate.

Malfunction	Frequency	Treatment
True Malfunction:		
1. Power source failing (see Table 1)	OOOO	O or nP
2. Timing circuit		
– component maturation – rate drift over first year post implant		
• rise – high temperature effect during manufacturer's testing	OOOO	O
• fall – carbon resistor	OOOO	O
– inadvertent reprogramming of programmable pulse generator	OO	gP
– random component failure		
• runaway pulse generator	O	nP
• slow	O	nP
Pseudo-malfunction:		
4. Misinterpretation		
– lack of understanding of rate changes with:		
• temperature change – room to body at implant	OOO	
– body increase, e.g. fever	O	
• power source depletion	OO	
• activation of reed switch (magnet or test rate)	OO	
5. Faulty recording		
– asynchronous and synchronous testing confused	OO	
– ECG paper output inaccurate speed	OO	
6. Testing equipment problem		
– equipment faulty	OO	

Frequency: OOOO=common; OOO=uncommon; OO=rare; O=very rare. *Treatment*: n: replace with new component; r: repair; p: reposition; g: reprogramme; o: observe. *Equipment:* P: pulse generator; P (vt): ventricular triggered pulse generator; P (vi): ventricular inhibited pulse generator; P (asy): asynchronous pulse generator; P (hvo): high voltage output pulse generator; P (prog)) programmable pulse generator; L: electrode-lead system; A: adapter.

maturation changes in the power source or timing circuit. Such rate drifts need to be observed carefully, but replacement of the pulse generator should only be undertaken after consultation with the manufacturers. In contrast, marked changes in the pulse generator repetition rate may represent impending timing circuit component failure. In these cases, a new pulse generator is indicated.

Pseudo-malfunctions include faulty ECG paper delivery and faulty test equipment. Unnecessary confusion may occur if there is a lack of understanding of the normal rate changes that occur with a particular pulse generator as the power source depletes.

Synchronous output irregular or slowed

If pulse generator output in the synchronous mode is irregular or slowed, this implies oversensing by the pacemaker system, and no problem can be detected in the asynchronous mode (Table 4). Intermittent oversensing produces an irregular output, whereas persistent oversensing may appear as a decreased rate or total inhibition of synchronous output.

True malfunctions do not as a rule imply malfunction of the pulse generator. Rather, the pacemaker system is sensing inappropriate intracardiac or extra-

Table 4. Pacemaker malfunctions: synchronous output irregular or slowed – oversensing.

Malfunction	Frequency	Treatment
True Malfunction:		
1 Inappropriate or concealed sensing		
– skeletal muscle myopotential inhibition		
• muscle beneath implanted pulse generator	○○○	○ or nP (asy or vt)
• diaphragm	○	nP (asy or vt)
– P or T wave sensing		
• abnormally large P or T waves	○○	nP (asy or vt)
• shifted electrode	○	pL
• sensing circuit too sensitive	○	nP (less sensitive)
– electromagnetic interference	○○	remove patient
– inactive lead	○○	cap terminal pin
– fractured lead	○	nL or rL or pL
– after potential sensing	○	nP (asy)
– concealed ectopic beat sensing	○	antiarrhythmics
Pseudo-malfunction:		
2. Misinterpretation – ECG		
– normal sensing with ventricular triggered rhythms interpreted as pacing	○○	
– low voltage marker spike (Telectronics, Edwards)		
– interpreted as fusion	○○	
– hysteresis interpreted as persistent oversensing	○○	
– partial recycling of pulse generator	○○	
3. Faulty recording		
– monitoring equipment undersensitive and does not detect weaker signals, e.g. trans-telephonic recording	○○	
– ECG strip chart		
• speed variable	○○	
• intermittent sticking of paper	○○	

Frequency: ○○○○=common; ○○○=uncommon; ○○=rare; ○=very rare. *Treatment*: n: replace with new component; r: repair; p: reposition; g: reprogramme; o: observe. *Equipment:* P: pulse generator; P (vt): ventricular triggered pulse generator; P (vi): ventricular inhibited pulse generator; P (asy): asynchronous pulse generator; P (hvo): high voltage output pulse generator; P (prog)) programmable pulse generator; L: electrode-lead system; A: adapter.

cardiac electrical potentials. These may include P waves (Figure 9), T waves, after potentials, concealed ectopic beats, diaphragm and anterior chest wall muscle myopotentials (Figure 6), and electromagnetic interference. Apart from anterior chest wall myopotentials, inappropriate or concealed oversensing is unusual or very rare. Troublesome oversensing can be treated where necessary by replacement of the pulse generator with an asynchronous or synchronous ventricular triggered type. Antiarrhythmic therapy is indicated for concealed ectopic beat sensing.

Pseudo-malfunctions may be due to ECG misinterpretation or faulty recording equipment. An example of irregular ECG paper delivery is illustrated in Figure 10.

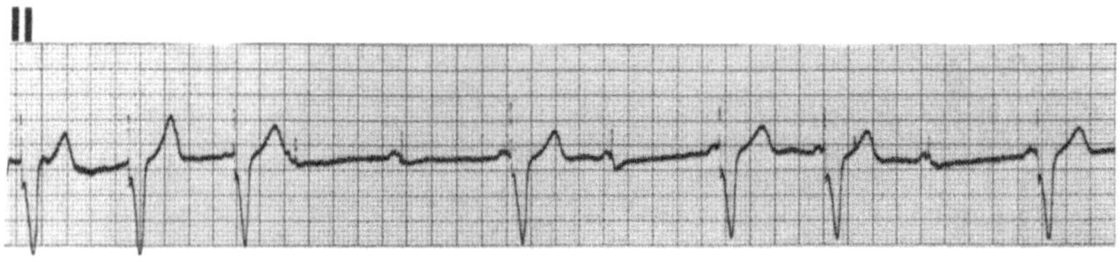

Figure 9. ECG showing P-wave sensing and pulse generator inhibition. In this example, the pulse generator, Telectronics 120, has a marker spike to identify pulse generator sensing and inhibition. Thus, on the P waves, small marker spikes can be seen. The problem was rectified with an asynchronous pulse generator.

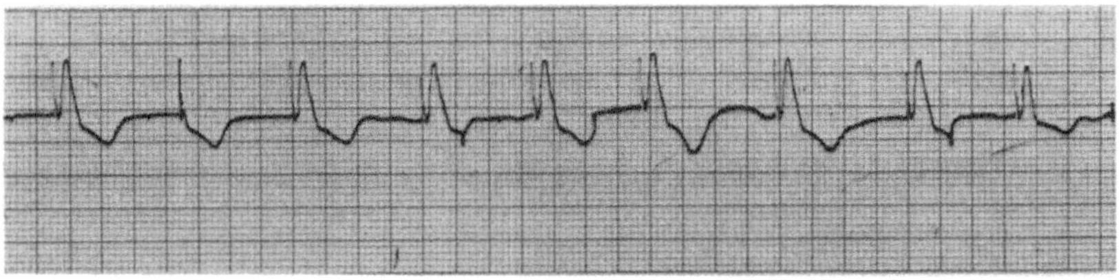

Figure 10. ECG showing erratic paper delivery due to intermittently sticking rollers in the ECG machine. Complex 2 shows a pulse artefact not followed by a QRS, but a T wave is present. In complexes 4 and 5, the QRS is present, but the T waves have been markedly deformed. These deformities have occurred with changes in the ECG paper delivery speed.

Output undesirably competitive

When pulse generator output is undesirably competitive the usual problem is undersensing of spontaneous intracardiac potentials (Table 5). More frequent causes of undersensing include a failing power source, reed switch lodged in the asynchronous mode, small or poorly transmitted intracardiac potentials, and the

Table 5. Pacemaker malfunctions: output undesirably competitive.

Malfunction	Frequence	Treatment
True Malfunction:		
1. Failure to sense R wave (undersensing)		
– power source failure (Table 1)	○○○	
– reed switch lodged in asynchronous mode after magnet removed	○○○	○ or nP
– asynchronous pulse generator	○○○	○ or nP (vi)
– reduced sensing		
• myocardial infarction	○○○	pL or nL
• fibrosis	○○	○ or pL or nL
• clot	○○	○ or pL or nL
• severe metabolic imbalance	○	treat
– broad QRS (poor slew rate)	○○	○ or pL or nL
– sensing circuit – random component failure	○○	○ or nP
– improper electrode-lead position		
• incorrectly placed at implant, e.g. coronary sinus	○○	○ or pL or nL
• displacement	○○	pL or nL
• retraction of electrode from endocardial surface	○○	○ or pL or nL
• perforation	○○	pL or nL
– loss of insulation (Table 1)	○○	
– electrode-lead system fracture with ends in contact with body fluids retaining pacing	○	nL
2. Persistent electromagnetic interference – pulse generator acting in asynchronous mode.	○	remove patient
Pseudo-malfunction		
3. Misinterpretation – ECG		
– fusion beats	○○○	
4. Faulty recording		
– magnet applied during test of synchronous mode	○○○	
– asynchronous testing labelled as synchronous mode	○○○	

Frequency: ○○○○ = common; ○○○ = uncommon; ○○ = rare; ○ = very rare. *Treatment*: n: replace with new component; r: repair; p: reposition; g: reprogramme; o: observe. *Equipment:* P: pulse generator; P (vt): ventricular triggered pulse generator; P (vi): ventricular inhibited pulse generator; P (asy): asynchronous pulse generator; P (hvo): high voltage output pulse generator; P (prog)) programmable pulse generator; L: electrode-lead system; A: adapter.

use of asynchronous pulse generators in patients whose spontaneous discharge rate exceeds that of the pulse generator repetition rate. Undesirable competition in the presence of persistent electromagnetic interference may also occur. Chest wall stimulation may differentiate low voltage spontaneous intracardiac potentials (normal inhibition) from a pulse generator component problem (no inhibition).

In many cases, observation is sufficient treatment. However, competition in the presence of ischaemic heart disease may precipitate ventricular fibrillation.

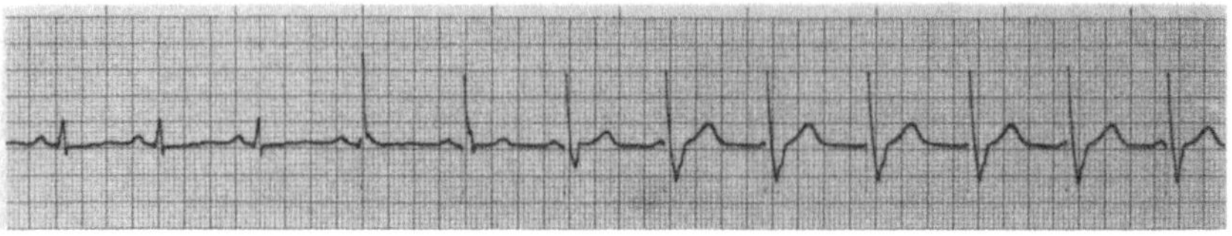

Figure 11. ECG showing fusion beats. The first three complexes are normal sinus beats. The last six complexes are paced beats. Complexes 4, 5 and 6 are fusion beats demonstrating and increasing contribution by the pacemaker.

In other situations, persistent competition may lead to a reduction in effective cardiac output. In all cases, unnecessary competition reduces the life of the power source. Surgical intervention is often necessary to determine the underlying problem. The lead may require repositioning or replacement; a new pulse generator may be indicated.

Pseudo-malfunctions include misinterpretation of fusion beats (Figure 11) and misinterpretation of results obtained from normally-functioning equipment.

Capture intermittent or absent

When the pulse generator in the synchronous mode demonstrates intermittent or absent capture (Table 6), true malfunctions include improper lead position, pulse generator voltage output below pacing threshold, and increased pacing threshold above a normal pulse generator voltage output (Figure 12). Intermittent capture may also be observed when the pulse artefact occurs during the refractory period of the previous spontaneous beat.

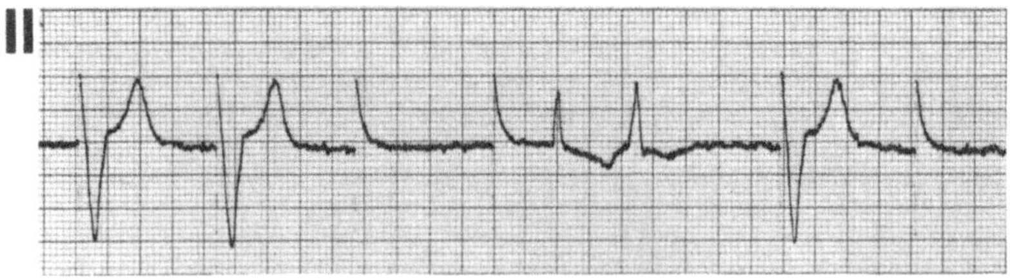

Figure 12. Pacing rhythm with intermittent failure of capture due to a high threshold of pacing. The first two complexes are normal paced beats. Complexes 3 and 4 are pulse artefacts not followed by a QRS, i.e. failed pacing. There is a marked delay before spontaneous ventricular escape beats occur (complexes 5 and 6). These are sensed by the pulse generator. Complex 7 is a normal paced beat that follows after an appropriate delay. Complex 8 again shows a pulse artefact without a QRS.

Table 6. Pacemaker malfunctions: capture intermittent or absent – sensing may be retained.

Malfunction	Frequency	Treatment
True Malfunction:		
1. Improper electrode-lead position (Table 5)	OOOO	
2. Pulse generator voltage output to heart below pacing threshold		
– power failing (Table 1)	OOOO	
– high resistance in electrode-lead system	OOO	nL ± nP
– current leakage		
• loss of insulation (Table 1)	OO	
• electrode-lead system fracture with ends in contact with body fluids	OO	nL ± nP
– voltage too low at implant (variable voltage pulse generator)	O	reset voltage
– output circuit – random component failure	O	nP
3. Increased pacing threshold		
– exit block		
• early: 4 to 6 weeks	OOO	nL or nP (hvo)
• late: fibrosis	OOO	n or nP (hvo)
– myocardial infarction	OO	nL or nP (hvo)
– severe metabolic imbalance	O	treat
4. Pulse artefact occurs during refractory period of previous spontaneous beat as a result of competition: failure to sense R wave (Table 5)	OOO	
Pseudo-malfunction:		
5. Misinterpretation – ECG		
– pulse artefact occurs during refractory period of previous spontaneous beat as a result of competition		
• asynchronous pulse generator	OOOO	
• magnet applied	OOOO	
– lack of understanding of 'vario' pulse generator function (threshold testing)	OO	
6. Testing equipment problem		
– ECG machine with automatic instow – pulse artefact instows stylus to baseline for 40 msec.	OO	

Frequency: OOOO = common; OOO = uncommon; OO = rare; O = very rare. *Treatment*: n: replace with new component; r: repair; p: reposition; g: reprogramme; o: observe. *Equipment:* P: pulse generator; P (vt): ventricular triggered pulse generator; P (vi): ventricular inhibited pulse generator; P (asy): asynchronous pulse generator; P (hvo): high voltage output pulse generator; P (prog)) programmable pulse generator; L: electrode-lead system; A: adapter.

When the pulse generator voltage output falls below pacing threshold, a new pulse generator is indicated. However, if the cause is accelerated power source discharge, then this problem must also be corrected, as well as implanting a new pulse generator. An increased pacing threshold may be treated by repositioning or replacing the electrode-lead system; this problem can also be overcome with the use of a high-output pulse generator.

Pseudo-malfunctions may be the result of ECG misinterpretation or lack of understanding of testing equipment; ECG machines with automatic instow (return to baseline whilst changing leads) may be particularly troublesome (Figure 13).

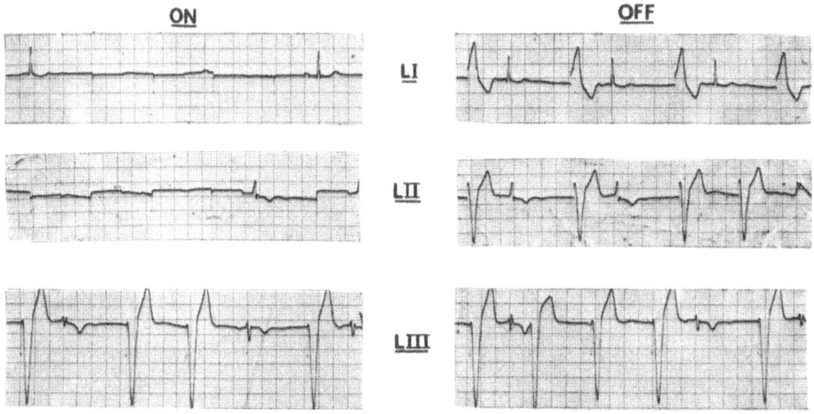

Figure 13. ECG showing pseudo-malfunction due to activation of automatic instow in an ECG machine (Nihon Kohden). The stylus of the machine returns to the baseline and is inactivated for 400 msec after the pulse artefact. Thus, paced beats are represented as a pulse artefact followed by 400 msec where the ECG machine is unresponsive to any electrical stimulus. Although leads I and II stimulate the automatic instow, lead III does not. The automatic instow can be inactivated by turning off the appropriate switch on the machine, and now the ECG shows pacing beats with intermittent spontaneous beats.

Side effects

Side effects caused by an otherwise normal pacemaker system can be divided into two categories: physical and psychological (Table 7). Physical side effects include: the pacemaker system causing erosion, infection, migration, or pain; pacing causing undesirable stimulation, the pulse repetition rate being inappropriate for the patient; and surgical diathermy creating an induction current along the lead causing intracardiac burning. Treatment is directed towards the cause.

The problem of pulse generator erosion and the incidence of infection has diminished significantly in recent years. Migration and subsequent erosion can, in many cases, be prevented by the use of the Parsonnet pouch. Good surgical technique and the routine use of antibiotics should prevent infection. If erosion occurs, direct suturing is inadvisable; both erosion and infection require a new pulse generator in a new site.

Pain at the site of the pulse generator is uncommon following normal recovery

Table 7. Pacemaker side effects.

Side effects	Frequency	Treatment
Physical side effect:		
1. Placement of pacemaker system causing:		
– erosion or pre-erosion		
• migration of pulse generator	○○○	nP and pP ± nL
• arm rub	○○○	nP and pP ± nL
– infection	○○○	nP and pP ± nL
– pain		
• local	○○	○ or pP
• remote		
– anginal	○○	treat ± gP or nP (Prog)
– pericardial (epicardial lead)	○○	± corticosteriods
– venous thrombosis	○○	anticoagulants
– pulmonary emboli	○○	anticoagulants
– pacemaker twiddler synchrome (lead displacement may occur)	○	caution patient
2. Pacing causing undesirable stimulation		
– skeletal muscle stimulation		
• local		
– indifferent electrode unipolar system	○○○	○ or pP
– loss of insulation (Table 1)	○○	
• diaphragmatic		
– direct	○	○ or pL or nL
– via phrenic nerve	○	section nerve or rL or nL
– ventricular fibrillation – asynchronous pacing procedures R on T phenomenon	○○	nP (vi)
3. Pulse generator characteristics		
– inappropriate programming	○○	gP
– hysteresis – slow intrinisic rate	○	nP
4. Surgical diathermy creating an induction current along the lead causing cardiac burning	○	care ± nL
Psychological side effect:		
5. Frequent self-detection of ectopic beats or hysteresis upsetting the patient	○○○	reassurance ± antiarrhythmics
6. Enforced reliance on pacing system by patient causing a psychological disturbance	○○○	reassurance

Frequency: ○○○○ =common; ○○○ =uncommon; ○○ =rare; ○ =very rare. *Treatment*: n: replace with new component; r: repair; p: reposition; g: reprogramme; o: observe. *Equipment:* P: pulse generator; P (vt): ventricular triggered pulse generator; P (vi): ventricular inhibited pulse generator; P (asy): asynchronous pulse generator; P (hvo): high voltage output pulse generator; P (prog)) programmable pulse generator; L: electrode-lead system; A: adapter.

from the surgical incision, and usually denotes infection, pre-erosion, or pressure on surrounding structures. Careful observation is necessary and, on occasion, repositioning of the pulse generator is required. The sudden onset of severe pain in elderly patients in the area of the pulse generator may denote pre-eruptive Herpes Zoster.

Skeletal muscle stimulation may result from the indifferent electrode lying directly on muscle, or it may occur, with loss of insulation, along the electrode-lead system. Loss of insulation should be rectified, as accelerated discharge of the power source will occur and result in premature depletion. An intact system need not be repositioned unless the patient suffers continual disturbance.

Direct diaphragmatic pulsation, following endocardial electrode insertion, is usually transient. However, persistent diaphragmatic stimulation may require the lead to be repositioned or replaced. Indirect diaphragmatic pacing occurs as a result of stimulation of the phrenic nerve by an epicardial electrode. In difficult situations, the problem can be rectified by sectioning the nerve in the neck, otherwise, the epicardial lead requires repositioning or replacement.

Psychological side effects following pacemaker system implantation can be minimized through careful explanation to the patient before and after the procedure. Some patients are disturbed by alteration in pacing rate brought about by sensing of ectopic beats. In most of these situations, reassurance is all that is required, although antiarrhythmic therapy may be helpful. More seriously, conflicts over loss of self-determination may cause depression. The patient may fear that the inevitable battery failure will introduce a further crisis into his life, or he may feel he is being run by an artificial device and hence he is, by association, less real.

CONCLUSION

All implanted pacemaker systems will fail with power source depletion. On occasion, systems will develop a defect before the expected end of life is reached. To expediate the determination of cause, the physician not only must be conversant with the range of malfunctions that may arise, but must also have a clear understanding of the numerous design idiosyncrasies of pacemaker models and the testing techniques used in order to distinguish pseudo-malfunctions from real malfunctions. It is hoped that the flow diagram, tables, and discussion, by covering these areas in some detail, will be valuable aids to any physician new to the field of pacing.

REFERENCES

1. Kosowsky DB, Barr I: Complications and malfunctions of electrical cardiac pacemakers. *Prog Cardiovasc Diseases* 14:501, 1972.
2. Furman S: Cardiac pacing and pacemaker VI: analysis of pacemaker malfunction. *Am Heart J* 94 (3):378, 1977.

3. Smith D, McDonald R, Sloman G: Implanted cardiac pacemakers: experience with electronic testing. *Cardiovasc Res* 5:236, 1971.
4. Sloman JG, Mond HG, Vohra JK, Hunt D: Pacemaker electrocardiography: the importance of QRS and T wave configuration. In: *To pace or not to pace*, (eds), The Hague, Martinus Nijhoff, 1978, p 289.
5. Anderson ST, Pitt A, Whitford JA, Davis BB: Interference with function of unipolar pacemaker due to muscle potentials. *J Thor Cardiovasc Surg* 71 (5):698, 1976.
6. El Gamal M, Van Gelder B: Suppression of an external demand pacemaker by diaphragmatic myopotentials: a sign of electrode perforation? *PACE* 2:191, 1979.
7. Peter T, Harper R, Sloman G: Inhibition of demand pacemakers caused by potentials associated with inspiration. *Br Heart J* 38:211, 1976.
8. Stillman MT, Richards A McD: Perforation of the interventricular septum by transvenous pacemaker catheter: diagnosis by change in pattern of depolarisation on the electrocardiogram. *Am J Cardiol* 24: 269, 1969.
9. Waxman MB, Berman ND, Sanz G, Downar E, Mendler P, Taylor KWG: Demand pacemaker malfunction due to abnormal sensing. *Circulation* 50:389, 1974.
10. Barold SS, Pupillo GA, Gaidula JJ, Linhart JW: Chest wall stimulation in evaluation of patients with implanted ventricular-inhibited demand pacemakers. *Br Heart J* 32:783, 1970.
11. Mond, HG, Stuckey JG, Sloman G: The diagnosis of right ventricular perforation by an endocardial pacemaker electrode. *PACE* 1:62, 1978.
12. Blacher R, Basch S: Psychological aspects of pacemaker implantation. *Arch Gen Psychiat* 22:319, 1970.
13. Kramp R: Cause and effect of rate drift in implanted pulse generators. *Impulse*, February 1976, p 7, Cardiac Pacemakers Inc.

11. A REVIEW OF PACEMAKER SURVEILLANCE, 1978

VICTOR PARSONNET, GEORGE H. MYERS, and MARJORIE MANHARDT

Methods for the systematic follow-up of patients with implanted pacemakers have not changed in recent years, but this year there are certain innovations and socioeconomic forces that promise to bring about new follow-up systems. The ever-broadening indications for pacemaker implantation, and some simplified operative techniques, will probably increase substantially the number of patients to be followed (1, 2). New pacemakers, most of them programmable, and some capable of transmitting information about their functional status, will add to the complexity of an already complex record-keeping system. A follow-up centre will be forced to adjust to the intricacies of programmable pacers, a particularly challenging task when the variable functions may have been altered elsewhere either accidentally or intentionally. Furthermore we must take into account the growing private and governmental efforts to contain medical costs, and the desires of third parties to limit what they consider to be widespread indulgence and needlessly expensive surveillance systems.

It is the intent of this review to summarize the present state of the art, and to identify essential features of patient care that require surveillance and study. This analysis is based in part upon the response of 300 physicians throughout the country to a comprehensive questionnaire, circularized in the fall of 1978, regarding pacemaker practices.[1] The survey has provided much factual and some subjective information from which meaningful conclusions can be drawn. Virtually every pacemaker user in the state of New Yersey has responded to the questionnaire, thereby generating a sample from within the United States. Trends have been identified by a comparison of present survey results with those of similar surveys conducted in 1969, 1972, and 1975 (3, 4, 5).

MEASURABLE PACEMAKER FUNCTION

Before discussing the ways that a follow-up service may be conducted one must inspect the features of pacemaker performance that can be analyzed. Table 1 lists

[1] Data to be published in the proceedings of the sixth international symposium, Montreal, 1-5 October 1979.

Table 1. Parameters of pacemaker performance.

		Pulse Generator Integrity		Lead and electrode Integrity		Functional information			
	Test performed or parameter measured	Battery voltage	Component or capsule	Wire	Insulation	1:1 capture	1:1 sensing (over or under sensing)	Threshold	Underlying ECG (pacer dependency; appropriate modes; and so on)
Output	Interval	+	+	±	±				
	Pulse duration	+	+	±	±				
	Amplitude	±	±	+	+			inf.	
	Wave shape	inf.	±	+	+			inf.	
ECG	Rhythm strip	±	±	±	±	+	+	±	±
	External overdrive	inf.	±	inf.	inf.				+
Programming	Output	±	±	inf.	inf.	+		inf.	+
	Rate	inf.	inf.	inf.	inf.	±	+		+
	Sensitivity	inf.	inf.	inf.	inf.		+		±
	Refractory period	inf.	inf.			inf.	inf.		+
Interrogation	Battery voltage	+	inf.	inf.	inf.			inf.	
	Load impedance			+	+			inf.	
	Moisture		+						
	Output suppression	+	inf.	inf.	inf.			+	+
Special analysers		inf.		inf.	inf.			+	+
Chest X-ray				+				inf.	

+ = valuable; ± = occasional or possible; inf. = valuable by inference when weighted with other findings.

Table 2. Parameters of pacemaker performance.

Test performed or parameter measured	How measured*	Transmittable by phone	Ease of performance (1-4): 1 = most difficult	Value in follow-up (1-4): 4 = most valuable
Output				
Interval	Digital counter	+	4	4
Pulse duration	Digital counter Oscilloscope display	+**	3	4
Amplitude	Oscilloscope display	+	2	2
Wave shape	Oscilloscope display		3	2
ECG – Standard	Rhythm strip or 12 lead	+	4	4
Vector	VCG		1	1
External overdrive	External pacer on skin plus rhythm strip		3	3
Programming	Varies with specific models	***	3	4
Interrogation	Varies with specific models		3	4
Chest X-ray			3	2
Special analysis system	Specific models		2	1

* Information digitalized can also be inserted on-line into a computer.
** Sometimes as pulse area.
*** One complex new pacer: manufacturer-operated.

these parameters, and indicates our views on how each may be useful in identifying certain groups of pacing system failures. The basic premise of this analysis is that the pacemaker must do what is expected of it, namely, pace the appropriate chamber(s) of the heart; sense the appropriate intracardiac electrocardiographic event(s), if so designed; and maintain stability of these functions. Table 2 indicates how these parameters are measured, whether or not the test can be performed routinely by a diagnostic centre, and how we appraise the importance of each test. A detailed description of these tests can be found elsewhere (6, 7); the following discussion is only a brief resumé.

The *output waveform* has a repetition rate (interval), duration, amplitude, and shape; the interval, and in some, the duration are designed to increase as the battery becomes exhausted. Some of these parameters are easily transmitted by phone, and all are measurable on oscilloscopic analysis. Interval and pulse duration are measured most easily. Defects in a pacing system, other than battery voltage, may affect the interval, depending on the circuit design. Output analysis is useful for evaluation of pulse generator function, and cognizance of the stability (or change) of any of the parameters is useful both directly and inferentially in diagnosing other types of system failure.

The *electrocardiogram*, usually a rhythm strip, is the other most useful test for signs of system failure, and is directed primarily to analysis of the interaction between the pacemaker and the heart. The application of external overdrive (EOD), will give additional information about the integrity of the sensing circuit, provide an approximation of the pacemaker refractory period, and display the unpaced electrocardiogram (in the case of inhibitory units). Again a more accurate definition of the cause of pacing system failure can be obtained by melding the known pacemaker output signs with the findings on ECG and EOD. The vector cardiogram, used by some as a diagnostic aid, has proved too cumbersome to use in our setting (8).

Programming of the implanted unit has been extremely useful in the diagnosis of impending pacing failure, in the evaluation and correction of clinical symptoms, and in providing an unpaced electrocardiogram. In fact, these 'trouble-shooting' features may yet prove to be the most persuasive reason for using programmable pacemakers.

Two new pacemakers that may be *interrogated* about their function are now in the validation stage. Interrogation will be the most specific way of evaluating an implanted pacemaker, because mearusement of its critical parameters, such as battery voltage and lead impedance, will be direct rather than indirect.

An overpenetrated *chest X-ray*, taken in several projections, may reveal a break, kink, dislocation, or malposition of a wire. By contrast an X-ray of the pulse generator is useless as a test of battery function or reserve.

Some pacemaker models provide *special test modes* and test devices to estimate the output/threshold ratio, i.e. the Siemens Elema Variopacer and Vitatron threshold Analyzer.[2] Although these devices are useful, they are not widely accepted in the United States.

A final, and perhaps one of the most important ingredients of pacemaker evaluation, is an *interview and examination* of the patient.

METHODS FOR TESTING AND EVALUATING PACEMAKERS

No follow-up. Throughout the country physicians provide a mixture of follow-up programs for their patients depending upon their personal attitudes, the geographical area in which they practice, and the intensity of their interest. There is still a group of physicans who believe that surveillance is not necessary and that pacemakers should be changed at a fixed date, presumably at the time recommended by the manufacturer, or else when a clinical problem becomes manifest. Although this attitude had a certain merit in the era when pacemakers lasted 18 to 22 months, it can no longer be justified. Formerly, if pacemakers were

[2] Siemens Elema, Stockholm, Sweden; Vitatron Medical B.V., Dieren, The Netherlands.

removed routinely at 18 months, when the average pacemaker lasted only 22 months, the saving of four or five months, although a significant percentage of the total pacemaker life, was not great in terms of a patient's paced lifetime. Today, however, if one were to remove a pacemaker at a set time, when many pacemakers will last eight or ten years, it would be impossible to find a satisfactory arbitrary date. if one chose six years, for example, and it turned out later that most of the pacemakers actually last ten years, the difference of four years would represent a substantial waste.

There are still other flaws in this technique. According to our own data as well as the recent survey, at least 30-40 percent of the problems that arise are not related to the battery or electronic components and are wholly unrelated to any manufacturer's prediction (Table 3, Table 4). And again, lack of patient contact makes it impossible to address any of the patient's medical, emotional, or financial needs.

Self-monitoring. An early system for pacemaker follow-up, and one that is still advocated by 15 percent of the respondents, is that of self-monitoring by the patient. When there were no other means of follow-up it was essential to teach the patient or a family member how to count the pulse rate accurately. Recently this has been simplified with the use of a portable electronic pulse monitor, of which there are now various kinds on the market (Appendix A). Although this system has the advantages of simplicity and moderate cost, it is not entirely satisfactory because there is no electrocardiographic analysis and it fails to provide for doctor-patient contact. Moreover, measurement of the pulse rate by the patient or his family is often difficult nowadays, when most patients have competing intrinsic rhythms. Finally, many patients cannot monitor themselves because they are incapable of complying with even the simplest instructions, and appropriate help at home or in a nursing facility may not be available.

Transtelephonic monitoring. The transmission of the pacemaker impulse interval and an electrocardiograpic rhythm strip, the basic pieces of information now being sent by telephone, has been accepted as an adequate monitoring system (9). The devices available for phone monitoring (Appendix B) can actually transmit not only the interval and electrocardiogram, but also the rate, impulse area, and even battery voltage, lead impedance, and capsular humidity.

These monitoring tests are performed by the treating physician in a private office or clinic, or by the pacemaker manufacturer, or by an intermediary proprietary service. Telephone may be the sole system of follow-up, or more often may be interspersed with an interview and examination and a more detailed waveform analysis at a clinic.

How phone transmission alone compares in effectiveness with phone transmission combined with waveform analysis remains a debatable issue. Phon

Table 3. Reasons for removal of pacemakers implanted before 1 July 1974.

Indication	Number		Percent	
Related to pulse generator	742		75.6	
Battery		589		60.0
Component		148		15.1
Battery/component		5		0.5
Unrelated to pulse generator	211		21.5	
Lead system		64		6.5
Extrusion		30		3.1
Death or LFU		9		0.9
Other		11		1.1
Elective		94		9.6
Recall		3		0.3
Undetermined or incomplete	28		2.9	
Totals	981		100	

Source. Joint pacemaker registry of Newark Beth Israel Medical Center (v. Parsonnet), Montefiore Hospital (S. Furman), and University of Southern California School of Medicine (M. Bilitch).

Table 4. Newark Beth Israel Medical Center: reasons for replacement of pacemakers in 1978.

Indication	Number		Percent		Not detected
Related to pulse generator	89		70.1		
Battery		75		59.1	
Component		11		8.7	4
Batt/Comp		3		2.3	1
Unrelated to pulse generator	38		29.9		
Wire fracture		10		7.9	8
Other lead system		4		3.1	2
Extrusion		5		3.9	
Change of mode		10		7.9	
Elective		2		1.6	
Recall		7		5.5	
Total	127		100		15* (11.8%)

*Nine of these were detected at zero output, through telephone surveillance.

transmission certainly desirable in areas where patients have to travel great distances to a pacemaker clinic. In other areas, where the patients can easily attend a clinic, phone monitoring alone is needlessly deficient. The recent survey indicated that most physicians in the United States choose the combined system. Phone monitoring lacks the direct patient-physician contact and the refinement of the other tests that can be provided by a clinic. No one, in fact, claims that phone monitoring alone is preferable to a complete surveillance system.

Proprietary phone monitoring companies (Appendix B) serve a useful function, especially in areas where caseloads are too small to justify establishment of a clinic. Some such services check thousands of pacemakers each week. They lack, however, not only the balance and thoroughness of a clinic, but also the systematic contact with patients. When follow-up is lost or the pacemaker fails they are not likely to know the precise reason.

Pacemaker clinics (waveform analysis). All follow-up systems designed to test pacemaker function depend upon the regularity of the pacemaker interval (rate) to indicate when the pacemaker is failing. The interval of the pacemaker may change (usually increase) as the only sign of battery exhaustion, or this may be associated with alteration in the pulse duration and amplitude. A pacemaker waveform analysis clinic provides facilities for a more complete analysis of all aspects of pacemaker function. The characteristics of the output impulse are studied with regard to interval, amplitude, pulse duration and shape, and the electrocardiogram is evaluated for consistent pacing and consistent sensing of the QRS complex by the pacemaker. At such a clinic many other procedures are performed, including history and physical examination, external overdrive (which tests the sensing circuit and measures the refractory period), chest X-rays, and pertinent laboratory tests – in short, a complete evaluation of the patient and the device.

The strongest objection to a pacemaker clinic is its cost, typically about $ 65 a visit as compared to $ 25 for a phone-monitoring call. Frequent clinic visits are therefore inconvenient and expensive. The schedules so far approved by third parties provide for clinic analysis two to four times a year; this leaves gaps of three to six months without any personal contact. Telephone monitoring which allowed contacts at more frequent intervals was a welcome innovation.

In some of the early, more elaborate, and well-funded clinics the computer was used as an aid in pacemaker analysis. Some of the computers merely provide record-keeping files, while others do more complete on-line analysis of the implanted pulse generator (10, 11). Because of the 'start-up' expense, however, only very few centres throughout the country have the advantage of this luxury.

Patients who attend pacemaker clinics appreciate the regular contact not only with the physicians but also with one another. In some areas they have organized pacemaker clubs that serve useful functions, particularly psychological support, transportation to and from clinics, and fund drives for research and service.

Obviously the number of people involved in the follow-up service varies greatly from centre to centre. In some instances follow-up can be done satisfactorily by the physician and his office nurse, while in others, particularly in pacemaker clinics, eight or nine individuals may be working simultaneously to process the great number of patients. The current survey indicates that 60 percent of the respondents believe that monitoring should be performed by the implanting physician; and 36 percent believe follow-up should be done through a pacemaker clinic, mostly in combination with phone monitoring, in which the implanting physician would play an active role.

BASIC (MINIMUM) OR OPTIMUM FOLLOW-UP: DEFINITION

An appraisal of pacemaker serveillance methods requires a thorough understanding of the information that is to be sought by the system. Selecting a method to use without taking the various pacemaker failure modes into account is certain to lead to an inadequate arrangement. Data collected from the Newark Beth Israel Medical Center over the past eight years (Figure 1) shows that battery exhaustion accounts for little more than half of the indications for reoperation. Therefore, an adequate surveillance system must also be able to identify and define rhythm disturbances, establish the integrity of the pacing system during modified forms of activity, and provide for examination of the wound and for evaluation of the patient's general medical condition (particularly the development of new medical problems).

With these considerations in mind, a *minimum* pacemaker follow-up system must provide an analysis of the pulse generator, specifically its 'magnet rate', and also the pacemaker-patient interface as represented by an electrocardiographic rhythm strip. At the other extreme, optimum (or complete) follow-up will take into account not only the pacemaker, but the whole pacing constellation which includes considerations of the patient as well.

SURVEILLANCE SCHEDULES

Schedules for pacemaker follow-up have developed over the years from independent decisions of individual clinicians. Eventually Medicare endorsed a schedule that provides for contact between the physician (or service) and the patient three or four times a year for the first two years, and more frequently thereafter, finally stabilizing with weekly contacts.

In order to define an appropriate schedule for follow-up contact (phone, clinic, and so on), one must know the answers to several pertinent questions. What is today's known reoperation rate? What are the chances of death should pacemaker failure occur suddenly? What are the consequences to the patient of sudden recurrence of the arrhythmia for which the pacemaker was implanted? Are additional medical and other expenses incurred by sudden and unanticipated failures? Will cardiac and other medical problems go undetected? Finally, is there any impact of new power sources and other technologies on the failure rates?

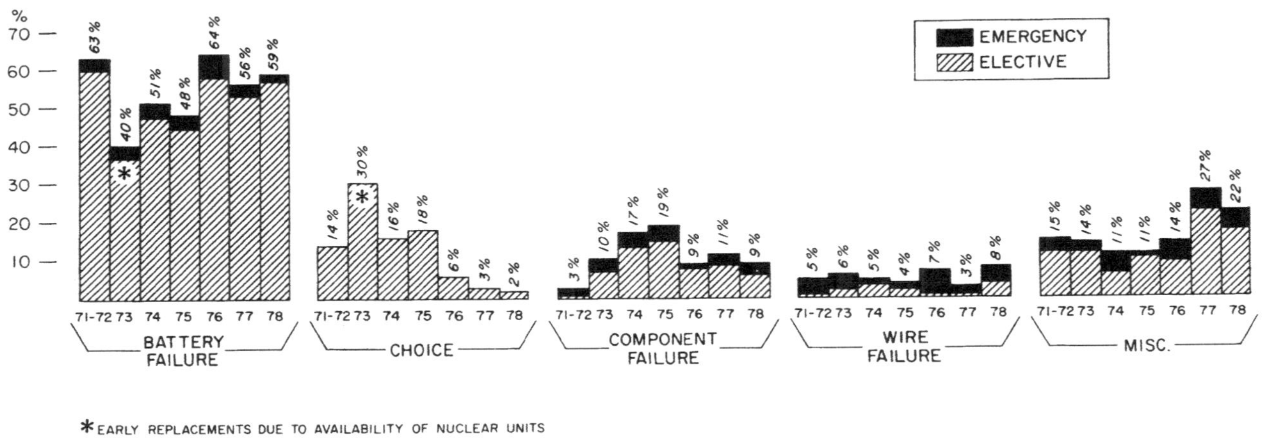

Figure 1. Indications for replacement of pulse generators over an eight-year period, 1971-1978, all causes, 998 cases (from the pacemaker center of the Newark Beth Israel Medical Center).

Unfortunately there are no firm data available on the frequency of reoperations on which definite schedules may be based, because there is wide variation of results among institutions. For example, the recent survey shows that early electrode malfunctions occur in 8 percent of cases, on the average, but range from 0 percent to more than 20 percent. In those institutions in which early malfunctions are frequent it would be necessary to provide weekly checkups in the first month, or perhaps even more often in pacemaker-dependent patients. On the other hand, in those centres in which malfunctions occur in less than 3 percent of cases in an entire year, weekly follow-up in the first month would hardly appear to be justifiable. Therefore, a certain amount of individualization and latitude is warranted.

There has been no statistical analysis of the risk to the patient who is never seen for any type of checkup. An early report by Bilitch (personal communication, March 1979), however, was disturbing in that on retrieving pacemakers from the Medical Examiner in Los Angeles County from patients who had died without follow-up care, he found that 5 percent of the pacemakers were not functioning. It is unfortunate that no comparable study has been done more recently when so few patients are dependent upon the pacemaker. It is unlikely that sudden failure of a pacemaker will result in sudden death, because the heart rate will usually return to its prepaced rhythm which was, obviously, life-sustaining. Sudden pacemaker failure is a more serious event in a pacemaker-dependent patient, although in the 1975 survey only 25 cases were reported in which there was even a suspicion that pacemaker failure had led to a patient's death (5). Still, even the non-dependent patient, whose original arrhythmia, though not lethal, required a pacemaker to improve his cardiac situation, will suffer a sudden or gradual return to the *status quo ante*, and logically this type of trauma should be avoided. In short, failure to detect signs of impending pacemaker malfunction and to correct the defect *before* overt failure of the system occurs will at worst result in the patient's death, or at best in an urgent, unplanned, and physically and emotionally traumatic experience.

At the end of pacemaker life (EOL) evaluations must be made more frequently, just as physical checkups should be more frequent in older people. Modern pulse generators (sometimes simplistically referred to as 'lithium' pacemakers), have already been shown to have a much longer life than the older models which had mercury-zinc cells, discrete components, and epoxy encapsulation. The lithium battery is not the only advancement that accounts for improved pacemaker reliablility, and therefore to discuss pacemakers in terms of 'lithium' and 'mercury-zinc' is fallacious. Almost all pacemakers manufactured in the United States today contain lithium batteries, but all pacemakers powered by lithium cells do not behave in the same way. One such pacemaker, for example, has performed badly as compared to others, while at least three or four brands have almost perfect records at 56 months (Figure 2). Therefore, it may

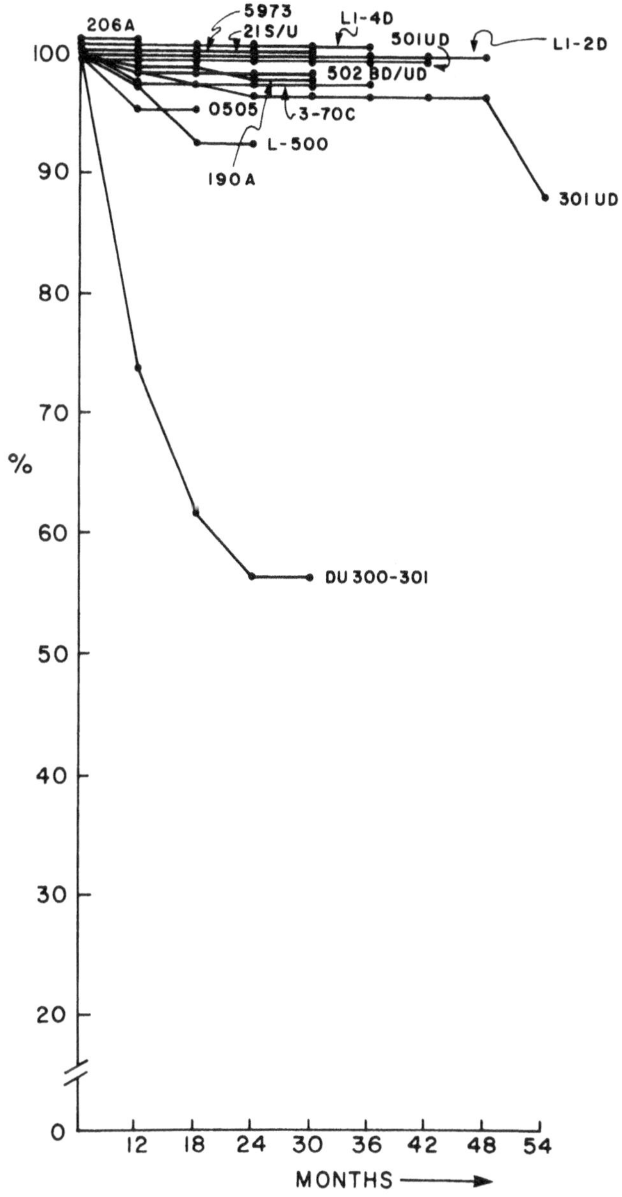

Figure 2. Actuarial survival of lithium pacemakers, collected by three-centre study group, March 1979.

not appear necessary to use the same follow-up schedule for each of these systems, but neither is it practical to devise an individual surveillance schedule for each model. Not knowing what the future will bring, we must select a schedule that will take these differences into account, and adjust it from time to time as experience (but not prediction!) dictates.

An acceptable schedule for follow-up must be one that reduces the chance of undetected pacemaker failure, and at the same time does not increase cost unreasonably. Adoption of such a schedule depends upon one's perception of the risks of missed pacemaker failure and one's definition of reasonable cost. As mentioned before, the incidence of undetected failure is continually changing. In the past pacemakers constructed with modern components and techniques, and touted to last a decade have had to be recalled. There already have been several 'advisories' on 'lithium' pacemakers, and three lithium batteries have shown rapid current drain that will shorten the lives of the pulse generators (Table 5).

Past experience has taught that when a sign of early battery failure is detected, 10 days to 2 months may elapse before the pacemaker output ceases (12). Therefore, for *battery failures* alone, a reasonable schedule would provide for a checkup every month once battery failure begins to manifest itself.

Further analysis of pacemaker failures, with both old and new units, shows that *non*-battery problems tend to occur randomly during the entire pacemaker life; at three years this will have resulted in reoperations in about 20 percent of patients (Figure 3). Battery and non-battery problems combined produce a monthly rate of 0.5 percent failure. Therefore, after the initial month or two when electrode stability will have been the major problem, a checkup of some

Table 5. Lithium Battery Problems.

Company	Model	Problem	Action taken
CPI	505	10kHz crystal failure, sudden zero output	Advisory on 700 units
ARCO	Li 2, 3, 4	Feed-through insulator short, possible lost capture	Advisory on 269 units
Intermedics	223	Double pulse output	Advisory on 200 units
Edwards	Early 20 series	Connector interface, possible intermittent capture	Advisory on 300 units
AMTECH	DU 300, 301 701, DB 400, 401, 800	Capacitor failure, sudden zero output	Advisory on 400 units
Battery			
SAFT		Faulty weld, 2-cell system, short life	Up to manufacturer
CRC 801		1975 – short life	Up to manufacturer
Mallory LSA-900-6 (in Coratomic)		Cell fracture	No action, 19 failed

Note: Advisory = Class 2 FDA recall.

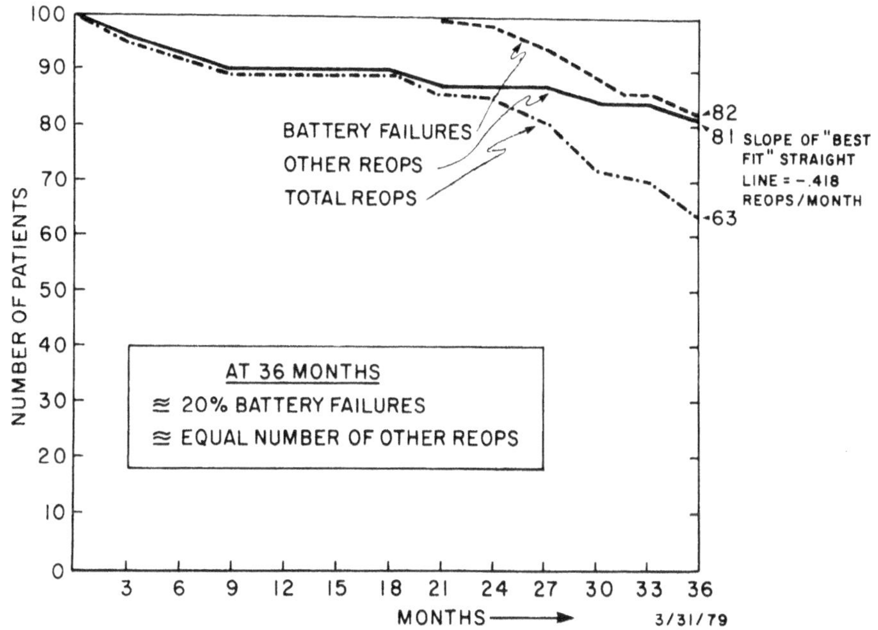

Figure 3. Failure rate of pulse generators of all types of 100 consecutive patients followed for three or more years (only the first three years are displayed).

sort at least every three months, and at most every month, would seem to be a reasonable schedule. Near the *predicted* EOL, when battery exhaustion will become increasingly frequent, tests should be performed at least monthly, and in some cases weekly, *depending on precisely how pulse generator failure tends to manifest itself.*

The schedule for follow-up should be changed if it is discovered with experience that failure modes are different from those anticipated, presenting, for example, as sudden output failure, or worse yet, with a 'runaway' rate. Data of this sort may be available from the manufacturers, but usually it has been slow in coming, and at times has been 'stonewalled' for a period before being made public. More reliable information has been obtained from local and national surveys, the best known of which is the FDA-supported three-centre study, active since 1974, Hauser's study of all major centres in Chicago (13), and the monthly systematic failure reports prepared by Professor Welti for AREC in France.[3] Information form the FDA study is published every two months in *PACE.* These ongoing evaluations will detect new pacemaker failure modes, their incidence, and the speed with which they occur in sufficient time to vary follow-up schedules accordingly. None of the surveys is complete enough to

[3] Association de Recherche et d'Entraide Cardiologiques, Hôpital Fernand-Widal 75010 Paris.

provide all the information that may be needed to establish optimum schedules, but it is clear that information such as this will be needed indefinitely so that changes in nationally approved schedules for reimbursement can be based upon facts.

With regard to the predictability of pacemaker failure, early studies of failure modes seen at the NBIMC Pacemaker Clinic show that most failures are predictable; this includes even some cases of wire fracture (Figure 1). Most of the failures that were not detected in impending stages were nevertheless identified in the clinic or on the phone before the patient had become symptomatic, and when appropriate semi-emergent action could still be taken. Less than 5 percent of failures were found by the patient himself, by the family, or by another physician. Consequently virtually all of our reoperations were elective or semi-elective.

During the past year, out of 127 reoperations for pacemaker system failure, there were 6 instances in which failures were missed by our detection method but were found by the patient or his physician. All required emergency admission to the hospital. Two needed a temporary pacing wire, and therefore required two operations instead of one. The average length of hospital stay was two days longer than for patients admitted electively, and overall costs were higher. Failure to detect early signs of pacing problems clearly has a measurable price.

The cost of pacing must take into account all expenses to the patient and the public, such as the price of the pacemaker, fees for surgery and hospitalization, and surveillance. A recent study at the NBIMC compared the monthly cost of mercury-zinc, 'lithium', and 'nuclear' pacemakers over a 10-year period, taking

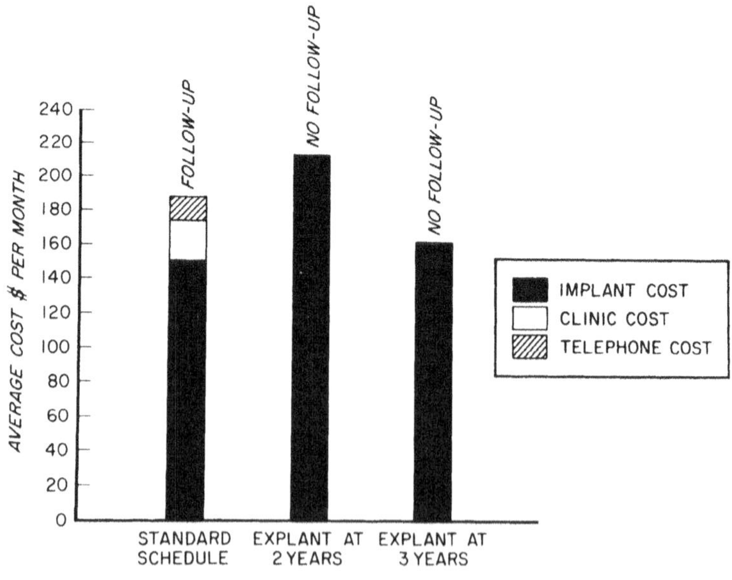

Figure 4. Cost of implantation and follow-up of various types of pacemakers.

into account a variety of follow-up schedules, as well as 10 percent non-battery reoperations and an appropriate number of replacements for battery exhaustion (Figure 4). It was shown that for lithium pacemakers elective replacement *without* any follow-up system was actually the most expensive, $ 214 per month, while follow-up according to Medicare's schedule was the least costly ($ 138 per month). Differences such as these were evident for all types of pacemakers, but the differences were larger for those with shorter life (14).

IMPACT OF NEW TECHNOLOGIES

As mentioned earlier, new follow-up systems will provide computer technology for physicians or services with small caseloads. Such sophistication may indeed prove necessary as more programmable pacemakers are implanted. At the NBIMC, where there are more than 450 patients with pacemakers programmable for rate and output, a reporting system has been established just to keep track of the programmed data. A computer-generated list is posted in the clinic office, with the pacemaker physicians, and the emergency room, so that it can be located without delay in an emergency. Without this information any follow-up service would be hard pressed to make reasonable judgements; it would be more difficult yet in proprietary services where there is even less contact between the service and the treating physician.

The pacemaker of the future will be interrogable to provide a direct print-out of its actual status – two such pacemakers are now in clinical validation.[4] Presumably follow-up will then be by periodic interrogation of the pacemaker, recording of the data, and serial comparison of data to all past readings.

Even with these exciting advances it will still be necessary to maintain follow-up services, for who, after all, will do these interrogation procedures but a competent individual or service? Moreover, it will *still* be necessary to interview and examine the patients and to perform a variety of specific tests to identify pacemaker system problems. New pacemakers therefore will *not* eliminate surveillance, but will merely change and probably further complicate the system.

SUGGESTED SCHEDULES

Based upon the various considerations discussed, it is appropriate to suggest a follow-up schedule that will provide patient contact at sufficiently frequent intervals to detect the mixture of problems that relate to the pulse generator and

[4] Intermedics, Inc., Freeport, Texas (Cyberlith model); and Pacesetter Systems, Inc., Sylmar, California.

to the patient's cardiac and other medical problems. It should be re-emphasized that periodic revision of this schedule will be needed as information on actual failure modes accrues.

In the schedule shown in Table 6, frequent contacts have been suggested during the first month of pacemaker life in order to detect electrode malfunction in patients with new electrode insertions. This would not be needed in replacement units, or by the experienced clinicians whose malfunction rates are extremely low. Although few are now being implanted, a schedule for mercury-zinc cells is also shown because we must still follow to EOL those implanted 3-6 years ago.

Table 6. Suggested schedules for frequency of surveillance contacts.*

Battery	Months	Primary implant or complete system replacement	Pulse generator replacement
	0-1	Weekly	–
Mercury-zinc	2-18	Every 2 months	Every 2 months
	19-24	Monthly	Monthly
	25-30	Twice monthly	Twice monthly
	31+	Weekly	Weekly
	0-1	Weekly	–
Lithium	2-24	Every 2 months	Every 2 months
	25-48	Monthly	Monthly
	49+	To be determined	To be determined

*A 'contact' includes telephone call or a pacemaker clinic visit (half of the contacts may be clinic visits except when scheduled contacts become very frequent). Extra contacts may be justified under the following conditions:

1. Documented or suspected arrhythmia;
2. Suspected faulty pacing or sensing;
3. Erratic pacemaker behaviour (suspected wire or component failure);
4. Manufacturer's or FDA advisory (alert or recall);
5. Panic call from patient (no more than two per year?).

PACEMAKER FOLLOW-UP TO THE FUTURE

Pacemaker follow-up of the future, contrary to intuitive expectations, will probably become more rather than less complex. Several developments lead to this prediction:

1. There are new indications for pacing, particularly supraventricular and ventricular tachycardias. These add to the complexity of ECG interpretation.

2. Pacemakers for arrhythmias, even for automatic defibrillation, will be exceedingly complicated, and will exhibit more intricate and perhaps dangerous failure modes.

3. Two-chamber pacing will be more commonplace, perhaps accounting for 20-50 percent of the new implants. These devices are already difficult to study, and their interaction with the normal and abnormal ECG, with and without failure of an integral piece of the system, may make accurate interpretation taxing to even the most learned expert.

4. Programming presents new problems in diagnosis and record keeping.

5. Patients loads will continue to grow. With these future developments in mind, we can predict that follow-up will become more demanding and will be relegated to the pacing expert. Future follow-up systems should contain the following characteristics and capabilities:

A. A physician must be involved in diagnosis and interpretation of the findings.

B. There should be provision for interview and examination of the patient at the time the test is performed.

C. A service should be available 24 hours a day

D. The tests should be sufficiently thorough to evaluate all pacemaker functions.

E. The system must include a capability of testing and programming specific pacemakers, and of interrogating telemetered functions.

F. Specific devices must be available for special tests, such as threshold analysis, EOD, 2-lead ECG, exercise tests, and so on.

G. Records must be detailed and serially recorded, preferably computerized, and available to pertinent areas of the hospital at all times (E.R., CCU, treating physicians).

H. It must be possible to compare the test results with all previous findings.

I. All pertinent test equipment must be available (programmers, EOD).

J. Phone transmission facilities must be available. Transmission of rate and ECG are essential.

K. There should be written plans for management of problems, such as sudden or unusual failure modes, pacemaker recalls, and so on.

L. The organization should provide for systematic filling, record-keeping, inventories, patient schedules, billing services, and counselling.

ACKNOWLEDGEMENT

The authors wish to express their appreciation to Mr. Todd Rodgers for collection and verification of the information in the appendices, and to Dr. Mia Parsonnet for her review of the manuscript.

REFERENCES

1. Littleford PO, Parsonnet V, Spector DS: Method for the rapid and atraumatic insertion of permanent endocardial pacemaker electrodes through the subclavian vein. *Am J Cardiol* 43: 980-982.
2. Parsonnet V, Werres R, Atherley T, Littleford PO: A new atraumatic technique for transvenous insertion of double sets of permanent electrodes for atrial synchronous (VAT) and atrio-ventricular sequential (DVI) pacemakers. *J Am Med Ass* (in press).
3. Parsonnet V: The status of permanent pacing of the heart in the United States and Canada. *Ann de Cardiol et d'Angéiol* 20 (4):287, 1971.
4. Parsonnet V: A servey of cardiac pacing in the United states and Canada. In: *Cardiac pacing: proceedings of the fourth international symposium*, Thalen HJTh (ed), Assen, Van Gorcum, 1973, p 41-48.
5. Parsonnet V, Manhardt M: Round table: world survey. In: *Cardiac pacing: proceedings of the fifth international symposium*, Watanabe Y (ed) Amsterdam, Excerpta Medica, 1977, p 569-571.
6. Parsonnet V, Myers GH, Gilbert L, Zucker IR, Shilling E: Follow-up of implanted pacemakers. *Am Heart J* 87:642-653, 1974.
7. Parsonnet V: Follow-up of implanted pacemakers: an evaluation of surveillance methods. In: *Diagnostic methods in cardiology*, Fowler NO (ed), Philadelphia: Davis, 1975, p 431-446.
8. Thomas DL Green GD: A vectorcardiograph for assessing implanted cardiac pacemakers. *Med Biol Eng* 12:593, 1974.
9. Furman S, Escher DJW Transtelephone pacemaker monitoring: five years later. *Ann Thor Surg* 20:326, 1975.
10. Hanson JS, Grant ME: Comprehensive cardiac pacemaker information system: basis for a regional follow-up network. *PACE* 1:327, 1978.
11. Black JL, Collins DWK: Computerized assessment of cardiac pacemaker performance. *Int J Biomed Comput* 7:163, 1976.
12. Parsonnet V, Myers GH: Residual function of explanted pulse generators. *AAMI* 7:203-207, 1973.
13. Hauser RG, Belic N, Casas R, et al: Clinical reliability of cardiac pacemaker: abstract *Circulation* 55-56 (suppl 3):12, 1977.
14. Myers GH, Parsonnet V: How much does a pacemaker cost? (In preparation).

APPENDIX A

Available phone devices	Information conveyed
ARCO Medical Products, PO Box 546, Leechburg, Pennsylvania 15656	interval, pulse width, ECG
Cardiac Pacemakers, Inc. 4100 N. Hamline Ave. St Paul, Minnesota 55165	interval, pulse width, ECG
Cordis Corp., PO Box 370428, Miami, Florida 33137	interval, pulse width, ECG
Edwards Pacemaker Syst., 1923 S.E. Main St., Irvine, California 92713	interval, pulse width, ECG
ESB, Inc., 5920 Rodman St., Hollywood, Florida 33023	interval, pulse width, ECG
Instromedix, Inc., Greentree Bus. Pk., 10950 S.W. Fifth, Beaverton, Oregon 97005	interval, pulse width, ECG

Intermedics, Inc., PO Box 617, Freeport, Texas 77541	interval, ECG, battery voltage, battery impedance, lead impedance
Medtronic, Inc., Teletrace, 3055 Old Hwy. Eight, Minneapolis, Minnesota 55418	interval, pulse width ECG
Pacesetter Systems, Inc., 12740 San Fernando Rd., Sylmar, California 91342	interval, pulse width, ECG
Survival Technology, Inc., 7811 Woodmont Ave., Bethesda, Maryland 20014	interval, pulse width, ECG, pseudo-waveform

APPENDIX B

Phone services	Information transmitted
Cardiac Datacorp, Inc., 1705 Walnut St., Philadelphia, Pennsylvania	interval, pulse width, ECG, peripheral pulse
Cardio Care, 425 E 61st St., New York, New York 10021	interval, ECG, pulse width
Cardio-Pace Evaluation, Inc., 9999 S.W. Wilshire, Portland, Oregon 97225	interval, pulse width, ECG
Medalert Corp., 1 Pennsylvania Plaza, New York City	interval, pulse width, ECG
Pacemaker Diagnostic Clinic of America, 4020 West Newberry Rd., Gainesville, Florida 32607	interval, amplitude, pulse width, ECG, pseudo waveform

INDEX OF SUBJECTS

A-H- interval 90
Action potential 79
Acupuncture 5
Adams-Stokes attacks 4, 5, 57, 58, 59, 72, 217
Ajmaline 67, 69
Amyloidosis 28, 37
Analyser, pacemaker 212, 239
Analysis, pacemaker (see also Follow-up and Photoanalysis) 172, 211-235
Anatomy, conduction system 23-55
Anesthesia 70, 140, 154, 162
Angina pectoris 72
Angiography 122
Antibiotics 164
Anticoagulants 75, 133, 162, 164, 233
Aorta-coronary bypass surgery 161
Aortic stenosis 59, 70, 71
AREC 249
Arrhythmias (see also Brady- and Tachycardia and Block)
  diagnosis 82-90, 127, 128
  genesis 79-82
Atrial contraction, synchronous 115-121
Atrial pathway, see Internodal pathway
Atrial systole 115, 118, 119, 120
Atrio-ventricular block, see Block
Atrio-ventricular bundle, see His bundle
Atrio-ventricular bundle branch 5,.23, 44-51, 81
  left 44, 46, 47, 48, 81
  right 44, 46, 47, 81
Atrio-ventricular conduction system 23-55
Atrio-ventricular node 32-44
  histology 34, 35, 38, 40-41, 45-47
Atropine 90
Automaticity (focal) 79-80, 93-94, 97

Bachmann's bundle 29
Baroreceptor reflex 115, 124
Battery, pacemaker 189-210
  Lithium 13, 16, 193, 199-203, 210, 247, 248, 250, 252
    end-of-life 201, 246, 249
  Mercury Oxide-Zinc 13, 16, 185, 191-195, 246, 250, 252
  Nuclear 193, 195-199, 250
  Rechargeable (nickle-cadmium) 13, 15, 193, 199
Betablockers 69, 71
Bio-engineer 168
Block, Atrio-ventricular
  complete 2, 5, 40, 57-72, 109, 114, 115
    congenital 37, 66
    paroxysmal 59, 71, 72
  incomplete 59-63
    first degree 60, 61, 68, 89
    second degree 66, 67
      Mobitz II 59, 66, 70, 89
      Wenckebach 59, 60, 67
Block, Atrio-ventricular bundle branch 48, 49, 57, 62, 67, 68
  bifascicular 68
  left 59, 60, 70
  left ant. hemi 60, 61, 68
  right 59
  right + L.A.H. 59, 68, 70
  trifascicular 59, 68
Block, Atrio-ventricular nodal 63, 64, 67, 69
Block, Intra-Hissian 61, 70
Block, Sino-atrial 72
Bradycardia 4, 57, 72, 79, 109, 123, 127
  Sinus 58, 61, 64, 79
Brady-Tachycardia syndrome 74-75, 127
Bundle of His, see His bundle

Can, pacemaker 172, 186-188
Cardiac arrest 59, 74, 127
Cardiac glycosides 69
Cardiac output 109-126
Cardiomegaly 65, 69
Cardiomyopathy 63
Cardioversion 71, 93
Carotid sinus syndrome 59
Catecholamines 112, 114, 115
Cerebrovascular insufficiency 65
Chestwall stimulation 218, 240

Chip 183, 185
Circuit, pacemaker 181-185
  design 12
  discrete 181-182
  efficiency 181
  hybrid 16, 182-185
Circus movement, see Re-entry
Clinic, pacemaker patient follow-up 17, 167, 213, 237-255
Computer, follow-up by 244
Concealed conduction 71
Connection, pacemaker-electrode 174
Coronary (ischaemic) heart disease 102, 119, 120, 179
Coronary sinus 29, 129, 144, 147, 148, 215, 219
Cost of pacing 248, 250
Current of injury 219, 220

Defibrillation 93
Diaphragmatic contraction 234
Diastolic filling time 111, 119, 120
Digitalis 71, 90
Diphenylhydantoïn 90
Dislocation, electrode 12, 57, 127, 128, 141, 154
Dizziness 58, 62
Dynamic electrocardiography 17, 58, 60, 218

Echocardiography 120
Ectopic ventricular beat 39, 89, 93, 101
Ejection fraction 119, 120, 121
Electrocardiography
  endocardial 60-68, 70, 71, 73, 179, 217, 218
  pacemaker 74, 213-216, 238, 241
Electrode
  indifferent 10, 128, 172
  stimulation 171-180
    atrial 154, 174
    epicardial 12, 133, 189
    endocardial (transvenous) 11, 12, 20, 128-130, 174-175, 189
      balloon 174
      bipolar 20, 128, 172, 191
      helifix 174
      ring 12, 20
      semi-floating 128, 130
    intramural 12, 172-174
      corkscrew 12, 20, 173, 174
      needle 10
      suture 11
  skin 12
  temporary vs. permanent 171-172
Electrode impedance 177
Electrode implantation 128-155
  endoscopic 154-155
  transthoracic 130-133
    atrial 133, 159
    epicardial 137
  transvenous 128-130, 134-154
    brachial route 129
    cephalic vein 129, 134, 135-137
    femoral vein 128-129
    jugular vein 128, 134, 135, 137, 138, 139
    subclavian vein 127, 128, 129-130, 134, 137
Electrode surface area 12, 177
Elisabeth 5, 6, 70
Embolism 75, 131, 154, 233
Emergency pacing 127, 128
Enddiastolic pressure 119
Enddiastolic volume 109-114, 117
Endoscopy 154-155
Endsystolic volume 109-114, 117
Energy, pacemaker 10, 12, 13, 189-210
Epoxy encapsulation, pacemaker 181, 182, 185-186, 246
Escape rhythm
  junctional 39
  nodal 74
European Working Group on Cardiac Pacing 18
Excercise 109, 114-115, 123
Exit block 154, 157, 178
Extrastimulus technique in electrophysiology 65, 66, 73, 74, 75, 84, 85

Facility for pacemaker implantation 127
Failure, pacemaker 239, 242, 245, 246, 248-250
  detection of 211-235
  reporting of 18, 167, 249
Fainting 58
Fibrillation
  atrial 61, 71, 74, 75, 89, 93, 102, 120, 121
  ventricular 93, 101, 229
Fibroma 39
Fibromuscular dysplasia 37, 38
Flutter
  atrial 74, 93, 94, 102
  ventricular 101
Fracture, lead 12, 171, 225, 227, 229, 231, 245
Frank-Starling law 109
Follow-up of pacemaker patients 167, 168, 237-255
  schedule 244-252
Foramen ovale 149
Fusion beats 227, 229, 230

Generator, see Pacemaker

H-V interval 57, 60, 61, 62, 63, 68, 69, 70, 72
Haemochromatosis 24, 37
Haemodynamics and pacing mode 109-126
Haemorrhage 129
Haemostasis 162
Haematomas 162
Heartblock, see Block
Heart failure 65, 72, 111, 120, 123, 124, 217
Helium leakage test 187, 201
Helmholtz layer 176
Hermetical sealing of pacemaker 16, 182, 186-188, 201
Herpes zoster 234
His bundle 5, 23, 33, 36, 37, 44-51, 60, 68, 81
  electrocardiography 60, 61, 83, 89-90, 128
  histology 34, 35, 38, 42, 43, 45-47, 50, 51
History of cardiac pacing 1-22, 189-191
Holter monitoring, see Dynamic electrocardiography
Hospitalisation of pacemaker patient 163, 250
Hypertension 65
Hypertrophy, ventricular
  left 110, 115
  right 141
Hypotension, orthostatic 58, 217
Hysteresis of pacemaker circuit 92, 123, 124, 125, 227, 233

Identification, pacemaker 18
Identification card, pacemaker patient 18
Implantation
  electrode, see Electrode
  pacemaker 162-164
  pacemaker system 212-213
Impulse analysis, see Analysis
Impulse duration 13, 177, 217, 221, 238, 239
Impulse output 13, 224-231
Impulse shape 229
Indications for pacemaker therapy 57-78
Infection 57, 127, 137, 162, 167, 232, 233
Insulation, electrode 12, 172, 234
Interface, electrode-heart 171, 176-180
Interference
  electromagnetic 172, 179, 221, 229
  muscle 172, 218
Internodal pathways 5, 23, 28-32, 33, 37
  anterior 28-29
  middle 29-30
  posterior 29, 32
Isoprenaline 90, 127
Isovolumetric systole 110, 122

Jan Jaap 5, 28, 69
Junctional escape rhythm, see Escape rhythm

Kent bundle 75

Lead 12, 171-172
Legal aspects of cardiac pacing 18, 168
Lenegre's disease 48
Lev's disease 48-49
Lifetime
  battery 193
  pacemaker 13, 123, 187
Lithium battery, see Battery
Lown-Ganong-Levine syndrome 36, 89
Lupus erythematosus 24, 28, 37

Maarten 12, 28, 71
Magnet test 164, 216-217, 223, 224
Mahaim fibers 44, 75
Malfunction, pacemaker 211-235
Mediastonostomy 154
Mercuryoxide-zinc battery, see Battery
Mesothelioma 39, 40-43, 52
Microcalorimeter 203
Migration, pacemaker 162, 232
Misinterpretation of pacemaker malfunction 224, 226, 227, 229, 231
Mitral stenosis 117, 121
Mobilisation of pacemaker patient 128
Mobitz II block, see Block
Monitoring of pacemaker impulse 172
Myocardial contractility 112
Myocardial infarction 71, 102
Myocarditis 99
Myocyte 28, 36, 48

Nernst equation 22
Nodal escape rhythm, see Escape rhythm

Orthorhythmic pacing 99, 100, 101
Oscilloscopic analysis, see Photo analysis
Ottel 12, 15, 79
Overdrive pacing 93, 97
  atrial 61, 73

P cell 24, 28, 36
P-R interval, prolonged 59, 61, 68, 89
PACE 17, 249
Pacemaker 12-17
  atrial inhibited 13, 91, 121, 125, 179
  atrial triggered 13, 90, 91, 121, 125, 17
  A-V sequential 91, 92-116, 117, 118, 1 125
  bifocal demand 13, 121, 125, 179
  fixed rate 13, 91, 92, 99, 121, 125
  ideal 122, 125-126
  patient controlled 95
  Ph-triggered 126

programmable 13, 123, 237
radio-frequency 76, 157
R-wave inhibited 3, 13, 91, 92, 121, 125
R-wave triggered 13, 91, 92, 121, 125
scanning 97
Pacemaker input 179
Pacemaker malfunctioning, see Failure and Malfunctioning
Pacemaker patient
activities 162
follow-up schedule 222, 244-252
hospitalisation 163, 250
mobilisation 128
Pacemaker pocket 162-167
Pacemaker positioning 156, 162-167
Pacemaker programming 13, 59, 240
Pacemaker systems 90-92
Pacing, cardiac
coupled 93
modes 91, 121, 122-125, 167
permanent 134-164
programmed 63, 83, 99, 103, 122-124, 164
temporary 127-133
Patient self-monitoring 241
Perforation 129, 153, 154, 215, 217
Pericarditis 37
Photoanalysis 172, 213, 218, 239, 243-244
Plutonium 238 196,198
Pneumothorax 130
Polarisation, electrode 172
Polyarteritis nodosa 28
Positioning of endocardial electrode 140-153
Postimplantation protocol 130
Postoperative pacing 70
Pre-excitation, ventricular 36, 93
Preoperative pacing 70
Printed circuit board 181, 182, 183
Promethium 147 196
Prophylactic pacing 58, 67, 68, 69
Propranolol 90
Pseudomalfunctioning, pacemaker 211, 223, 224, 225, 226, 227
Pulmonary oedema 117
Pulse counting 3
Pulsilogon 1
Purkinje fibers 5, 36, 44, 48, 80, 101

Q-U interval 64

R-H histogram 71
R-R interval histam 72
Radiation 196
Rapid filling phase 115
Reconditioning, pacemaker 18
Recycling, pacemaker 177
Re-entry arrhythmia 39, 75, 79-82, 83, 94, 97, 99
circuit 102
Refractory period
cardiac cycle 80-81, 97
pacemaker 13, 177, 221, 240
Replacement, pacemaker 17, 162, 241, 242, 245
Reliability
lead 57, 171
pacemaker 57, 193
Retrograde conduction 118
Röntgen, see X-ray
Runaway pacemaker 249

Scleroderma 25, 27, 37
Seat belts, automobile 162
Selection of pacing system 90-91, 122-125, 128
Sensing
ectopic 121, 125, 234
P-wave 123, 227
R-wave 221, 227, 229
T-wave 227
Septal defect, ventricular 70
Sick sinus syndrome 17, 52, 72-76, 83-88, 124-125
Sino-atrial conduction time 73, 74, 83, 84, 85, 86, 87, 88
Sinus arrest 74
Sinus node 5, 23-28, 115
blood supply 23
cells 24
dysfunction, see Sick sinus syndrome
histology 25, 26, 27
Sinus node recovery time 73, 83, 85, 86, 87, 88
Skin erosion 185, 232
Slew rate 179
Society, Pacing 17-18
International 17
Sphygmographic recording 2, 3, 5
Sphygmology 1
Standardization, pacemaker 18
Stroke volume 109, 110, 113, 114
Stylet, electrode 171
Subclavian vein, see Electrode implantation
Sudden death 37, 39, 44, 57, 75, 179, 246
Sudden failure, pacemaker 12, 246, 248
Surgery, cardiac 70, 133, 161
Surgical techniques in pacing 127-169
Sympathetic stimulation 112, 113, 114
Syncope 39, 57, 58, 70, 72, 74, 218
cough 58
vago vasal 58
effort 59

T-wave inversion 219
Tachycardia
  nodal 94
  pacemaker 75-76, 94-104
  paroxysmal 61, 74, 75
  supraventricular 74, 75, 93, 94, 96, 97
  therapy of 92-104
  ventricular 76, 93, 98
Tamponade, cardiac 133, 154
Technology, pacemaker 181-188
Testing, pacemaker 211-213, 240-244
  explanted 221
Tetralogy of Fallot 70, 89
Threshold
  fibrillation 97
  potential of 79
  stimulation 11, 133, 154, 157, 177-179, 212, 231
Thrombosis 133, 137, 233
Torsade de pointes 59, 64
Transitional cell 24, 36, 48
Transoesophagal stimulation 97
Transtelephone analysis of pacemaker 17, 218, 241-242, 252, 255
Transthoracic electrode implantation, see Electrode implantation
Transvenous pacing, see Pacing
Trendelenburg's position 130
Tritium 196, 198
Twitching, muscle 162, 172, 234

Vagal nerve 7
Vector cardiography 17
Venous return 109, 113-114, 118
Ventricular filling 115
Verapamil 90
Vertebro-basilar insufficiency 58, 217
Vertigo 58
Vulnerable period 93, 172

Warburg resistor 176
Wenckebach block, see Block
Wenckebach point 62
Whipple's lipodystrophy 24
Wolff-Parkinson-White syndrome 36, 75, 89
World Symposium on Cardiac Pacing 10, 12, 17, 18, 22, 155

X-ray analysis of pacemaker batteries 191-195
X-ray picture
  electrode position 142-153
  pacemaker 16

GPSR Compliance

The European Union's (EU) General Product Safety Regulation (GPSR) is a set of rules that requires consumer products to be safe and our obligations to ensure this.

If you have any concerns about our products, you can contact us on ProductSafety@springernature.com

In case Publisher is established outside the EU, the EU authorized representative is:

Springer Nature Customer Service Center GmbH
Europaplatz 3
69115 Heidelberg, Germany

Batch number: 10761599

Printed by Printforce, the Netherlands